Like many people, you may be confused by herbal manufacturers' unproven claims.

If you turn to your family doctor for answers, you're not likely to get them. Most mainstream health care practitioners lack the knowledge needed to counteract herbal manufacturers' claims or provide guidance on herbs.

We know this from experience. As clinical pharmacists, we often field questions from both the general public and health care professionals. For the last few years, we've been virtually bombarded with questions about herbal medicines. "What's gossypol?" someone will ask. "How does myrtle work?"

THE COMPLETE GUIDE TO HERBAL MEDICINES contains extensively referenced, unbiased information . . . written in language that anyone can understand. We wrote it to give you the scientific facts about herbs—not to confuse or distract you with the myths or folkl[illegible] them.

—FROM THE PREFACE

For information regarding special discounts for bulk purchases, please contact Simon & Schuster Special Sales at 1-800-456-6798 or business@simonandschuster.com

The Complete Guide to

Herbal Medicines

Charles W. Fetrow, PharmD
Juan R. Avila, PharmD

POCKET BOOKS
New York London Toronto Sydney

POCKET BOOKS, a division of Simon & Schuster, Inc.
1230 Avenue of the Americas, New York, NY 10020

Published by arrangement with Springhouse Corporation

For information address Springhouse Corporation,
1111 Bethlehem Pike, Springhouse, PA 19477

ISBN 13: 978-0-7434-0070-1
ISBN 10: 0-7434-0070-4

First Pocket Books mass market paperback printing September 2000

30

POCKET and colophon are registered trademarks of
Simon & Schuster, Inc.

Cover design and illustration by William Sloan / Three

Printed in the U.S.A.

CONTENTS

CONTRIBUTORS AND CONSULTANTS

SPECIAL CONSULTANT

Christine K. O'Neil, PharmD
Assistant Professor Clinical Pharmacy
Duquesne University
Clinical Pharmacist
St. Francis Medical Center
Pittsburgh

Reem A. Abo-Zena, PharmD
Pharmacy Practice Resident
The Cleveland Clinic Foundation
Cleveland

Jorge G. Avila, PharmD
Oncology Pharmacy Specialist
H. Lee Moffitt Cancer Center & Research Institute
Tampa, Fla.

Erica A. Barnum, PharmD
Pharmacy Resident
Moses H. Cone Memorial Hospital
Greensboro, N.C.

Cathy L. Bartels, PharmD
Assistant Professor, Director of Drug Information
School of Pharmacy and Allied Health Sciences
University of Montana
Missoula

Stephanie Beckman, PharmD
Clinical Pharmacist
Western Missouri Mental Health Center
Adjunct Clinical Instructor
University of Missouri–Kansas City

Hildegarde J. Berdine, PharmD
Clinical Assistant Professor
Duquesne University
School of Pharmacy
Pittsburgh

Keith Berndtson, MD
Medical Director
American WholeHealth/Lincoln Park
American WholeHealth, Inc.
Chicago

Donna Bey, PharmD
Clinical Specialist, Drug Information
Medical University of South Carolina Medical Center
Charleston

Riccardo L. Boni, PhD
Assistant Professor of Pharmaceutical Chemistry
Duquesne University
Mylan School of Pharmacy
Pittsburgh

Paula McFadden Bortnichak, MD
Freelance Medical Consultant; Psychiatrist
Sparta, N.J.

Mary L. Brubaker, PharmD, FASHP, BCPS, BCNSP, CHES
Clinical Assistant Professor
Northern Arizona University
Flagstaff

Hope E. Campbell, PharmD, BCPS
Clinical Research Pharmacist
Vanderbilt University Medical Center
Nashville, Tenn.

Paula J. Ceh, PharmD
Assistant Professor of Pharmacy Practice
Butler University
College of Pharmacy and Health Sciences
Indianapolis

M.L. Champion, PharmD
Clinical Pharmacist
University of Pittsburgh Medical Center
Southside Hospital

Mary L. Chavez, PharmD
Director of Didactic Education
Midwestern University
College of Pharmacy–Glendale, Ariz.

Umberto Conte, PharmD
Clinical Pharmacist
The Mount Sinai Medical Center
New York

Jason C. Cooper, PharmD
Assistant Professor Clinical Specialist, Drug Information
Medical University of South Carolina
Charleston

Virginia L. Cronin, RN, MSN, MBA
Associate Professor
Northern Virginia Community College
Annandale

Melissa Crouthamel, PharmD
Clinical Pharmacist
University of Pittsburgh Medical Center

Eric Culley, RPh, PharmD Candidate
Duquesne University
Pittsburgh

Christine M. Damico, MSN, CPNP
Pediatric Nurse Practitioner
Central Bucks Pediatric Associates
Doylestown, Pa.

Linda M. Dean, RN, MSN, CRNP, ACRN, CS
Clinical Nurse Coordinator
MCP Hahnemann University
Section HIV/AIDS Medicine
Partnership Comprehensive Care Practice
Philadelphia

Brent Ednie, MD
Indiana (Pa.) Hospital
Department of Internal Medicine

Rachael M. Fantz, PharmD
Psychiatric Pharmacy Resident
Medical University of South Carolina
Charleston

Suzanne E. Fecik, PharmD
Clinical Pharmacist
Behavioral Health Pharmacy
Scripps Mercy Hospital
San Diego

Sandra S. Feldman, PharmD
Pharmacy Practice Resident
Buffalo (N.Y.) General Hospital

Emily F. Grandey, MD
Internal Medicine
St. Francis Medical Center
Pittsburgh

Michelle A. Gravlin, PharmD
Clinical Pharmacist
Cox Medical Center North
Adjunct Clinical Instructor
University of Missouri–Kansas City
Springfield

Amy L. Gruel, PharmD
Visiting Faculty
School of Pharmacy & Allied Health Sciences
University of Montana
Missoula

Peggi Guenter, RN, PhD, CNSN
Editor-in-Chief
Nutrition in Clinical Practice
American Society of Parenteral and Enteral Nutrition
Silver Spring, Md.

Stacy L. Haber, PharmD
Clinical Assistant Professor
The University of Arizona
College of Pharmacy
Tucson, Ariz.

William R. Hamilton, PharmD
Assistant Professor
Creighton University
School of Pharmacy and Allied Health Professions
Omaha

Fred Harchelroad, MD, FAAEM, FACMT
Director, Medical Toxicology Treatment Center
Allegheny General Hospital
Pittsburgh

Jennifer Harkins, RN
Coram Health Care
Winston-Salem, N.C.

Jane Holmes, PharmD
Clinical Coordinator Pharmacy Services
Allegheny University Hospitals: Allegheny Valley
Natrona Heights, Pa.

Jamie L. Holowka, PharmD
Clinical Pharmacist
University of Pittsburgh Medical Center

Pamela A. Hucko, PharmD
Pharmacy Practice Resident
West Virginia University Hospital
Morgantown

Anne-Marie Jefferson, PharmD
Department of Pharmacy
University Medical Center
Jacksonville, Fla.

T. M. Jenkins, PharmD
Senior Masters of Pharmacy Administration Resident
The Ohio State University Medical Center
Columbus

Kirk Jones, PharmD
Clinical Pharmacist
University of Pittsburgh Medical Center: Beaver
Pittsburgh

April M. King, PharmD
Clinical Pharmacist
In-Home Health, Inc.
Pittsburgh

Robert V. Laux, PharmD
Assistant Professor
Duquesne University
Pittsburgh

Mandy C. Leonard, PharmD
Drug Information Specialist
The Cleveland Clinic Foundation
Cleveland

David Lippman, MD
Internal Medicine
St. Francis Medical Center
Pittsburgh

Scott F. Long, RPh, PhD
Assistant Professor of Pharmacology and Toxicology
School of Pharmacy
Southwestern Oklahoma State University
Weatherford

Kevin J. Lynch, PharmD
Clinical Manager
Stadtlander's Managed Services
Pittsburgh

Barbara L. Martinelli, RPh, BCNSP, MBA
Clinical Pharmacist/Coordinator
Metabolic Support Team
St. Francis Medical Center
Pittsburgh

Laura K. McCoy, MS, PharmD
Manager, Patient Care Services
Children's Hospital
Columbus, Ohio

Lee Ann McDowell, PharmD
Clinical Pharmacy Specialist
University of Pittsburgh Medical Center Health System

Pamela S. Messer, RN, MSN
Global Safety Surveillance and Epidemiology
Wyeth Ayerst Laboratories, Inc.
Radnor, Pa.

Brian J. Moore, RPh
Clinical Pharmacist
Ohio State University Medical Center
Columbus

Heather C. Murren, PharmD
Staff Pharmacist
Magee-Women's Hospital
Pittsburgh

Linda M. Nicolaus, PharmD
Staff Pharmacist
Eckerd Drug, Inc.
Pittsburgh

Brian N. Peters, PharmD
Pharmacy Practice Resident/Graduate Research Associate
The Ohio State University Medical Center
Columbus

T.W. Prasthofer, PhD
Associate Professor, Biopharmaceutical Sciences
Shenandoah University School of Pharmacy
Winchester, Va.

Harry S. Rafkin, MD
Head, Clinical Investigation for Critical Care Medicine
Director, Department of Research
St. Francis Medical Center
Pittsburgh

Holly Roche, PharmD
Staff Pharmacist
University of Pittsburgh Medical Center: Presbyterian
Pittsburgh

Catherine Romanos, PharmD
Pharmacy Practice Resident
Ohio State University Medical Center
Columbus

J.P. Rose, PharmD
Clinical Pharmacist
Allegheny University Hospitals: Allegheny General
Pittsburgh

Paul L. Schiff, Jr., PhD
Professor of Pharmaceutical Sciences
School of Pharmacy
University of Pittsburgh

Pazit Shaked, PharmD
Resident, Pharmacy Practice
Albert Einstein Healthcare Network
Philadelphia

Douglas Slain, PharmD
Clinical Fellow
Clinical Instructor
Virginia Commonwealth University Medical College
Richmond, Va.

Adam Sohnen, MD
Internist, Department of Internal Medicine
St. Francis Medical Center
Pittsburgh

Joan Stachnik, PharmD, BCPS
Drug Information Specialist
University of Illinois College of Pharmacy
Chicago

S.B. Tanna, PharmD
Specialty Practice Resident
The Ohio State University Medical Center
Columbus

S.E. Taylor, PharmD
Critical Care Resident
University of Pittsburgh Medical Center Health System

James A. Tjon, PharmD
Drug Information Pharmacist
University of Pittsburgh Medical Center

Theresa M. Wadas, RN, MSN, CCRN, CRNP
Nurse Practitioner
Advanced Heart Failure & Transplant Service
University of Alabama Hospital
Birmingham

Mathew Wallack, MD
Medical Resident in Neurology
Wake Forest University Medical Center
Winston-Salem, N.C.

Mary Grace S. Wilson, PharmD
Staff Pharmacist
Children's Hospital
Pittsburgh

Eric Wright, PharmD
Clinical Pharmacist
VA Pittsburgh Healthcare System
Clinical Instructor
University of Pittsburgh School of Pharmacy

Chris A. Yeschke, RPh
Supervisor, Sterile Products
Pharmacy Services
St. Francis Medical Center
Pittsburgh

Acknowledgments to the Springhouse Corporation staff:

PUBLISHER: Donna O. Carpenter; EDITORIAL DIRECTOR: William J. Kelly; CLINICAL DIRECTOR: Ann M. Barrow, RN, MSN, CCRN; CREATIVE DIRECTOR: Jake Smith; ART DIRECTOR: John Hubbard; MANAGING EDITOR: Kathy E. Goldberg; DRUG INFORMATION EDITOR: Lisa Truong, RPh, PharmD; EDITORS: Marcia Andrews, Kevin D. Dodds, Catherine Harold, Peter H. Johnson; COPY EDITORS: Karen C. Comerford (manager), Colleen P. Coady, Leslie Dworkin, Karen Stover; DESIGNERS: Arlene Putterman (associate art director), Elaine Kasmer Ezrow, Joseph John Clark, Donald G. Knauss, Donna S. Morris; TYPOGRAPHERS: Diane Paluba (manager), Joyce Rossi Biletz; MANUFACTURING: Deborah Meiris (director), Pat Dorshaw (manager), Otto Mezei (book production manager); EDITORIAL ASSISTANTS: Carrie R. Cameron, Carol A. Caputo, Arlene Claffee; INDEXER: Barbara Hodgson

Pocket Books edition designed by Pagesetters/a division of Stratford Publishing Services, Inc.

FOREWORD

Each year, more than 60 million Americans use herbal remedies and other types of alternative medical care. In fact, more people seek help from alternative health care providers than from conventional health care practitioners. Perhaps most telling of all, nearly three out of four patients who use alternative medicines never tell their doctors about it.

Without question, herbal medicines are here to stay. Those that have been proven safe and effective deserve to be considered valid treatment options. The truth is, though, the effectiveness of many herbs remains largely unproved.

Unfortunately, you wouldn't know that if you visited a bookstore or community library. Today, a large bookstore may have a few dozen books on herbal remedies; a large Internet book outlet may have a hundred or more. Yet nearly every herbal resource available is either incomplete or strongly biased for or against herbal medicines. Anyone who uses such a resource—even a health care professional—has trouble discerning fact from myth and answering with certainty the many questions he or she has about herbal therapy.

What's more, only a handful of these resources cover more than a few dozen of the most commonly available herbs. Fewer still give a complete picture of the potential dangers of herbal remedies—especially the risks of using herbs while taking prescription or nonprescription drugs.

Suppose, for instance, a friend urges you to drink a few cups of chamomile tea in the evening to help you fall asleep at night. Her comments pique your interest in herbal remedies, but you have a history of blood clots—in fact, you're taking a blood thinner. So you decide to read up on the topic before taking your friend's advice. In the health section of your local library, you randomly pick up one of the many books on herbal medicine and turn to the chamomile section. Here you read a paragraph about the folklore and another on the purported benefits of this herb. Perhaps you also read that people with certain plant allergies should avoid chamomile. Chances are, you *won't* find a warning that people on blood thinners shouldn't use chamomile.

But if you were lucky enough to have picked up *The Complete Guide to Herbal Medicines,* you *would* find that warning under a clearly labeled "Interactions" section. You'd also find a complete list of other precautions under the heading "Important points to remember." This book goes beyond the often entertaining folklore to give a balanced picture of the herb's medicinal value. Perhaps most importantly, it summarizes the pros and cons of using each of more than the 300 herbs and related medicines it covers.

And, unlike virtually all other herb books on the market, *The Complete Guide to Herbal Medicines* provides references for each entry. The authors, both widely respected and highly experienced, have pored over dozens of books, hundreds of journal articles, and thousands of pages of government documents to compile this most comprehensive resource.

If you decide to use herbs for medicinal purposes, I strongly urge you to consult your health care practitioner first. Remember, too, that herbs are no substitute for a healthy lifestyle and good nutrition.

Above all, keep *The Complete Guide to Herbal Medicines* handy. You won't find a more detailed and reliable resource on herbal medicine anywhere. Nor will you find one that places more emphasis on the *facts* about herbs, not just the folklore.

Simeon Margolis, MD, PhD
Professor of Medicine and Biological Chemistry
The Johns Hopkins University School of Medicine
Baltimore

PREFACE

Over the last decade, more and more people have turned to herbs instead of—or in addition to—their doctors to help cure or prevent disease. We can think of several reasons why. For one thing, some people have lost faith in mainstream medicine—especially if it has failed them and if herbalists or herbal product manufacturers offer hope of a cure. For another, many people think any "natural" treatment is inherently safer or better than one produced in a lab or high-tech manufacturing facility.

A third reason for the herbal resurgence is the herbal industry's high profile. Most of us have seen or heard advertisements for herbal products on television, in magazines and newspapers, or on the Internet. Unlike pharmaceutical companies, herbal manufacturers don't have to provide evidence to support their claims, supply information about their products' contents or side effects, or prove that their products are safe or effective.

Like many people, you may be confused by herbal manufacturers' unproven claims. If you turn to your family doctor for answers, you're not likely to get them. Most mainstream health care practitioners lack the knowledge needed to counteract herbal manufacturers' claims or provide guidance on herbs.

We know this from experience. As clinical pharmacists, we often field questions from both the general public and health care professionals. For the last few years, we've been virtually bombarded with questions about herbal medicines. "What's gossypol?" someone will ask. "How does myrtle work?"

While researching these questions, we discovered that this area of health care is poorly understood and even less well documented. Most information on herbal products comes from herbal manufacturers or advocates. Peer-reviewed medical journals rarely publish articles on clinical trials or side effects involving herbs, and those that do aren't easily accessible. Also, much of the clinical literature on alternative medicine comes from foreign journals that aren't written in English. And some of the studies they publish predict people's responses to herbs based only on animal experiments. Seeking unbiased resources, we turned to textbooks. Although some were excellent, many covered only the most commonly used herbal products.

These obstacles made our research time consuming and cumbersome. Realizing we weren't the only ones having trouble getting information on alternative therapies, we decided to fill the herbal information gap ourselves by creating a comprehensive, objective resource for health care professionals. That book, *Professional's Handbook of Complementary & Alternative Medicines*, was so warmly received that the publisher asked us to adapt it for the general public.

The Complete Guide to Herbal Medicines, which you hold in your hands, is the result of that effort. It contains the same extensively referenced, unbiased information as our first book but is written in language that anyone can understand. We wrote it to give you the scientific facts about herbs—not to confuse or distract you with the myths or folklore that surround them. We hope you'll turn to our book first when deciding whether to use any herbal medicine.

Charles W. Fetrow, PharmD
Juan R. Avila, PharmD

ABOUT THIS BOOK

The Complete Guide to Herbal Medicines goes beyond the headlines and the hype to take a close, *unbiased* look at herbal remedies. Written by pharmacists in simple, everyday language, it takes herbal medicine seriously—but doesn't give it a free ride.

This book presents both the scientific facts and the folklore on more than 300 commonly used herbal medicines. Unlike other herbal medicine guides, *The Complete Guide to Herbal Medicines* is fully referenced to help you evaluate claims made by herbalists and manufacturers of herbal products.

The first chapter briefly reviews the history of herbal medicines from their first known use in ancient times to the current herbal revival. It recounts efforts to regulate herbal medicine throughout the 20th century in the United States and Europe. Next, it describes the major medicinal uses of herbs and explains how herbal medicine research is conducted. After the chapter identifies the different forms of herbal preparations (such as capsules, extracts, tablets, tinctures, and teas), it discusses how to take herbs safely and effectively.

Herbal entries

Next, you'll find entries for more than 300 herbs and 11 nonherbal alternative medicines, arranged alphabetically by the product's most commonly used name. Each entry starts with basic information about the herbal or alternative medicine, including its source, botanical name, folklore, and other general information.

Then come clearly marked headings, which appear in the same sequence in all entries: Common doses, Side effects, Interactions, Important points to remember, Other names for the herb, and Selected references.

Common doses

This section identifies the known forms of the herb—for example, teas, tinctures, or capsules. It also lists standardized strengths (when these are known).

Then it gives the recommended dosage for each form based on herbal literature, anecdotal reports, and available clinical data. Keep in mind, though, that not all uses for each herb have specific dosage information. If experts disagree on the dosage, the authors have no dosage information, or the herb is considered too dangerous for anyone to take, those facts are mentioned here. Be aware that the dosages in this section reflect current clinical trends—not recommendations of the authors or publisher.

Side effects

This section lists, in alphabetical order, the undesirable side effects the herb may cause. In some cases, these effects haven't been reported but are listed here because the authors believe they *could* occur based on the herb's chemical composition or action in the body.

Interactions

Here you'll find an alphabetical list of drugs and foods that the herb might interact with to cause discomfort or harm. As with side effects, some of the listed interactions haven't been proven but are theoretically possible. When a particular drug shouldn't be taken with the herb at all, the authors state this.

Important points to remember

This section lists important warnings about the herb; contraindications to using it (such as diseases); instructions on preparing, administering, or storing the herb; steps you can take to help prevent side effects; and other points of interest.

Other names for the herb

Here you'll find alphabetical lists of the herb's alternative names and commercial products containing the herb. (Some of these products may contain combinations of the herb with other agents.) Mention of a trade name doesn't imply that the authors or publisher endorse that product or guarantee that it's legal.

Selected references

This section lists key clinical studies of the herb. As you'll see from these citations, the authors and reviewers conducted an exhaustive review of literature from around the world, including many foreign publications and hard-to-find research studies.

Featured information

For each herb and nonherbal alternative medicine, you'll find two boxes that feature important facts.

Why people use this herb

This box lists both traditional and modern uses for the herb. Keep in mind that these uses aren't recommendations but unproven claims for use.

What the research shows

In this box, the authors separate myth from fact, evaluating all available evidence to let you know exactly where each herb stands from a scientific viewpoint. As appropriate, they also offer recommendations for the herb's use.

Glossary

The glossary clearly and concisely defines more than 160 key terms used in this book, helping to enhance your understanding of herbal medicine.

Where to get more information

Here you'll find the names, addresses, phone numbers and, in many cases, Web addresses of organizations and agencies that can provide further information on herbs and nonherbal alternative medicines.

Index

This extensive, user-friendly index lists each herb's common name and alternative names as well as all medicinal uses of the herbs described in the book.

Understanding and Using Herbal Medicines

Most people are familiar with herbs as foods—for example, basil and oregano in sauces, parsley as a garnish. However, for thousands of years many cultures around the world have used herbs and plants not just to eat but to treat illness. Archaeological evidence shows that even prehistoric man used plants to heal. Today, the World Health Organization estimates that 80% of the world's population uses some form of herbal medicine.

Many of the drugs now prescribed come from plants that ancient cultures used medicinally. (The word *drug* comes from the Old Dutch word *drogge,* meaning "to dry," because pharmacists, doctors, and ancient healers often dried plants to use as medicines.) About one-fourth of all conventional pharmaceuticals—including roughly 120 of the most commonly prescribed modern drugs—contain at least one active ingredient derived from plants. The rest are chemically synthesized. (See *Common drugs made from plants*.)

Common drugs made from plants

Many drugs in common use today have botanical origins. Here's a selected list.

- Aspirin (salicylic acid)—from white willow bark and meadowsweet plant
- Atropine, used to treat irregular heartbeats—from belladonna leaves
- Colchicine, used for gout—from autumn crocus
- Digoxin (Lanoxin), the most widely prescribed heart medication—from foxglove, a poisonous plant
- Ephedrine, used to widen or relax the airways—from the ephedra plant
- Morphine and codeine, potent narcotics—from the opium poppy
- Paclitaxel (Taxol), used to treat metastatic ovarian cancer—from the yew tree
- Quinine, a drug for malaria—from cinchona bark
- Vinblastine (Velban) and vincristine (Oncovin), anticancer drugs—from periwinkle

Potentially dangerous herbs

Herbs can harm as well as heal. The herbs below may pose special risks.

- *Bloodroot,* promoted as an expectorant, purgative, stimulant, and plaque and cavity preventer, is used in such a range of doses that it can be dangerous. It has caused death when used to induce vomiting.
- *Chan su,* a topical aphrodisiac also known as stone, love stone, and rockhard, has been fatal when mistakenly ingested.
- *Chaparral tea*, claimed to be an antioxidant and pain reliever, has caused liver failure, necessitating liver transplantation.
- *Coltsfoot*, used for respiratory problems, has caused liver problems.
- *Comfrey*, used to promote wound healing (and formerly to relieve ulcers of the bowel, stomach, liver, and gallbladder), has caused liver problems and cancer.
- *Indian herbal tonics* can lead to lead poisoning.
- *Jin bu huan*, an ancient Chinese sedative and analgesic, contains morphine-like substances and has caused hepatitis.
- *Kombucha tea*, made from mushroom cultures and used as a cure-all, has caused death from a blood acid disorder.
- *Lobelia*, used to treat respiratory congestion, has led to respiratory paralysis and death.
- *Ma huang, or ephedra*, an ingredient in many diet pills, can cause psychotic behavior, seizures, irregular heartbeats, heart attack, stroke, and death. It's also sold under such names as Herbal Ecstasy, Cloud 9, and Ultimate Xphoria to induce a "high" associated with illegal drugs.
- *Pennyroyal*, used to induce menstruation and treat colds, fevers, and the flu, has caused liver failure, kidney failure, coma, and death.
- *Sassafras*, used as a diuretic and a treatment for skin disorders and rheumatism, has caused liver damage. It has also been linked to narcotic poisoning and miscarriage. The Food and Drug Administration has banned sassafras volatile oil and the component safrole as food additives and flavor enhancers.
- *Yohimbe bark*, used as an aphrodisiac and hallucinogen, has caused psychotic behavior.

Misleading claims

The herbs below have been misrepresented as cures for serious illnesses.

- *Mistletoe* has been falsely touted as a cure for cancer.
- *Pau d'Arco tea* has been falsely touted as a cure for cancer and AIDS.

Some herbs and plants have value not just for their active ingredients but for other substances they contain, such as:

- minerals
- vitamins

- volatile oils (used in aromatherapy)
- glycosides (sugar derivatives)
- alkaloids (bitter organic bases containing nitrogen)
- bioflavonoids (colorless substances that help maintain collagen and blood vessels).

In the United States, many traditional health care providers lack knowledge about herbal remedies, and their patients may be reluctant to reveal their use of such remedies. But renewed interest in all forms of alternative medicine has led consumers, health care providers, and drug researchers to reexamine herbal remedies. Medicinal herbs have been touted in magazines, books, and television shows, sometimes with advocates making amazing claims for their benefits.

Unfortunately, herbs don't have magical or mystical properties. Like all drugs, they must be taken in the right doses for the right length of time—and for the right purpose—to produce a benefit. While some herbs are safe and effective, others can cause lasting harm and even death. (See *Potentially dangerous herbs*.)

Still other herbs are neither harmful nor effective.

History of herbal medicine

Herbal medicine, also called *phytotherapy* or *phytomedicine,* has been practiced since the beginning of recorded history. Specific remedies have been handed down from generation to generation.

In ancient times, medicinal plants were chosen for their color or the shape of their leaves. For example, heart-shaped leaves were used for heart problems, while plants with red flowers were used to treat bleeding disorders. This primitive approach is called the *Doctrine of Signatures*. Practitioners determined the best use for each plant by trial and error.

The formal study of herbs, called *herbology*, dates back to the ancient cultures of the Middle East, Greece, China, and India. These cultures revered the power of nature and developed herbal remedies based on the plants found in their home environments. Written evidence of the medicinal use of herbs has been found on Mesopotamian clay tablets and ancient Egyptian papyrus.

The first known compilation of herbal remedies was ordered by the king of Sumeria around 2000 B.C. and included 250 medicinal substances, including garlic. Ancient Greece and Rome produced their own compilations, including *De Materia Medica*, written in the 1st century A.D. Of the 950 medicinal products described in this work, 600 come from plants and the rest from animal or mineral sources.

The Arabs added their own discoveries to the Greco-Roman texts, resulting in a compilation of more than 2,000 substances. Eventually, this work was reintroduced to Europe by Christian doctors traveling with the Crusaders. Herbal therapy is also a major component of India's Ayurvedic medicine, traditional Chinese medicine, Native American medicine, homeopathy, and naturopathy.

In the United States, herbal remedies handed down from European settlers and learned from Native Americans were a mainstay of medical care until the early 1900s. The rise of technology and the biomedical approach to health care eventually led to the decline of herbal medicine.

The herbal revival that we're seeing today has several causes:

- general disillusionment with modern medicine
- the high cost and side effects of prescription drugs
- widespread availability of herbal medicines
- the belief that natural remedies are superior to manmade drugs.

Regulating herbal medicine

In the 19th century, many fake remedies were sold to gullible, desperate Americans. The federal government finally took action against disreputable purveyors of phony remedies by passing the Food and Drug Act of 1906. This law addressed problems of mislabeling and adulteration of plant remedies—but not safety and effectiveness.

Today, herbal remedies remain largely unregulated. The Food and Drug Administration (FDA) regulates herbal products only as dietary supplements, not drugs. This means that the FDA can recall herbal products that are shown to be harmful, but manufacturers aren't required to provide information about their products' contents or side effects or to prove their safety or efficacy. They need only provide "reasonable assurance" that the product contains no harmful ingredients.

What's more, although manufacturers can't claim a particular product cures or prevents a specific disease, they can make any other claim about the supposed benefits without providing supporting evidence. They need only add the following disclaimer: "This statement has not been evaluated by the FDA. This product is not intended to diagnose, treat, cure or prevent any disease."

In essence, herbal remedies in the United States are sold on a buyer-beware basis. This highlights the importance of learning everything you can about any herbal products you plan to use.

European standards

In Europe, where millions of people use herbal and homeopathic remedies, governments and the scientific community are much more open to natural remedies, especially those with a long history of use. In Great Britain and France, traditional medicines that have been used for years with no serious side effects are approved for use under the "doctrine of reasonable certainty" when scientific evidence is lacking.

The European Economic Community has established guidelines that standardize the quality, dosage, and production of herbal remedies. These guidelines are based on the World Health Organization's *Guidelines for the Assessment of Herbal Medicines,* a 1991 publication that addressed concerns about the safety and effectiveness of herbal medicines.

Therapeutic uses of herbs

A plant's leaves, flowers, stems, berries, seeds, fruit, bark, roots, or any other part may be used for medicinal purposes. Most herbal remedies are used to treat minor health problems, such as nausea, colds, cough, flu, headache, aches and pains, stomach and intestinal disorders (such as constipation and diarrhea), menstrual cramps, insomnia, skin disorders, and dandruff.

Some herbalists have reported success in treating certain chronic conditions, including peptic ulcers, inflammation of the colon, rheumatoid arthritis, high blood pressure, and respiratory problems. Some use herbal remedies for illnesses usually treated only with prescription drugs, such as heart failure.

However, if you have a serious disorder and are considering an herbal remedy, *don't* discontinue ongoing medical treatment. Also be sure to tell your health care practitioner about any prescribed drugs you're taking, because these may interact with herbal remedies. (See *Taking herbal remedies safely,* pages 6 and 7.)

Research on herbal remedies

Numerous studies on herbal remedies have been done in Europe and Asia. European studies have shown benefits from such herbs as ginkgo, bilberry extract, and milk thistle in treating various chronic disorders. Chinese researchers have extensively studied many herbs, such as ginseng, fresh ginger rhizome, foxglove, licorice root, and wild chrysanthemum. Indian researchers using modern scientific methods have recently studied various Ayurvedic herbs, including Indian gooseberry and turmeric.

Taking herbal remedies safely

Many people take for granted the safety of the drugs and foods they buy. But unlike drugs, herbal remedies aren't reviewed by any government agency for quality, dosage, safety, or efficacy. If you're thinking about taking an herb, know that the vast majority of botanical products sold in the United States haven't been scientifically tested. Their alleged benefits are based largely on word-of-mouth.

How herbal products are regulated

The Food and Drug Administration regulates herbal products as food supplements, not drugs. The labels on these products don't tell you about their ingredients, risks, side effects, or possible harmful interactions with other substances. Nor do they guarantee that the herb is in a form your body can absorb or that the recommended dosage has been tested on animals or humans.

Also, herbal products may contain ingredients other than those indicated on the label. For example, Siberian ginseng capsules were found to contain a weed full of male hormone-like chemicals. What's more, the amount of active ingredient in an herb varies from brand to brand and possibly from bottle to bottle within a particular brand.

To help prevent problems caused by herbal medicine, follow these guidelines.

General precautions

- Check with your health care practitioner before using any herbal product, especially if you're taking a prescription drug. Tell your practitioner about all drugs you're taking, including nonprescription medications and vitamins. Many herbal remedies can interact with other drugs.
- Make sure your health care practitioner is aware of your medical history, including allergies.
- When taking an herb, follow the instructions exactly. If you take too much of an herb or take it inappropriately, you may get no benefit from taking it—or put yourself at risk for potentially dangerous side effects.
- Never ignore symptoms you're experiencing. Contact your health care practitioner if you experience side effects of an herbal agent or if you have other health concerns that would normally require medical attention.
- Be sure to call your health care practitioner if you experience abdominal cramping, abnormal bleeding or bruising, changes in your pulse or heart rhythm; vision changes, dizziness or fainting; hair loss; hallucinations, inability to concentrate or other mental changes, hives, itching, rash, or other allergic symptoms, appetite loss, or dramatic weight loss.
- Don't use herbal agents to delay seeking more appropriate therapy. Keep in mind that herbs aren't necessarily a substitute for proven medical therapy.

Taking herbal remedies safely *(continued)*

- If you're a parent or other caregiver, consider each of the preceding precautions before giving herbal medicines to a child or an elderly or debilitated person.
- Discontinue herbs at least 2 weeks before surgery. They can interfere with anesthesia and cause heart and blood vessel problems.

When to avoid herbs

- Avoid herbal preparations if you're pregnant or breast-feeding. Most herbs' effects on the fetus are unknown. If you're a woman of childbearing age, use birth control when taking herbs.
- Don't use herbs for serious or potentially serious medical conditions, such as heart disease or bleeding disorders.
- Never let other people take your herbs or other medicine. Store herbal agents out of reach of children and pets.
- If you have questions about the herb you're taking, seek advice from a qualified health care provider. If your practitioner isn't knowledgeable about herbs, ask for a referral to someone who is.

Buying herbal products

- Be wary of products that promise to cure specific health problems.
- Read labels carefully when buying herbal products. Check for the term *standardized* on the label. *Standardized* means that the dose of medicine in each tablet or capsule in that package is the same. Also make sure the label states specific percentages, amounts, and strengths of active ingredients.
- Avoid herbal "cocktails" that contain more than one ingredient. Experts know little about the effects of combining herbs.
- Buy your herbs from reputable companies. Avoid products sold through magazines, brochures, the broadcast media, or the Internet.
- Consider buying organically grown herbs. Some people believe herbs that grow naturally in the wild are subject to contamination from pesticides, polluted water, and automobile exhaust fumes.
- Remember that the clerk at the health food store is a salesperson, not a trained health care practitioner.

The United States lags behind other countries in herbal medicine research for several reasons. Until the Office of Alternative Medicine (OAM) was established in 1992, such research lacked federal support. Also, pharmaceutical companies have no financial incentive to develop herb-based drugs because botanical products can't be patented. That means the companies could never recoup their research investment.

The inherent difficulty in studying herbs according to Western pharmaceutical standards has posed another obstacle to herbal research.

Western standards favor isolating a single active ingredient. However, herbs may contain several active ingredients that work together to produce a specific effect.

Although large gaps remain in research, many clinical trials of herbs used as medication are currently underway. Since 1995, the OAM has collected more than 60,000 research citations on complementary and alternative health care practices, including 2,500 clinical trials that have been compiled in a computer database system.

Forms of herbal preparations

Herbs come in various forms, depending on their medicinal purpose and the body system involved. You can buy herbs individually or in mixtures formulated for specific conditions. Herbs may be prepared as tinctures or extracts, capsules or tablets, lozenges, teas, juices, vapor treatments, or bath products. Some herbs are applied topically with a poultice or compress. Others are rubbed into the skin as an oil, an ointment, or a salve.

Tinctures and extracts

An herb placed in alcohol or liquid glycerin is called a *tincture* or an *extract.* (Tinctures contain more alcohol than extracts.) Alcohol draws out the herb's active properties, concentrating them and helping to preserve them. Alcohol is cheap, is easily absorbed by the body, and allows the herb's full taste to come through. Alcohol-based tinctures and extracts have an indefinite shelf life.

Liquid glycerin extracts, called *glycerites,* are an alternative to alcohol extracts and preferred by some people. Most glycerites taste sweet and feel warm on the tongue. They're processed by the body as fat, not sugar—important to diabetics and others who must limit sugar intake.

Glycerin extracts have certain drawbacks. Taking more than 1 ounce (30 milliliters) of glycerin can have a laxative effect. Also, glycerin isn't an efficient solvent for some herbs that contain resins and gums. Such herbs need alcohol for extraction.

Extracts should contain at least 60% glycerin with 40% water to ensure preservation. Glycerin-based extracts have shorter shelf-lives than alcohol-based extracts. An extract that contains citric acid can last for more than 2 years if stored properly.

Tinctures or extracts may be taken as drops in a tea, diluted in spring water, used in a compress, or applied during body massage. If the tincture's alcohol content is a concern—for example, if the remedy is meant for a child—a few drops may be placed in one-quarter cup (60 milliliters) of very hot water and left to stand for 5 minutes. As the tincture stands, most of the alcohol evaporates and the mixture becomes cool enough to drink.

To make an herbal tincture, a glass bottle or jar is filled with herbal parts (cut fresh herbs or crumbled dry herbs), pure spirits, such as vodka, are added, and the container is sealed and placed in a warm area (70° to 80° F [21° to 26.6° C]) for 2 weeks. The mixture should be shaken daily. After 2 weeks, the herbs can be strained out and the residue squeezed out.

Extracts are made with alcohol or water to bring out the herb's essence. (The product label should indicate which base was used.) Extracts have the same advantages and disadvantages as tinctures but are more concentrated and therefore more cost-effective. Because of their strong herbal taste, they're usually diluted in juice or water.

Capsules and tablets

Capsules and tablets contain the ground or powdered form of the raw herb. They are easier to transport and typically are tasteless. The capsule or tablet should be made within 24 hours of milling the herb because herbs degrade quickly.

The best products use fresh herbs, which should be indicated on the label. Capsules can be a hard gel or soft gel made of animal or vegetable gelatin. Most people find capsules easier to swallow than tablets.

Both capsules and tablets may contain a large amount of filler, such as soy or millet powder. Filler makes the herb hard to identify in the powdered form, and an herb of poorer quality may be substituted without your knowledge. Tablets also may contain a binder, such as magnesium stearate or dicalcium phosphate, which in turn may contain lead. Binders help the herb absorb water and break down more readily for easy absorption in the body.

Capsules or tablets can be swallowed whole, as indicated, or can be mixed with a spoonful of cream-style cereal or applesauce. They also may be dissolved in sweet fruit juice.

Lozenges

Herbal lozenges are nutrient-rich, naturally sweetened preparations that dissolve in the mouth. They come in various formulas, such as cough suppressant, decongestant, or cold-fighting. Most lozenges are boosted with natural vitamin C. The horehound lozenge, one type that has become popular, is used to relieve coughs and minor throat irritation.

Lozenges should be taken as directed by a health care practitioner or herbalist. For self-treatment, follow the directions on the package.

Teas

Herbal teas can be made from most herbs. Teas are used for a wide range of purposes, with formulations aimed at specific conditions or desired effects.

Usually, you prepare the tea by infusion or decoction. Decoction is preferred for denser plant materials, such as roots or bark. To prepare an *infusion,* let the dried herb steep in hot water for 3 to 5 minutes. To make a *decoction*, put the herb in a rolling boil of water for 15 to 20 minutes. You may steep teas in a muslin or conventional tea bag or tea ball or use them in their loose form for their fragrant, aromatic flavor.

Some teas taste bitter because they contain alkaloids (for example, goldenseal root) or highly astringent tannins (for example, oak bark). You may want to add honey to sweeten the tea, but don't give honey to a child younger than 18 months because of the risk of infant botulism.

For an infant, you may mix the tea with breast milk or formula and then put it into a bottle, an eyedropper, or an empty syringe (without a needle) and gently squirt the tea into the infant's mouth. *Caution:* If you're breast-feeding and taking an adult dose of an herbal remedy, keep in mind that the herb may pass through your breast milk to your child. Also remember that, as with any drug, you must use care when deciding whether to give these medicines to an infant or a child.

The Chinese teach that the heat of the water and the taste of the herb enhance its effectiveness. Steeping an herb in hot water draws out its therapeutic essence. With dried herbs, you'll probably want to use 2 heaping tablespoons of herb for every cup of tea, unless the product label directs otherwise. Place the dried herbs in a china or glass teapot or cup (plastic or metal containers aren't suitable for steeping). Immerse in 8 ounces (237 milliliters) of freshly boiled water for each cup and cover.

When using leaf or flower herbs, steep for 5 to 10 minutes. With roots or bark, simmer or boil for 10 minutes, and then steep for 5 minutes longer. After steeping, strain the tea and let it cool to a comfortable temperature before drinking. If you're going to place a tincture or extract in the tea, let the cup of hot water sit for 5 minutes so the alcohol will evaporate. You can drink herbal teas hot, cold, or iced, depending on the purpose and instructions.

When using fresh herbs, remember that three parts of a fresh herb generally equal one part of a dried herb. Bark, root, seeds, and resins must be powdered (to break down the cell walls) before they're added to water. Seeds should be slightly bruised to release the volatile oils. You may infuse an aromatic herb in a pot with a tight lid to reduce the loss of volatile oil through evaporation. Because roots, wood, bark, nuts, and certain seeds are tough, they should be boiled in water to release their properties.

Juices

Juices are made by washing fresh herbs under cold running water, cutting them with scissors into suitable pieces, and running them through a juice extractor until they turn into a liquid. Usually, herbal juices are taken by placing a few drops in tea or spring water. They also may be applied externally by dabbing them on the affected body part.

Ideally, you should drink fresh juices immediately after extraction. However, you also may store them in a small glass bottle, corked tightly, and refrigerate for several days to minimize breakdown of ingredients.

Vapor and inhalation treatments

Many herbalists recommend herbal vapor and inhalation treatments for respiratory and sinus conditions. The treatment helps open congested sinuses and lung passages, promote mucus discharge, and ease breathing.

One inhalation method requires a sink and an herbal oil. Fill the sink with very hot water and add 2 to 5 drops of the herbal oil. Let the hot water trickle into the sink to keep the water steaming. As the mixture becomes diluted, you may need to add a few more drops of the herbal oil. Then inhale the steam for 5 minutes.

Another method involves heating a large, wide pot of water, adding a handful of dried or fresh herbs, and bringing the pot to a boil. After the herbs have simmered for 5 minutes, remove the pot from the heat and place it on a trivet to cool slightly. (If you're using an aromatic oil, first heat the water to just short of boiling and then remove it from the heat.) With the pot on a trivet, add 4 to 5 drops of the oil. Then drape a towel over your head to form a tent and lean over the pot, inhaling the steam for 5 minutes. Remember, though—if the vapor is too hot, it can burn your nasal passages.

Herbal baths

An herb that's in a soluble agent, such as baking soda or aloe gel, may be dissolved in hot bath water. An herb in an oatmeal-type preparation may be finely milled or whirled it into a powder in a blender. You may also bag fresh or dried herbs in a square of cheesecloth or place them in a washcloth and tie the cloth securely. The goal is maximum release of the herbal essence without having parts of the herb floating in the bath water. Full baths require about 6 ounces (170 grams) of dried or fresh herbs.

As the tub fills with water, place the bagged herbs under a forceful stream of comfortably hot water, and then drag them through the bath water to better distribute the herbal essence. Squeezing the bag releases a rich stream of essence that you can direct to the affected body part. You may also gently rub the bag over itching skin. *Caution:* Herbs with pointy or rough edges may be too irritating to use this way.

You can also add an herbal infusion to bath water. To make the infusion, soak 6 tablespoons (57 grams) of dried or fresh herbs overnight in 3 cups (710 milliliters) of hot water. The next morning, pour the strained infusion directly into the bath water.

Poultices and compresses

A *poultice* is a moist paste made from crushed herbs that's applied directly to the affected area, or wrapped in cloth to keep it in place and then applied. Poultices are useful for treating bruises, wounds, and abscesses.

Use only fresh herbs for poultices. One preparation method involves wrapping the herbs in a clean white cloth (such as gauze, linen, cotton, or muslin), folding the cloth several times, and crushing the herbs to a pulp with a rolling pin. (Pulping the herb directly onto the poultice cloth helps retain its juices and makes the poultice more effective.) Then expose the pulp and apply it to the affected area. To trap the herbal juices and hold them in place, wrap the entire area with a woolen cloth or towel. This type of poultice can remain in place overnight.

You can also prepare the herbs by placing them in a steamer, colander, strainer, or sieve over a pot of rapidly boiling water and allowing the steam to penetrate and wilt the herbs. After 5 minutes, spread the softened, warmed herbs on a clean white cloth (such as loosely woven cheesecloth) and apply the cloth to the affected area. To help retain the heat, wrap the poultice with a woolen cloth or towel. You can leave this type of poultice on for 20 minutes or overnight if you find the wrap comforting and soothing.

Compresses are effective for bleeding, bruises, muscle cramps, and headaches. They may be hot or cold, depending on the herb and the purpose for using it. To make a *compress*, soak a soft cloth in a strong herbal tea, a tincture or glycerite, an oil, or aromatic water. Then wring it out and apply it to the affected area. You may use a bandage or plastic wrap to hold the compress in place.

Oils, ointments, salves, and rubs

Herbal oils usually are expressed from the peels of lemons, oranges, or other citrus fruits. Because they may irritate the skin, they're commonly diluted in fatty oils or water before being topically applied. Essential oils are used in massage and aromatherapy. They may be diluted to prevent skin irritation.

To make an herbal oil, wash fresh herbs and let them dry overnight. Then slice the herbs (or crumble them if you're using dry herbs), place them in a glass bottle or jar, and cover them with about 1 inch (2.5 cm) of light virgin olive oil, almond oil, or sunflower oil. Cover the container tightly and let it stand in a warm area, such as on a stove or in the sunshine, for 2 weeks. Strain the oil before use.

Herbal ointments, salves, and rubs are applied topically for a variety of conditions. Examples include:

- calendula ointment for broken skin and wounds
- goldenseal applied to infections, rashes, and skin irritations
- aloe vera gel for minor burns
- heat-producing herbs for muscle aches and strains.

Commercial varieties of ointments, salves, and rubs usually are more appealing than homemade concoctions.

You can make an ointment in a ceramic or glass double boiler by heating 2 ounces (60 milliliters) of vegetable lanolin or beeswax until it liquefies. Once the lanolin or wax melts, add 80 to 120 drops of tincture and mix the compound together. Then pour the formula into a glass container and refrigerate it until it hardens. You can substitute a strong herbal tea made from fresh or dried herbs for a store-bought tincture.

Visiting an herbalist

If you decide to visit an herbalist, expect to start with an evaluation, including a review of your medical history. The herbalist may check your pulse and tongue to assess you and may perform a more thorough physical examination. Some herbalists assess the iris, a technique known as iridology, to aid diagnosis. This procedure involves correlating minute markings on the iris with specific parts of the body.

Most herbalists also ask if you're taking prescription or nonprescription drugs to avoid an interaction with an herb or to prevent a cumulative effect. For example, St. John's wort, an herb used as an antidepressant, shouldn't be taken with a prescription antidepressant. If you're a female, the herbalist will ask if you're pregnant or breastfeeding because certain herbs can cause miscarriage, harm the fetus, or pass to the infant in breast milk, causing side effects.

After the evaluation, the herbalist may suggest individual herbs or herbal combinations to treat a particular condition. Medicinal plants may be combined to increase their therapeutic effect, alter the individual actions of each herb, or minimize or negate toxic effects of stronger herbs. An herbal combination, or compound, may make the remedy more effective. (The art of herbal compounding has been practiced for over 5,000 years and is the basis of today's herbal practice.)

Herbal dosages

No dosages for herbal remedies have been established. Manufacturers' guidelines must be adjusted to each person based on such factors as age, weight, and whether he or she is using other herbs or drugs.

Keep in mind that herbal remedies take time to work. The length of therapy depends on the specific herb, whether you're using it as a therapy (to relieve symptoms), a tonic (to build strength), or both. If you're using an herb for therapy, you may need to take it only for a brief period—typically, 1 to 4 weeks. If you're using an herbal remedy as a tonic, expect to take it for a longer period—usually 4 to 6 months or longer. For example, hawthorn, a tonic for the heart and blood vessels, is most effective when used for 6 to 12 consecutive months.

As with other drugs, be sure to take the herb at the appropriate times of the day. Some herbs are more effective when taken in the morning; others, in the evening.

Also, some herbs work best if used with a resting cycle. For example, an herbalist might recommend that you take an herb for 6 days followed by 1 day off, 6 weeks on and 1 week off, 6 months on and 1 month off, or a similar pattern. According to advocates of the resting cycle, each period of rest from the herb treatment allows its effect to become integrated into the body. If the desired effect doesn't appear in the specified time or if side effects develop, the dosage or herb may be changed.

Avoiding problems

Although their overall risk to public health appears to be low, some traditional herbal remedies have been associated with potentially serious side effects. For example, ma huang, an ingredient in numerous diet pills, contains the same active ingredient that's in the bronchodilator ephedrine and can cause irregular heartbeats, seizures, and even death. A few other herbs have also been linked to death and other serious complications.

To promote safer and more effective herbal therapy, follow these guidelines:

- Before you start the herbal regimen, make sure you understand the potential risks involved in self-treatment. These include misdiagnosing your ailment, taking the wrong herb, worsening your condition by delaying conventional treatment, taking an herb that counteracts or interacts with prescribed medical treatment, and aggravating other disorders.
- Familiarize yourself with the herb's actions and side effects before you start taking it. Possible symptoms of sensitivity or side effects include headache, upset stomach, and a rash. Also, some people are predisposed to react to particular herbs. For example, if you're feeling depressed, taking certain herbs used to treat insomnia may heighten your depression. This warning may appear on the herbal remedy package, but the lack of federal regulation means there's no guarantee that remedies will carry adequate warnings.
- Discontinue the herb if you develop a side effect, such as headache, an upset stomach, or a rash.
- If you respond favorably but too intensely to an herb, decrease the dosage or stop taking it altogether. For example, if you're taking a laxative herb to treat constipation, stop taking it if you experience diarrhea.
- If you experience side effects, you may be taking the herb too often or continuing therapy for too long. Sometimes symptoms stem from an incorrect dosage. For instance, eating large amounts of black licorice on a daily basis can lead to high blood pressure.

Aconite

Aconite comes from the leaves, flowers, and roots of *Aconitum napellus,* an erect perennial with tuberous roots. This herb is native to the mountainous regions of North America, Europe, Japan, China, and India.

Aconite was first used medicinally in the 1800s. However, because it can be toxic, it's not recommended for any medicinal use. In fact, this herb was once used as a poison in arrows and has been linked to many suicides.

Common dose

Aconite is available as a tincture, a tea, and a liniment. However, experts warn against using this herb in any form.

Side effects

If you or someone you're with has taken aconite, get immediate medical help if any of these side effects occurs:

- blurred vision
- diarrhea
- increased salivation
- irregular heartbeats
- nausea
- numbness and tingling of the arms and legs
- numbness around the mouth
- slow heartbeat
- throat closure
- vomiting
- weakness.

Why people use this herb

- Fever
- Headache
- High blood pressure
- Inflammation
- Severe stabbing pains

Aconite also can cause low blood potassium, resulting in irregular heartbeats, weakness, and flaccid muscles.

Interactions

Combining herbs with certain drugs may alter their action or produce unwanted side effects. Don't use aconite while taking:

- drugs for irregular heartbeats
- drugs that lower blood pressure.

Important points to remember

- Know that death can result from using as little as 5 milliliters of aconite tincture, 2 milligrams of pure aconite, 1 gram of crude plant parts, or 6 grams of cured aconite.
- Don't use aconite to treat any condition, especially if you have heart disease, irregular heartbeats, blood vessel disease, poor circulation, or a known allergy to this herb.
- Don't use aconite if you're pregnant or breast-feeding.
- Don't consume any part of the aconite plant.
- If you grow aconite, restrict it to the garden. Handle the plant only when wearing gloves that slow absorption of plant oils through the skin.

Other names for aconite

Other names for aconite include friar's cap, helmet flower, monkshood, soldier's cap, and wolfsbane.

No products containing aconite are available commercially in the United States.

WHAT THE RESEARCH SHOWS

Information linking aconite with death points out the danger of using this herb. Aconite has no therapeutic value and poses a grave threat to anyone who uses even small amounts.

Selected references

But, P., et al. "Three Fatal Cases of Herbal Aconite Poisoning," *Veterinary and Human Toxicology* 36:212-15, 1994.

Fatovich, D. "Aconite: A Lethal Chinese Herb," *Annals of Emergency Medicine* 21:309-11, 1992.

Tai, Y., et al. "Cardiotoxicity After Accidental Herb-Induced Aconite Poisoning," *Lancet* 340:1254-56, 1992.

Agrimony

The Greeks supposedly used agrimony to treat eye problems. The Anglo-Saxons, who called the herb *garclive,* apparently used it for wounds. One early herbal remedy for internal bleeding involved swallowing a mixture of agrimony, human blood, and pulverized frog parts. Today, some herbalists recommend agrimony as a throat-soothing gargle for speakers and singers.

Sometimes used as a dye, agrimony comes from the leaves, stems, and flowers of the dried herb *Agrimonia eupatoria,* which grows in the western United States, Europe, and Asia. Pale yellow in September, this plant turns deep yellow later in the year. Some people use agrimony as a tea or poultice as well as a gargle.

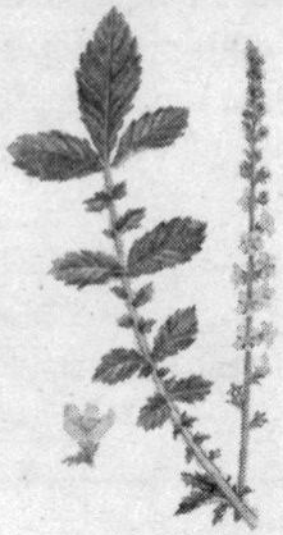

Common doses

Agrimony is available as tablets or teas. Experts know little about appropriate doses for any medicinal use. One source suggests adding 2 to 4 teaspoons of dried leaves per cup of water to make a tea to be taken once a day. Other sources suggest making a compress of agrimony to apply topically to sores.

Why people use this herb

- As a decongestant
- As a gargle
- As a sedative
- Asthma
- Back pain
- Corns
- Eye problems
- Fluid retention
- Gallbladder problems
- To thicken the blood
- Tumors
- Warts
- Weak heartbeat
- Wound healing

Side effects

Call your health care practitioner if you experience any of these possible side effects of agrimony:

- allergic reaction
- skin sensitivity to sunlight.

Interactions

Combining herbs with certain drugs may alter their action or produce unwanted side effects. Tell your health care practitioner about any prescription or nonprescription drugs you're taking.

Important points to remember

- Don't use agrimony if you're allergic to rose plants.
- Avoid this herb if you're pregnant or breast-feeding.
- Watch for skin reactions if you apply agrimony to your skin.
- Avoid strong sunlight because agrimony increases the risk of sunburn.

Other names for agrimony

Other names for agrimony include church steeples, cocklebur, liverwort, philanthropos, sticklewort, and stickwort.

A product containing agrimony is sold as Potter's Piletabs in England.

> **WHAT THE RESEARCH SHOWS**
>
> Experts have little information about agrimony's safety and effectiveness. Thus, they don't recommend the herb for medicinal purposes.

Selected reference

Swanston-Flatt, S. K., et al. "Traditional Plant Treatments for Diabetes: Studies in Normal and Streptozotocin Diabetic Mice," *Diabetologia* 33:462-64, 1990.

Allspice

Because of its pleasant aroma and flavor, allspice is a popular ingredient in food recipes, toothpastes, and other products. The Food and Drug Administration deems it safe for external use.

Active chemicals in allspice come from the dried, unripened berries of *Pimento officinalis* or *Eugenia pimenta*. This tree is native to Central America, Mexico, and the West Indies.

Why people use this herb

- Bruises
- Common cold
- Diabetes
- Diarrhea
- Fatigue
- Hysterical spasms
- Intestinal gas
- Indigestion
- Menstrual cramps
- Sore joints and muscles

Common doses

Allspice is available as:

- a powdered fruit (10 to 30 grains)
- a fluid extract (essential oil)
- pimento water (aqua pimentae), which contains 1 fluid ounce of pimento oil.

Some experts recommend the following doses:

- As a *laxative ingredient,* 1 to 2 fluid ounces (5 parts bruised pimento to 200 parts water, distilled to 100 parts).
- For *indigestion,* mix 1 to 2 teaspoons of allspice powder per cup of water; take up to 3 cups daily.
- For *intestinal gas,* place 2 to 3 drops of allspice oil on sugar and take orally.
- For *toothache pain,* apply 1 to 2 drops of allspice oil to the painful area no more than four times daily.
- For *muscle pain,* mix allspice powder with enough water to make a paste; apply topically to the affected area.

Side effects

Call your health care practitioner if you experience any of these possible side effects of allspice:

- nausea, vomiting, stomach discomfort, diarrhea, and appetite loss (from stomach and bowel inflammation)
- seizures (with excessive use)
- skin rash
- vomiting.

Interactions

Combining herbs with certain drugs may alter their action or produce unwanted side effects. Don't take allspice when using iron and other mineral supplements.

Important points to remember

- Don't use allspice if you have a chronic digestive disease, such as duodenal ulcers, reflux disease, ulcerative colitis, irritable bowel, diverticulosis, or diverticulitis.
- Don't use this herb if you have a history of cancer or an increased risk for cancer. Eugenol, a substance in allspice, may pose a cancer risk.
- Avoid allspice if you're pregnant or breast-feeding.
- Know that allspice may cause allergic skin reactions when used topically.
- Be aware that some experts caution against consuming more allspice than the amounts normally found in foods, toothpastes, and similar products.

WHAT THE RESEARCH SHOWS

Although allspice is safe to consume in small amounts (such as in foods and dental products), controlled clinical trials must be done to validate herbalists' medicinal claims. Right now, scientists have too little information about allspice to recommend medicinal uses.

Other names for allspice

Other names for allspice include clove pepper, Jamaica pepper, pimenta, and pimento.

Allspice is sold as a condiment.

Selected references

Kanerva, L., et al. "Occupational Allergic Contact Dermatitis from Spices," *Contact Dermatitis* 35:157-62, 1996.

Moleyar, V., and Narasimham, P. "Antibacterial Activity of Essential Oil Components," *International Journal of Food Microbiology* 16:337-42, 1992.

Oya, T., et al. "Spice Constituents Scavenging Free Radical and Inhibiting Pentosidine Formation in a Model System," *Bioscience Biotechnology Biochemistry* 61:263-66, 1997.

Suarez, U.A., et al. "Cardiovascular Effects of Thanolica and Aqueous Extracts of *Pimenta dioica* in Sprague-Dawley Rats," *Journal of Ethnopharmacology* 5:107-11, 1997.

Aloe

Aloe has a long history of popular use. It comes from the aloe vera plant (also called *Aloe barbadensis, A. vulgaris hybrids, A. africana, A. ferox, A. perryi,* and *A. spicata*). The plant's large, bladelike leaves are the source of aloe gel. Aloe preparations for oral use contain either the colorless juice that comes from plant's top layer or a solid yellow latex obtained by evaporating the juice.

Aloe comes as both topical and oral preparations. Topical preparations contain the colorless aloe gel or aloe vera gel (sometimes mistakenly called "aloe juice"). Aloe gel can be prepared by various methods. Some people prefer to obtain fresh gel directly from the aloe vera plant.

Common doses

Aloe comes as:

- capsules (75, 100, or 200 milligrams of aloe vera extract or aloe vera powder)
- gel (98%, 99.5%, 99.6%)
- juice (99.6%, 99.7%)
- cream, hair conditioner, jelly, juice, liniment, lotion, ointment, shampoo, skin cream, soap, sunscreen, and in facial tissues.

Some experts recommend the following dose:

- For *skin irritation, itching, burns, and other wounds,* apply an external form of aloe liberally as needed.

Although internal use isn't recommended, some people suggest 100 to 200 milligrams of aloe or 50 to 100 milligrams of aloe extract orally, taken in the evening.

Side effects

Call your health care practitioner if you experience any of these possible side effects of aloe:

Why people use this herb

- Acne
- AIDS
- Arthritis
- Asthma
- Bleeding
- Blindness
- Bursitis
- Cancer
- Common cold
- Colitis (inflammation of the large intestine)
- Constipation
- Depression
- Diabetes
- Glaucoma
- Hemorrhoids
- Lack of menstruation
- Seizures
- Skin conditions (abrasions, cuts, irritations, minor burns, frostbite, sunburn, and wounds)
- Stomach ulcers
- Varicose veins

- delayed healing of deep wounds (with topical forms)
- dehydration (with frequent use)
- intestinal spasms
- reddish urine (with frequent use)
- skin irritation (from direct contact).

Aloe also can cause:

- blood build-up in the pelvis (with large doses)
- low blood potassium, resulting in irregular heartbeats, weakness, and flaccid muscles
- severe diarrhea, kidney damage, and possible death (from overdose)
- spontaneous abortion or premature birth if taken during late pregnancy.

Interactions

Combining herbs with certain drugs may alter their action or produce unwanted side effects. Don't use aloe internally if you're taking:

- digoxin (Lanoxin)
- drugs that cause potassium loss, such as Bumex, Demadex, Edecrin, Lasix, and Sodium Edecrin
- diuretics
- drugs for irregular heartbeats
- steroids.

Important points to remember

- Don't use external aloe preparations if you're allergic to aloe or plants in the Liliaceae family (garlic, onions, and tulips).
- Don't take aloe internally if you're pregnant, breast-feeding, or menstruating.
- Don't give aloe to children.
- Avoid aloe if you have kidney disease or heart disease.
- Don't use aloe vera gel or aloe vera juice internally. You may experience severe stomach discomfort and serious problems from body salt imbalances.
- Be aware that four people have died after receiving aloe vera injections for cancer. Injecting aloe vera isn't recommended.

Other names for aloe

Other names for aloe include aloe barbadensis, aloe vera, Barbados aloe, burn plant, Cape aloe, Curacao aloe, elephant's gall, first-aid plant, hsiang-dan, lily of the desert, lu-hui, medicine plant, miracle plant,

plant of immortality, socotrine aloe, Venezuela aloe, and Zanzibar aloe.

Products containing aloe are sold under such names as All Natural Aloe Vera Gel, Aloe Grande, Aloe Vera Gel, Soft Gel Capsules; Aloe Vera Inner Leaf Capsules, Aloe Vera Jelly, Aloe Vera Juice, Aloe Vera Ointment, Aloe Vesta Perineal, Benzoin Compound Tincture, Dermaide Aloe, Skin Gel Aloe Life, and Whole Leaf Aloe Vera Juice.

WHAT THE RESEARCH SHOWS

Studies show that topical aloe gel application eases acute inflammation and itching, promotes wound healing, and reduces pain. Fresh aloe may have value in treating burns and minor tissue injury, although studies aren't well documented. The Food and Drug Administration considers topical aloe to be generally safe, although it doesn't recommend aloe for any specific condition.

No studies support internal consumption of aloe juice. Aloe laxatives that contain anthraquinone have dramatic effects, and most experts recommend less toxic laxatives.

A recent study found that aloe can alter the body's DNA. This finding may lead to research investigating aloe's possible role in treating cancer.

Selected references

Grindlay, D., and Reynolds, T. "The Aloe Vera Phenomenon: A Review of the Properties and Modern Uses of the Leaf Parenchyma Gel," *Journal of Ethnopharmacology* 16:117-51, 1986.

Heggers, J.P., et al. "Beneficial Effects of Aloe in Wound Healing," *Phytotherapy Research* 7:S48-S52, 1987.

Muller, S.O., et al. "Genotoxicity of the Laxative Drug Components Emodin, Aloe-Emodin, and Danthron in Mammalian Cells: Topoisomerase II-Mediated," *Mutation Research* 371:165-73, 1996.

American cranesbill

American cranesbill comes from *Geranium maculatum,* a perennial herb common to the eastern United States and Canada. Herb forms taken internally are prepared from the plant's dried rhizome (underground stem) and leaves. The flowers are used for topical preparations.

Common doses

American cranesbill comes as extracts, decoctions, tinctures, teas, and poultices. Some experts recommend the following doses:

- As an *infusion,* steep 1 ounce of plant material in 1 pint of water.
- As a *decoction,* use 1 to 2 teaspoons of the rhizome in 1 cup of water three times daily.
- As a *tincture,* use 2 to 4 milliliters three times daily.

Why people use this herb

- Abnormally long or heavy menstrual periods
- Birth control
- Bladder inflammation
- Burns
- Cancer
- Cholera
- Diarrhea
- Dysentery
- Hemorrhoids
- Kidney bleeding
- Lip or mouth inflammation
- Plague
- Sores
- Sore throat
- Uterine bleeding (other than menstrual)
- Vaginal discharge

Side effects

Call your health care practitioner if you experience unusual symptoms when using American cranesbill. This herb may cause liver damage.

Interactions

Combining herbs with certain drugs may alter their action or produce unwanted side effects. Tell your health care practitioner about any prescription or nonprescription drugs you're taking.

Important points to remember

- Don't use American cranesbill if you're pregnant or breast-feeding.
- Know that medical experts warn against consuming this herb because they know little about its effects. If you wish to do so despite this caution, watch for unusual symptoms and report these to your health care practitioner at once.

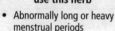

WHAT THE RESEARCH SHOWS

Information about this herb's safety and effectiveness isn't available. Without this crucial data, medical experts advise people to avoid American cranesbill.

Other names for American cranesbill

Other names for American cranesbill include alum bloom, alum root, American kino, chocolate flower, crowfoot, dove's-foot, *Geranium robertianum,* herb robert, old maid's nightcap, shameface, spotted cranesbill, stinking cranesbill, storksbill, wild cranesbill, and wild geranium.

No known products containing American cranesbill are available commercially.

Selected reference

Guevara, J.M., et al., "The In Vitro Action of Plants on *Vibrio cholerae,*" *Revista de Gastroenterologia del Peru* 14:27-31, 1994. Abstract.

Angelica

A perennial plant in the parsley family, angelica is a Chinese herb whose roots, rhizomes (underground stems), fruits, and leaves are used medicinally. The many *Angelica* species include *A. acutiloba, A. archangelica, A. atropurpurea, A. dahurica, A. edulis, A. gigas, A. keiskei, A. koreana, A. polymorpha, A. pubescens, A. radix,* and *A. sinensis.*

Some authorities believe angelica may cause cancer. Such concerns led the International Fragrance Commission to recommend a limit of 0.78% angelica root in commercial preparations of suntan lotions.

Common dose

Angelica is available as fluid extract, tincture, essential oil, or cut, dried, or powdered root. Experts disagree on what dose to take.

Why people use this herb

- Anemia
- Asthma
- Backache
- Eczema (skin inflammation)
- Gynecologic disorders
- Hay fever
- Headache
- Menstrual discomfort
- Osteoporosis
- Poor leg and arm circulation
- Postmenopausal symptoms

Side effects

Call your health care practitioner if you experience any of these possible side effects of angelica:

- dizziness or a faint feeling (from low blood pressure)
- unusual skin sensitivity to sunlight.

Interactions

Combining herbs with certain drugs may alter their action or produce unwanted side effects. Don't use angelica while taking Coumadin (a blood thinner).

Important points to remember

- Don't use angelica if you're pregnant or breast-feeding.
- Use this herb cautiously if you have diabetes.
- Call your health care practitioner if you notice unusual bleeding or bruising after using angelica—especially if you're taking a blood thinner such as Coumadin.
- Be aware that using angelica may pose a cancer risk.

- If you experience an allergic reaction after taking this herb, seek medical help promptly.
- Avoid direct sun exposure while using angelica.

Other names for angelica

Other names for angelica include angelica root, angelique, dong quai, engelwurzel, garden angelica, heiligenwurzel, root of the Holy Ghost, tang-kuei, and wild angelica.

The species *A. sinensis* (from which this herb gets its name) is sold as dong quai or tang-kuei.

WHAT THE RESEARCH SHOWS

In a study of young women with menstrual problems and vaginal discharge, angelica root extract (combined with several other Chinese herbs) helped regulate the menstrual cycle and reduce the amount of discharge. However, the herb hasn't been studied adequately in people. Although it's widely used in traditional Chinese medicine, Western medical experts don't recommend it for specific medicinal uses.

Selected references

Bergendorff, O., et al. "Furanocoumarins with Affinity to Brain Benzodiazepine Receptors In Vitro," *Phytochemistry* 44:1121-24, 1997.

Hoult, J.R., and Paya, M. "Pharmacological and Biochemical Actions of Simple Coumarins: Natural Products with Therapeutic Potential," *General Pharmacology* 27:713-22, 1996.

Kwon, Y.S., et al. "Antimicrobial Constituents of *Angelica dahurica* Roots," *Phytochemistry* 44:887-89, 1997.

Wang, Y., and Zhu, B. "The Effect of Angelica Polysaccharide on Proliferation and Differentiation of Hematopoietic Progenitor Cells," *Chung-Hua I Hsueh Tsa Chih* 76:363-66, 1996.

Anise

Used as a flavoring agent in foods and beverages, anise also is found in many cough drops, baked goods, and beverages. Anise comes from *Pimpinella anisum,* a Mediterranean plant.

Anise oil is extracted from aniseed (the plant's dried ripe fruit) by steam distillation. The oil also can be obtained from the Chinese star anise plant (*Illicium verum).* The Food and Drug Administration considers anise oil safe.

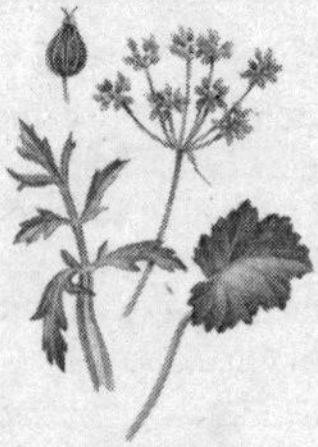

Why people use this herb

- As an expectorant
- Asthma
- Cough
- Intestinal gas
- Lice
- Muscle spasms
- Scabies
- To repel insects

Common dose

Anise comes as an extract and lozenges and in teas. It's also available in trace quantities as a flavoring agent in liqueurs, lozenges, and teas and as a fragrance in soaps, creams, perfumes, foods, and candies. Some experts recommend the following dose:

- For *intestinal gas,* 0.1 milliliter of anise oil taken orally three times a day.

Side effects

Call your health care practitioner if you experience any of these possible side effects of anise:

- allergic reaction
- mouth and lip inflammation (from anise-containing toothpaste)
- nausea, vomiting, and seizures (from ingesting as little as 1 to 5 milliliters of anise oil)
- skin irritation on contact.

Ingesting just 1 to 5 milliliters of anise oil may lead to pulmonary edema.

Intoxication with an anise-based beverage can cause pseudo-Conn's syndrome (hypermineralocorticism), an overgrowth of the adrenal glands that causes low blood potassium levels, muscle weakness, high blood pressure, and increased urination and thirst.

Interactions

Combining herbs with certain drugs may alter their action or produce unwanted side effects. Don't use anise while taking iron supplements.

Important points to remember

- Don't use anise if you're pregnant.
- Use this herb cautiously if you're prone to contact dermatitis or hypersensitivity reactions.
- Don't ingest pure anise oil except under a health care practitioner's supervision. It may be toxic.
- Store anise in a tightly sealed, light-resistant container at room temperature.
- Be aware that anise may cause weight gain from salt and water retention.

WHAT THE RESEARCH SHOWS

In a Russian study, aviation flight controllers who took a combination of anise, brandy mint, and lavender oils had reduced mental fatigue. Nonetheless, anise has limited therapeutic benefits. Until researchers know more about the herb, they caution against using it except as a flavoring agent or fragrance. They especially warn people not to ingest large amounts (several milliliters or more) of anise oil because this may cause serious digestive tract problems.

Other names for anise

Other names for anise include aniseed, anise oil, and sweet cumin.

Products containing anise are sold under such names as Beech Cough Drops and Bronhillor Natural Source Cough Candies & Throat Discs.

Selected references

el-Shobaki, F.A., et al. "The Effect of Some Beverage Extracts on Intestinal Iron Absorption," *Zeitschrift für Ernährungswissenschaft* 29:264-69, 1990.

Trono, D., et al. "Pseudo-Conn's Syndrome due to Intoxication with Non-alcoholic Pastis," *Schweizerische Medizinische Wochenschrift* 113:1092-95, 1983.

Arnica

Some herbalists believe arnica has exciting medical possibilities. The German government has approved it as a topical agent for relief of inflammation, pain, and bacterial infections. Nonetheless, the Food and Drug Administration considers arnica unsafe.

Arnica comes from the flowers and rootstocks of *Arnica montana, A. fulgens, A. sororia,* and *A. cordofolia*. Certain *Arnica* species are native to Alaska, the western United States, and Mexico. Others are native to Europe and Siberia.

Why people use this herb

- Joint aches
- Muscle aches
- Pain
- Wound healing

Common doses

Arnica comes as a spray for topical application and as tablets, teas, gels, tinctures, creams, ointments, and under-the-tongue preparations. Creams typically contain 15% arnica oil. Salves should contain 20% to 25% arnica oil.

Experts disagree on what dose to take. Homeopathic doses (trace amounts) seem to be most popular.

Side effects

Call your health care practitioner if you experience any of these possible side effects of arnica:

- allergic skin inflammation with topical use
- irregular heartbeats and headache (from high blood pressure)
- nausea, vomiting, stomach discomfort, diarrhea, and appetite loss (from stomach and bowel inflammation).

Arnica also can cause:

- liver failure
- muscle weakness, collapse, and possibly death
- nausea, vomiting, organ damage, coma, and possibly death in children who eat arnica flowers or roots
- nervous disorders.

Interactions

Combining herbs with certain drugs may alter their action or produce unwanted side effects. Don't use arnica while taking drugs that lower blood pressure.

Important points to remember

- Don't use arnica if you're pregnant. This herb may cause uterine contractions and has unknown effects on the fetus.
- Don't apply arnica to broken skin or open wounds.
- Keep arnica preparations out of children's reach.
- Know that when taken orally or applied on an open wound, arnica may cause high blood pressure, severe heart problems, vertigo, and kidney dysfunction.
- Avoid prolonged topical use because of the risk of allergic reaction.

WHAT THE RESEARCH SHOWS

Clinical studies don't bear out herbalists' claims that arnica has medical benefits. Studies of postoperative dental patients and hysterectomy patients suggest the herb isn't effective in treating pain. Also, a small study of marathon runners found that arnica didn't help relieve muscle stiffness or promote healing of muscle injuries. What's more, arnica carries a significant risk of allergic reactions.

Other names for arnica

Other names for arnica include arnica flowers, arnica root, common arnica, leopard's bane, Mexican arnica, mountain arnica, mountain daisy, mountain tobacco, sneezewort, and wolfsbane.

Products containing arnica are sold under such names as Arnicaid, Arnica Spray, and Arniflora (Gel).

Selected references

Baillargeon, L., et al. "The Effects of *Arnica montana* on Blood Coagulation: A Randomized, Controlled Trial," *Canadian Family Physician* 39:2362-67, 1993.

Hart, O. et al. "Double-Blind, Placebo-Controlled, Randomized Clinical Trial of Homeopathic Arnica C30 for Pain and Infection After Total Abdominal Hysterectomy," *Journal of the Royal Society of Medicine* 90:73-78, 1997.

Kaziro, G.S. "Metronidazole and *Arnica montana* in the Prevention of Post-surgical Complications: A Comparative Placebo-Controlled Trial," *British Journal of Oral and Maxillofacial Surgery* 22:42-49, 1984.

Avens

Since the 12th century, some Europeans have claimed avens can ward off evil spirits and repel poisonous creatures. A volatile oil, avens is extracted from the dried herb, rhizome (underground stem), or root of *Geum urbanum*, a member of the rose family (Rosaceae).

Why people use this herb

- As an antiseptic
- Chills
- Chronic bleeding
- Diarrhea
- Dysentery
- Inflammation
- Insect bites
- Intermittent fever
- Plague
- Sore throat
- Stomach problems
- Vaginal discharge
- Wound healing

Common dose

Avens comes in a tincture and a tea. Some experts recommend the following dose:

- 1 dram (fluid extract of the herb), ½ to 1 dram (fluid extract of the root), or 15 to 30 grains as a tonic (powdered herb or root) taken orally three times a day.

Side effects

Call your health care practitioner if you experience unusual symptoms when using avens.

Interactions

Combining herbs with certain drugs may alter their action or produce unwanted side effects. Tell your health care practitioner about any prescription or nonprescription drugs you're taking.

Important points to remember

- Don't use avens if you're pregnant or breast-feeding.
- Report unusual symptoms to your health care practitioner.

Other names for avens

Other names for avens include Benedict's herb, city avens, clove root, colewort, geum, goldy star, herb bennet, way bennet, wild rye, and wood avens.

No known products containing avens are available commercially in the United States.

WHAT THE RESEARCH SHOWS

Studies comparing avens to Tylenol or other drugs that contain acetaminophen and other drugs used to reduce inflammation suggest that the herb may have some anti-inflammatory effect. However, experts know little about its safety.

Selected reference

Tunon, H., et al. "Evaluation of Anti-inflammatory Activity of Some Swedish Medicinal Plants: Inhibition of Prostaglandin Biosynthesis and PAF-Induced Exocytosis," *Journal of Ethnopharmacology* 48:61-76, 1995.

Balsam of Peru

***Myroxylon pereirae (M. balsamum)*—the tree that balsam of Peru comes from—grows in Peru, Florida, and Central America. The herb is made from a boiled extract of the tree's battered and scorched bark.**

Balsam of Peru's vanilla-like scent and flavor make it useful in hair care products, lotions, chocolates, baked goods, gelatins, puddings, frozen dairy desserts, and other cosmetic and food products. The German government permits its use as a treatment for various skin conditions.

Common dose

Many commercial products, such as shampoos, conditioners, lotions, and salves, contain small amounts of balsam of Peru. Some experts recommend the following dose:

- For *hemorrhoids,* 1.8- to 3-milligram suppositories taken rectally.

Why people use this herb

- Anal itching
- As an expectorant
- Bedsores
- Cancer
- Dandruff
- Dental uses (to make dental impressions, to treat dry socket)
- Diaper rash
- Hemorrhoids
- Lice
- Pinworms, tapeworms, and other worm infections
- Scabies
- Skin sores
- Wound healing

Side effects

Call your health care practitioner if you experience skin inflammation or irritation. Balsam of Peru also can cause poisoning in breast-fed infants whose mothers applied the herb to their nipples.

Interactions

Combining herbs with certain drugs may alter their action or produce unwanted side effects. Don't use balsam of Peru when taking sulfur-containing products, such as Azulfidine or Bactrim.

Important points to remember

- Don't use this herb if you're pregnant or breastfeeding.
- Use balsam of Peru cautiously if you're prone to skin inflammation or irritation.
- Watch for allergic reactions if you're using a topical form of this herb.

Other names for balsam of Peru

Other names for balsam of Peru include black balsam, Indian balsam, and myroxylon.

No known medicinal products containing balsam of Peru are available commercially.

WHAT THE RESEARCH SHOWS

Little scientific evidence supports claims that balsam of Peru has medicinal value. What's more, the potential side effect of skin irritation limits medicinal uses. For these reasons, experts caution people not to use balsam of Peru except in manufactured cosmetic and pharmaceutical products.

Selected references

"Peruvian Balsam," in *Remington's Pharmaceutical Sciences.* Easton, Pa.: Mack Publishing Co., 1990.

"Peruvian Balsam," in *The United States Dispensatory.* Philadelphia: Lippincott, Williams & Wilkins Pubs., 1993.

Barberry

Barberry comes from the roots, wood, and bark of *Mahonia vulgaris* and *M. aquifolium* (also called *Berberis aquifolium* and *B. vulgaris).* Native to Europe and some parts of North America, *Mahonia* species are popular landscape shrubs. The plants have edible, red-orange, fruitlike berries. The rootwood of the barberry plant gets its bright golden-yellow color from berberine, which is added to some eyedrops and eyewashes.

Why people use this herb

- As an eye astringent
- Cough
- Diarrhea
- Fever
- Jaundice

Common dose

Barberry comes as:

- tablets (400 milligrams)
- liquid
- extract
- tea.

Some experts recommend the following dose:

- 400 milligrams taken orally daily.

Side effects

Call your health care practitioner if you experience any of these possible side effects of barberry:

- bloody urine, painful urination, flank pain, and fever (symptoms of kidney inflammation)
- diarrhea
- confusion
- poisoning symptoms (diarrhea, bloody urine, painful urination, fever, flank pain, confusion, and stupor).

Barberry also can cause miscarriage and stupor.

Interactions

Combining herbs with certain drugs may alter their action or produce unwanted side effects. Tell your health care practitioner about any prescription or nonprescription drugs you're taking.

Important points to remember

- Don't use barberry if you're pregnant because it can cause miscarriage.

- Use this herb cautiously if you're a female of childbearing age.
- Seek immediate medical help if you experience poisoning symptoms (diarrhea, bloody urine, painful urination, fever, flank pain, confusion, and stupor).
- Don't consume large amounts of barberry because it contains potentially toxic chemicals.

WHAT THE RESEARCH SHOWS

Medical experts don't have enough information about barberry to recommend it for treating diarrhea or other conditions. In one study, barberry proved more effective than a placebo in resolving diarrhea caused by cholera. However, it wasn't more effective than a placebo when diarrhea stemmed from other causes.

Other names for barberry

Other names for barberry include berberry, common barberry, European barberry, jaundice berry, Oregon grape, pepperridge bush, sourspine, sowberry, trailing mahonia, and wood sour.

A product containing barberry is sold as Oregon Grape Root.

Selected references

Farnsworth, N.R., et al. "Potential Value of Plants as Sources of New Antifertility Agents. I," *Journal of Pharmaceutical Sciences* 64:535-98, 1975.

Ivanovska, N., and Philipov, S. "Study on the Antiinflammatory Action of *Berberis vulgaris* Root Extract, Alkaloid Fractions, and Pure Alkaloids," *International Journal of Immunopharmacology* 10:553-61, 1996.

Maung, K.U., et al. "Clinical Trial of Berberine in Acute Watery Diarrhea," *BMJ* 291:1601, 1985.

Basil

A spicy herb prized by cooks, basil belongs to the mint family. It comes from a plant called *Ocimum basilicum* (sweet or common basil) or *O. sanctum* (holy basil).

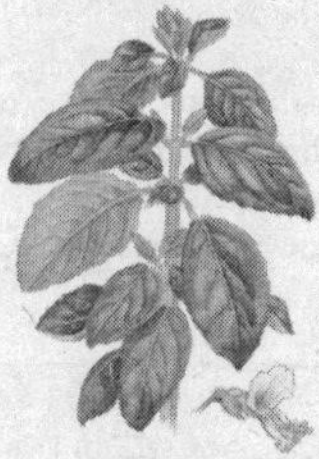

Why people use this herb

- As an antiseptic
- Inflammation
- High blood sugar
- Pain relief
- Stomach ulcers

Common dose

Basil comes as a tea and as powdered or chopped leaves. Some experts recommend the following dose:

- 2.5 grams of fresh dried leaf powder taken daily. To make a tea, place 2.5 grams of fresh dried leaf powder in ½ cup water, strain, and drink once or twice daily as needed.

Side effects

Call your health care practitioner if you experience dizziness, hunger, confusion, headache, trembling, heavy sweating, rapid pulse, and cold, sweaty skin (symptoms of low blood sugar).

Basil also may cause or contribute to liver cancer.

Interactions

Combining herbs with certain drugs may alter their action or produce unwanted side effects. Tell your health care practitioner about any prescription or nonprescription drugs you're taking, especially:

- insulin
- oral drugs used to treat diabetes (don't use basil medicinally when taking these drugs).

Important points to remember

- Don't use basil for medicinal purposes if you're pregnant or breastfeeding.
- If you have diabetes, use this herb only in the amounts typically found in foods.
- Avoid long-term medicinal use of basil.

WHAT THE RESEARCH SHOWS

Of the few human studies of basil's medicinal effects, one small study showed it significantly reduced blood sugar. This could make it useful in treating non-insulin-dependent diabetes. However, similar results must be duplicated in a large, controlled trial before medical experts can recommend the herb. Claims that basil is effective against other diseases remain unproven.

Other names for basil

Other names for basil include common basil, garden basil, holy basil, and sweet basil.

No known products containing basil are available commercially.

Selected references

Agrawal, P., et al. "Randomized Placebo Controlled, Single-Blind Trial of Holy Basil Leaves in Patients with Non-Insulin-Dependent Diabetes Mellitus," *International Journal of Clinical Pharmacology and Therapeutics* 34:406-09, 1996.

Akhtar, M.S., et al. "Antiulcerogenic Effects of *Ocimum basilicum* Extracts, Volatile Oils and Flavonoid Glycosides in Albino Rats," *International Journal of Pharmacognosy* 30:97-104, 1992.

Brinker, F. *The Toxicology of Botanical Medicines,* rev. 2nd ed. Sandy, Oreg.: Eclectic Medicinal Publications, 1996.

Bay

An ingredient in some natural toothpastes, bay usually is obtained from the leaves and berries of *Laurus nobilis,* a small tree native to the Mediterranean area. A different bay tree species that grows in California has a more bitter product used primarily in extracts. Because bay seems to enhance insulin's effects, some nutritionists recommend it for diabetic diets.

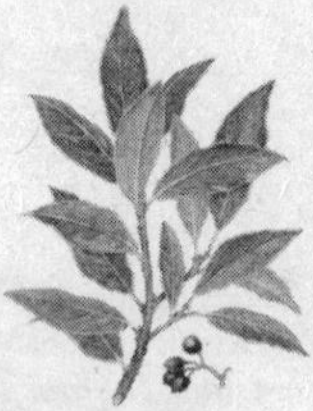

Common doses

Bay is available as leaves, berries, extracts, and essential oil.

Some people apply bay extracts topically or use them in baths and soaks. The leaves typically are used to season foods. *Before eating bay leaves, be sure to thoroughly dry and crush them.*

Why people use this herb

- As an antiseptic
- As a stimulant
- Common cold
- Fluid retention
- Muscle sprains and strains
- Rheumatism

Side effects

Contact your health care practitioner if you experience any of these possible side effects of bay:

- asthma
- skin irritation.

Eating bay leaves without crushing them first may cause bowel perforation.

Interactions

Combining herbs with certain drugs may alter their action or produce unwanted side effects. Tell your health care practitioner about any prescription or nonprescription drugs you're taking, especially insulin.

Important points to remember

- Don't use bay if you're pregnant or breast-feeding.
- Don't consume essential oil from bay leaves because of the risk of allergic reaction and an asthma attack.
- Don't ingest whole, intact bay leaves. Because of their sharp, serrated edges, they can become lodged in the esophagus or intestine. Some people have had to have surgery to remove them.

Other names for bay

Other names for bay include bay laurel, bay leaf, bay tree, and sweet bay.

Various manufacturers provide the entire leaf or crushed leaves as a condiment. No known medicinal products containing bay are available commercially.

> **WHAT THE RESEARCH SHOWS**
>
> Although bay leaf is a popular seasoning, scientists can't verify claims that it's effective in treating diabetes or any other disease.

Selected references

Hausen, B.M., and Hjorth, N. "Skin Reactions to Topical Food Exposure," *Dermatologic Clinics* 2:567-78, 1984.

Panzer, P.E. "The Dangers of Cooking with Bay Leaves," *JAMA* 250:164-65, 1983. Letter.

Rao, A.R. and Hashim, S. "Chemopreventive Action of Oriental Food-Seasoning Spices Mixture Garam Masala on DMBA-Induced Transplacental and Translactational Carcinogenesis in Mice," *Nutrition and Cancer* 23:91-101, 1995.

Bayberry

Medicinal extracts of bayberry usually are obtained from the dried root bark of *Myrica cerifera*, a shrub native to Texas and the eastern United States. Bayberry is best known for its small, bluish-white berries. Wax extracted from the berries is used in fragrances and candles.

Why people use this herb

- As a stimulant
- Diarrhea
- Jaundice
- To induce vomiting
- Wound healing

Common dose

Bayberry comes as:
- capsules (450 and 475 milligram)
- liquid
- tea
- extract.

Experts disagree on what dose to take. Most suggest consuming bayberry as a tea.

Side effects

Contact your health care practitioner if you experience any of these possible side effects of bayberry:
- nasal allergy symptoms
- other allergic reactions
- stomach discomfort
- vomiting.

Bayberry also can cause cancer and liver damage.

Interactions

Combining herbs with certain drugs may alter their action or produce unwanted side effects. Tell your health care practitioner about any prescription or nonprescription drugs you're taking.

Important points to remember

- Don't use bayberry if you're pregnant or breast-feeding.
- Avoid eating parts of the bayberry plant. Its high tannin content may cause stomach irritation and liver damage.
- Be aware that this herb may cause weight gain, high blood pressure, water retention, and body salt imbalances.
- Report allergic reactions to your health care practitioner.

Other names for bayberry

Other names for bayberry include candleberry, myrica, southern wax myrtle, spicebush, sweet oak, tallow shrub, vegetable tallow, waxberry, and wax myrtle plant.

A product containing bayberry is sold as Bayberry Bark.

> **WHAT THE RESEARCH SHOWS**
>
> Little evidence supports medicinal claims for bayberry. Its high tannin content (which can lead to stomach distress and liver damage) rules out oral use. Allergic reactions to the pollen extract further limit bayberry's medicinal value.

Selected references

Jacinto, C.M., et al. "Nasal and Bronchial Provocation Challenges with Bayberry *(Myrica cerifera)* Pollen Extract," *Journal of Allergy and Clinical Immunology* 90:312-18, 1992.

Paul, B.D., et al. "Isolation of Myricadiol, Myriciatrin, Taraxerol, and Taxerone from Myrica cerifera Root Bark," *Journal of Pharmaceutical Sciences* 63:958-59, 1974.

Bearberry

Bearberry comes from the dry leaves—not berries—of the low, trailing evergreen shrub *Arctostaphylos uva-ursi* (also *A. coactylis* and *A. adenotricha*).

Common dose

Bearberry comes as drops, tablets, and tea. Some experts recommend the following dose:

- 1 to 10 grams taken orally daily.

Side effects

Contact your health care practitioner if you experience any of these possible side effects of bearberry:

- bluish gray skin
- green urine
- nausea
- vomiting.

When taken in large doses (more than 20 grams as a single dose), bearberry may cause ringing in the ears, vomiting, seizures, and blood vessel collapse.

Why people use this herb

- Fluid retention
- To sterilize the urinary tract

Interactions

Combining herbs with certain drugs may alter their action or produce unwanted side effects. Don't use bearberry while taking:

- diuretics
- drugs that make the urine acidic, such as ascorbic acid and Urex.

Important points to remember

- Don't use this herb if you're pregnant or breast-feeding.
- Know that although some people have taken up to 20 grams of bearberry at a time with no side effects, others have experienced poisoning symptoms from as little as 1 gram.
- Be aware that bearberry may turn your urine green.

Other names for bearberry

Other names for bearberry include arctostaphylos, bear's grape, crowberry, foxberry, hogberry, kinnikinnick, manzanita, mountain box, rockberry, and uva-ursi.

Products containing bearberry are sold under such names as Arctuvan, Solvefort, Uroflux, and Uvalyst.

WHAT THE RESEARCH SHOWS

Bearberry may help relieve fluid retention and ease inflammation, but more studies are needed to verify these effects. Until medical experts have more information, they can't recommend bearberry for any condition.

Selected references

Jahodar, L., et al. "Investigation of Iridoid Substances in Arctostaphylos uva-ursi," Pharmazie 33:536-37, 1978.

Matsuda, H., et al. "Effects of Water Extract From Arctostaphyllos uva-ursi on the Antiallergic and Anti-inflammatory Activities of Dexamethasone Ointment," *Yakugaku Zasshi* 112:73-77, 1992. Abstract.

Swanston-Flatt, S.K., et al. "Evaluation of Traditional Plant Treatments for Diabetes: Studies in Streptozocin Diabetic Mice," *Acta Diabetologica Latina* 26:51-55, 1989.

Turi, M., et al. "Influence of Aqueous Extracts of Medicinal Plants on Surface Hydrophobicity of E. coli Strains of Different Origin," *APMIS* 105:956-62, 1997. Abstract.

Benzoin

A resin of balsam, benzoin has been used for over 100 years. It's obtained by wounding the bark of *Styrax benzoin* trees age 7 years or older. Benzoin can also be obtained from the bark of *S. paralleloneurus* and *S. tonkinensis*.

Common doses

Benzoin comes as compound benzoin tincture USP, which contains 10% benzoin, 2% aloe, 8% storax, 4% tolu balsam, and 75% to 83% alcohol. It's also an ingredient in some cold-sore lotions, creams, and ointments. Some experts recommend the following doses:

- By *steam inhalation,* add approximately 5 milliliters of compound benzoin tincture to 1 pint of hot water, and inhale. Or place the tincture on a handkerchief and inhale.
- For *mucous membrane protection* (adults and children over age 6 months), apply a few drops topically no more than once every 2 hours. Use in infants only under medical supervision.

Why people use this herb

- As an antiseptic
- As an expectorant
- As a wound adhesive
- Cough
- Pain from canker sores, inflamed gums, and oral herpes sores
- To protect the mouth's mucous membranes

Side effects

Contact your health care practitioner if you experience any of these possible side effects of benzoin:

- allergic reactions
- asthma (when inhaled)
- hives
- skin irritation

If ingested, benzoin can cause stomach inflammation or digestive tract bleeding.

Interactions

Combining herbs with certain drugs may alter their action or produce unwanted side effects. Tell your health care practitioner about any prescription or nonprescription drugs you're taking.

Important points to remember

- Don't inhale benzoin if you have asthma.
- Know that benzoin is poisonous if taken internally.
- Avoid benzoin if you have a history of allergic reactions, asthma, or skin irritation.
- Be aware that topical benzoin use can discolor the skin and cause skin irritation.
- Know that inhaling the volatile steam of benzoin isn't effective. Consider using unmedicated water vapor instead.

WHAT THE RESEARCH SHOWS

Most clinical information about benzoin comes from case reports and the herb's long history of use in numerous medical specialties. Such information shows that the herb is inferior to other products in protecting the skin and mucous membranes and as a wound adhesive.

Although people have been inhaling compound benzoin tincture for many years, the practice has never been studied systematically. Experts believe inhaling plain steam is probably just as effective—maybe more so.

As for benzoin's use in protecting the skin and mucous membranes, experts don't recommend the herb because it can cause allergic reactions and because many conventional antiseptics have proven to be effective.

Other names for benzoin

Other names for benzoin include benjamin tree, benzoe, benzoin tree, gum benjamin, Siam benzoin, and Sumatra benzoin.

Products containing benzoin are sold under such names as Balsam of the Holy Victorious Knight, Friar's Balsam, Jerusalem Balsam, Pfeiffer's Cold Sore Preparation, Turlington's Balsam Of Life, Ward's, and Balsam.

Selected references

Council on Dental Therapeutics. *Accepted Dental Therapeutics,* 40th ed. Chicago: American Dental Association, 1984.

Covington, T.R., ed. *Handbook of Nonprescription Drugs,* 11th ed. Washington, D.C.: American Society of Hospital Pharmacists, 1993.

James, W.D. "Allergic Contact Dermatitis to Compound Tincture of Benzoin," *Journal of the American Academy of Dermatology* 11:847-50, 1984.

Betel palm

Betel palm comes from the raw, sweetened leaves and nuts of *Areca catechu,* a member of the Palmaceae (Palm) family. The plant is native to India, China, Indonesia, Sri Lanka, the Philippines, and parts of Africa. Roughly 200 million people throughout the Pacific Rim, Southeast Asia, India, and Indonesia chew betel nuts and leaves, as much as some Americans chew tobacco.

Why people use this herb

- As a mild stimulant
- Cough
- Respiratory symptoms
- Sore throat
- To aid digestion

Common doses

Betel palm is available as betel oil, raw leaves, and nuts. Usually, the betel nut is sweetened with lime (calcium hydroxide), wrapped in the leaf of the betel vine, and then chewed. Chewing the "quid," as this habit is called, can take up to 15 minutes. Some users chew up to 15 quids daily.

Side effects

Call your health care practitioner if you experience any of these possible side effects of betel palm:

- anxiety
- blurred vision
- cold sweats
- constipation
- diarrhea
- fast or slow heartbeat
- facial flushing
- fever
- hallucinations
- insomnia
- muscle jerking or muscle paralysis
- nervousness
- pale skin
- restlessness
- stomach cramps
- unusually small or large pupils
- vomiting
- worsening of asthma.

Betel palm also can cause high blood pressure. With *prolonged* use, it may cause:

- calcium loss from the teeth
- increased risk of mouth and esophagus cancer
- inflammation of the gums and related tissues
- red staining of the teeth and inside of the mouth.

Excessive betel chewing can cause dizziness, nausea, vomiting, diarrhea, and seizures (similar to symptoms of excessive nicotine use).

Interactions

Combining herbs with certain drugs may alter their action or produce unwanted side effects. Don't use betel palm when taking:

- alcohol
- atropine
- drugs used to treat glaucoma
- heart drugs called beta blockers (such as Inderal or Betapace) or calcium channel blockers (such as Calan or Procardia).

Important points to remember

- Avoid betel palm if you have a high risk for cancer of the mouth or esophagus, squamous cell cancer, or oral leukoplakia (thick, white patches inside the mouth).
- Don't use betel palm if you're pregnant or breast-feeding.
- Be aware that prolonged betel nut chewing is linked to mouth and esophagus cancers.

WHAT THE RESEARCH SHOWS

No data support medicinal uses of betel palm. Chewing betel nut has been compared with using tobacco or alcohol—legal but potentially harmful.

Other names for betel palm

Other names for betel palm include areca nut, betal, betel nut, chavica betal, hmarg, maag, marg, paan, pan masala, pan parag, pinang, and supai.

Betel nuts are sold under various names in ethnic grocery stores in the United States.

Selected references

Chu, N.S. "Betel Chewing Increases the Skin Temperature: Effects of Atropine and Propranolol," *Neuroscience Letters* 194:130-32, 1995.

Huston, B. "Betel Nuts." Bureau of Food Regulatory, International and Intraagency Affairs, Health Canada. Field Compliance Guide. Citation 1991-01. Ottawa, Canada.

Ko, Y.C., et al. "Betel Quid Chewing, Cigarette Smoking and Alcohol Consumption Related to Oral Cancer in Taiwan," *Journal of Oral Pathology and Medicine* 24:450-53, 1995.

Merlidhar, V., and Upmanyu, G. "Tobacco Chewing, Oral Submucous Fibrosis and Anaesthetic Risk," *Lancet* 347:1840, 1996. Letter.

Bethroot

Native Americans used bethroot to reduce postpartum bleeding. For this reason, some people call it birthroot. Others call it stinking Benjamin because its dark purple flowers smell like rotting flesh. Following the early doctrine that "like cures like," the plant was applied to gangrenous wounds to try to halt the infection.

Bethroot's active agents come from the dried roots, rhizomes (underground stems), and leaves of *Trillium erectum*, a low-lying perennial of the Lily family (Liliaceae). The plant grows in Canada and Eastern and Central United States.

Common doses

Bethroot comes as a powder, powdered root, and fluid extract. Some experts recommend the following doses:

- 1 tablespoon of bethroot powder in a pint of boiling water taken "freely in wineglassful doses."
- 1 dram of powdered root taken orally three times a day.
- 30 minims of fluid extract as an astringent or tonic expectorant.

Why people use this herb

- Abnormally long or heavy menstrual periods
- As an expectorant
- Bleeding
- Bloody diarrhea
- During childbirth and delivery
- Skin irritation
- Snakebite
- To stimulate the uterus

Side effects

Call your health care practitioner if you experience any of these possible side effects of bethroot:

- stomach upset
- vomiting.

Bethroot also may cause toxic effects on the heart.

Interactions

Combining herbs with certain drugs may alter their action or produce unwanted side effects. Don't use bethroot while taking drugs used to treat heart problems.

Important points to remember

- Avoid bethroot if you're pregnant because it may stimulate the uterus.

- Don't use bethroot if you're taking drugs prescribed for a heart condition. This herb may affect heart function.
- Consider discontinuing the herb if you experience stomach upset.

WHAT THE RESEARCH SHOWS

Little scientific evidence supports bethroot's traditional uses in promoting childbirth and delivery, managing postpartum bleeding, or treating snakebites, skin irritation, and many other problems. Medical experts can't consider bethroot or its components medically useful until it has been studied carefully in humans.

Other names for bethroot

Other names for bethroot include birthroot, cough root, ground lily, Indian balm, Indian shamrock, Jew's harp, purple trillium, snake bite, squaw root, stinking Benjamin, trillium, trillium pendulum, and wake-robin.

A product containing bethroot is sold under the name Trillium Complex.

Selected reference

Hufford, C.D., et al. "Antifungal Activity of *Trillium grandiflorum* Constituents," *Journal of Natural Products* 51:94-96, 1988.

Betony

Betony comes from the flowers and leaves of *Stachys officinalis*, a plant found in Europe, Northern Africa, and Siberia. Folklore suggests many uses for this herb.

Common doses

Betony comes as capsules and tea. Typically, it's taken as an infusion or a tea.

Side effects

Call your health care practitioner if you experience stomach upset when using betony. Betony also can cause liver damage.

Interactions

Combining herbs with certain drugs may alter their action or produce unwanted side effects. Don't use betony when taking drugs that lower blood pressure.

Why people use this herb

- Asthma
- Bronchitis
- Diarrhea
- Heartburn
- Kidney disease
- Palpitations
- Roundworms
- Seizures
- Stomachache
- Toothache
- Wounds

Important points to remember

- Don't use betony if you're pregnant because it may stimulate the uterus.
- Use this herb cautiously because it may cause liver damage and stomach discomfort.

Other names for betony

Other names for betony include bishopswort and wood betony.

A product containing betony is sold as Wood Betony.

Selected reference

Lipkan, G.N., et al. "Primary Evaluation of the Overall Toxicity and Anti-inflammatory Activity of Some Plant Preparations," *Farmatsevtychnyi Zhurnal* 1:78-81, 1974.

WHAT THE RESEARCH SHOWS

Despite various claims, evidence doesn't support using betony for any medicinal purpose.

Bilberry

Native Americans used bilberry teas and tinctures to treat diabetes symptoms. During World War II, British pilots ate bilberry preserves to improve their night vision.

Bilberry's active components are extracted by a drying process from the *Vaccinium myrtillus* plant. Some people prepare a hydroalcoholic extraction of the leaf.

Why people use this herb

- Cataracts
- Diabetic retinopathy (a vision disorder caused by diabetes)
- Glaucoma
- Hemorrhoids
- Macular degeneration (a vision disorder related to aging)
- Poor circulation
- Poor night vision
- Varicose veins

Common doses

Bilberry comes as:

- capsules (60, 80, 120, and 450 milligrams)
- liquid
- tincture
- fluid extract
- dried roots, leaves, and berries.

Some experts recommend the following doses:

- To *improve night vision,* 60 to 120 milligrams of bilberry extract taken orally daily.
- For *poor vision* or *poor circulation,* 240 to 480 milligrams orally every day, taken in two or three equal doses.

Side effects

Call your health care practitioner if you experience unusual symptoms while taking bilberry. Long-term consumption of large doses of bilberry leaves may cause toxic reactions. Doses of 1.5 grams of bilberry per kilograms of body weight may cause death.

Interactions

Combining herbs with certain drugs may alter their action or produce unwanted side effects. Tell your health care practitioner about any prescription or nonprescription drugs you're taking, especially:

- Antabuse (don't use bilberry products containing alcohol when taking Antabuse)

- antiplatelet drugs such as aspirin
- blood thinners such as Coumadin.

Important points to remember

- Don't use bilberry if you're pregnant or breast-feeding.
- If you use bilberry when taking a blood thinner, be sure to report unusual bleeding or bruising to your health care practitioner.
- Know that experts recommend using only standardized bilberry products with 25% anthocyanoside content.

WHAT THE RESEARCH SHOWS

A study conducted in the 1960s found that bilberry improved night vision. Medical experts are intrigued with the possible use of bilberry extracts to treat fluid retention and blood vessel leakage, but can't support such use until more human studies are done. What's more, they know little about bilberry's potential toxicity—except that daily doses exceeding 480 milligrams may be dangerous.

Other names for bilberry

Other names for bilberry include bilberries, bog bilberries, European blueberries, huckleberries, and whortleberries.

Products containing bilberry are sold under such names as Bilberry Extract and Bilberry Vegicap.

Selected references

Laplaud, P.M., et al. "Antioxidant Action of *Vaccinium myrtillus* Extract on Human Low Density Lipoproteins in Vitro: Initial Observations," *Fundamental and Clinical Pharmacology* 11:35-40, 1997. Abstract.

Morazzoni, P., and Magistretti, M.J. "Effects of *V. myrtillus* Anthocyanosides on Prostacyclin-like Activity in Rat Arterial Tissue," *Fitoterapia* 57:11-14, 1986.

Birch

Active compounds of birch come from the dried bark and twigs of the birch species *Betula alba (B. pendula), B. verrucosa, B. pubescens,* and *B. lenta*. Several birch species are native to eastern North America, Europe, and parts of Russia.

In Germany, some people use *B. pendula* leaves as a diuretic to treat urinary tract infections. German researchers are evaluating betulin, a compound found in birch, for possible use against tumors.

Common dose

Birch comes as essential oil (bark, wood), dried bark, and tea. Some experts recommend the following dose:

- As an *extract* or *tea,* steep 2 to 3 grams of the bark in boiling water for 10 to 15 minutes and ingest up to several times daily.

Side effects

Call your health care practitioner if you experience any of these possible side effects of birch:

- acute skin irritation from exposure to birch leaves or sap
- allergies caused by cross-sensitivity to other plant allergens, such as celery and mugwort pollen
- nasal allergy symptoms.

Why people use this herb

- Bladder infections
- Digestive problems
- Gout
- Headache
- Kidney stones
- Pain relief
- Rheumatism
- Skin disorders

Interactions

Combining herbs with certain drugs may alter their action or produce unwanted side effects. Tell your health care practitioner about any prescription or nonprescription drugs you're taking.

Important points to remember

- Don't use birch if you're pregnant or breast-feeding.
- Use this herb cautiously if you have seasonal allergies or a known hypersensitivity to plant allergens.
- Keep birch preparations out of children's reach. Sweet birch oil contains

98% methyl salicylate, which has been fatal to children when applied topically to the skin. Poisoning has occurred with as little as 4.7 grams of methyl salicylate applied topically.

- Know that topical birch preparations may irritate the skin and mucous membranes. Report new or unusual skin problems to your health care practitioner.

WHAT THE RESEARCH SHOWS

Birch has some interesting chemical properties, but until more clinical research is available, the herb won't play a role in modern medicine. Also, the risk of allergic reactions gives cause for concern.

Other names for birch

Other names for birch include birch tar oil, birch wood oil, black birch, cherry birch, sweet birch oil, and white birch.

No known products containing birch are available commercially.

Selected references

Bisset, N.G., ed. *Herbal Drugs and Phytopharmaceuticals.* Boca Raton, Fla.: CRC Press, 1994.

Budavari, S., et al., eds. *The Merck Index,* 12th ed. Whitehouse Station, N.J.: Merck and Co., Inc., 1996.

Lahti, A., and Hannuksela, M. "Immediate Contact Allergy to Birch Leaves and Sap," *Contact Dermatitis* 6:464-65, 1980.

Bistort

Bistort comes from *Polygonum bistorta,* a member of the Buckwheat family (Polygonaceae). This plant is native to Europe and naturalized in North America. The most prized parts, the root and rhizomes (underground stems), are gathered in the fall. The leaves are gathered in the spring.

Rich in starch, bistort root has been roasted and eaten as a vegetable. Different folk cultures use different parts of bistort.

Why people use this herb

- As an antidote for certain poisons
- Bleeding from the respiratory tract or stomach
- Canker sores
- Dysentery
- Excessive respiratory secretions
- Gum problems
- Hemorrhoids
- Insect bites
- Irritable bowel syndrome
- Jaundice
- Laryngitis
- Measles
- Small burns or wounds
- Snakebite
- Sore throat
- Stomach ulcers
- Tapeworm, pinworm, and other worm infections
- To stop external and internal bleeding
- Ulcerative colitis
- Vaginal bleeding or discharge

Common dose

Bistort comes as a powder, dried or cut root, and tea. Some experts recommend the following dose:

- For *diarrhea,* 1 teaspoon of the powdered root combined with 1 to 1½ cups of boiling water, taken orally. Don't take more than 3 cups daily.

Side effects

Call your health care practitioner if you experience stomach upset. Bistort also may cause liver damage.

Interactions

Combining herbs with certain drugs may alter their action or produce unwanted side effects. Tell your health care practitioner about any prescription or nonprescription drugs you're taking.

Important points to remember

- Don't use bistort if you're pregnant or breast-feeding.
- Don't take this herb internally for more than 3 weeks at a time.

Other names for bistort

Other names for bistort include adderwort, common bistort, Easter ledges, Easter mangiant, knotweed, oderwort, osterick, patience dock, snakeroot, snakeweed, and twice writhen.

No known products containing bistort are available commercially.

WHAT THE RESEARCH SHOWS

Bistort shows some promise in easing inflammation, relieving arthritis symptoms, and treating diarrhea in children. It also may have value as an astringent to use in poultices. However, few scientific studies support these uses. Until clinical trials can precisely define bistort's therapeutic value, medical experts can't recommend it.

Selected references

British Herbal Pharmacopoeia, Consolidated ed. London: British Herbal Medicine Association, 1983.

Duwiejua, M., et al. "Anti-inflammatory Activity of *Polygonum bistorta, Guaiacum officinale,* and *Hamamelis virginiana* in Rats," *Journal of Pharmacy and Pharmacology* 46:286-90, 1994.

Black catechu

Black catechu was popular in the United States and abroad during the mid-1800s and early 1900s. In some parts of the world, people still use it to treat diarrhea and prevent pregnancy.

Black catechu is prepared as a dried extract from the heartwood of *Acacia catechu,* a tree native to Burma and Eastern India and naturalized in Jamaica. The extract is prepared by boiling heartwood pieces in water, evaporating the mixture to a syrup, and cooling it to molds, which are then broken into pieces.

Don't confuse black catechu with pale catechu, which comes from a different plant. Pale catechu is used in the dye industry and as a veterinary astringent.

Why people use this herb

- Birth control
- Chronic gonorrhea
- Cracked nipples
- Diarrhea and other digestive tract problems
- Mouth ulcers
- Nosebleed
- Painless ulcers
- Sore gums

Common doses

Black catechu is available as:

- dry powder
- dried extract or liquid for oral use (0.3 to 2 grams)
- tincture
- local injection for hemorrhoids.

Some experts recommend the following doses:

- For *oral use* or by *infusion* (as a tea), 0.3 to 2 grams of the dried extract.
- As a *tincture,* 2.5 to 5 milliliters of a 1:5 dilution in 45% alcohol.

Side effects

Call your health care practitioner if you experience any of these possible side effects of black catechu:

- constipation
- symptoms of low blood pressure, such as dizziness and weakness.

Using nonstandardized black catechu products that contain large amounts of inactive ash and aflatoxin (a fungal contaminant) can cause aflatoxin contamination, a condition associated with certain cancers.

Interactions

Combining herbs with certain drugs may alter their action or produce unwanted side effects. Don't use black catechu when taking:

- Calan
- Captopril
- drugs that lower blood pressure
- drugs that suppress the immune system, such as Atgam, Imuran, and Sandimmune
- narcotic pain relievers.

Also, tell your health care practitioner if you're taking iron-containing products, which aren't compatible with black catechu.

Important points to remember

- Don't use this herb if you're pregnant or breast-feeding.
- Don't use black catechu when taking drugs that suppress your immune system, such as Atgam, Imuran, and Sandimmune.
- Be aware that this herb is known to cause cancer when consumed in the diet.
- Be aware that medical experts don't know the long-term effects of chronic black catechu use.
- If have high blood pressure, take your blood pressure regularly when using this herb.
- Be aware that taking black catechu along with a drug that causes constipation (such as a narcotic pain reliever) may worsen constipation.
- If you have diabetes, be aware that this herb may cause your blood sugar to fall too low.
- Don't rely on black catechu to prevent pregnancy.

Other names for black catechu

Other names for black catechu include acacia catechu, acacia di cachou, acacie au cachou, amaraja, cake catechu, catechu, cutch, erh-ch'a, hai-erh-ch'a, kadaram, katechu akazie, katesu, khair, pegu katechu, and wu-tieh-ni.

Products containing black catechu are sold under such names as Diarcalm, Élixir Bonjean, Enterodyne, Hemo Cleen, Katha, Shanti Bori (used in rural Bangladesh as an oral contraceptive component), and Spanish Tummy Mixture.

WHAT THE RESEARCH SHOWS

Although black catechu has possible medical uses, medical experts can't recommend it for any condition until they know more about its risks and benefits. The herb hasn't been clinically tested in humans and its value in treating chronic diarrhea hasn't been proven. What's more, researchers don't know if black catechu is toxic.

Although some women with cracked nipples have used black catechu, scientists don't know if these women were breast-feeding at the time and thus couldn't determine whether the herb can harm breast-fed infants.

Selected references

Azad Chowdhury, A.K., et al. "Antifertility Activity of a Traditional Contraceptive Pill Comprising Acacia catechu, A. arabica, and Tragia involuceria," *Indian Journal of Medical Research* 80:372-74, 1984.

Morton, J.F. "Widespread Tannin Intake via Stimulants and Masticatories, Especially Guarana, Kola Nut, Betel Vine, and Accessories," *Basic Life Sciences* 59:739-65, 1992. Abstract.

Pharmaceutical Society of Great Britain, Department of Pharmaceutical Sciences, ed. *The Pharmaceutical Codex,* 11th ed. London: The Pharmaceutical Press, 1979.

Roy, A.K., et al. "Aflatoxin Contamination of Some Common Drug Plants," *Applied and Environmental Microbiology* 54:842-43, 1988.

Black cohosh

Black cohosh is extracted mainly from the dried roots and rhizomes (underground stems) of *Cimicifuga racemosa* (*Actaea racemosa*), a plant native to eastern North America. Because the herb's effects resemble those of the hormone estrogen, some people have used it to treat menopause symptoms.

Common dose

Black cohosh comes as:
- caplets (40, 400, or 420 milligrams)
- capsules (25 or 525 milligrams).

Some experts recommend the following dose:
- 8 to 2,400 milligrams taken orally daily.

Why people use this herb
- Diarrhea
- Fluid retention
- Inflammation
- Menopause symptoms

Side effects

Call your health care practitioner if you experience any of these possible side effects of black cohosh:
- nausea or vomiting
- symptoms of low blood pressure, such as dizziness.

When taken in large doses, black cohosh can cause miscarriage.

Interactions

Combining herbs with certain drugs may alter their action or produce unwanted side effects. Don't use black cohosh when taking drugs that lower blood pressure.

Important points to remember

- Don't use black cohosh if you're pregnant because it can cause miscarriage.
- Use this herb cautiously if you're taking drugs that lower blood pressure. Doing so may cause your blood pressure to fall too low.

Other names for black cohosh

Other names for black cohosh include black snakeroot, bugbane, bugwort, cimicifuga, rattleroot, rattleweed, and squawroot.

WHAT THE RESEARCH SHOWS

Findings from the few existing studies of black cohosh suggest that the herb's estrogen-like effects may help control menopause symptoms. However, most clinical data come from German studies involving only a small number of women. More well-controlled studies must be done to define the herb's possible role in estrogen replacement therapy.

Products containing black cohosh are sold under such names as Black Cohosh, CX, Estroven, FC With Dong Quai, Femtrol, GNC Menopause Formula, and Remifemin.

Selected references

Duker E., et al. "Effects of Extracts of *Cimicifuga racemosa* on Gonadotropin Release in Menopausal Women and Ovariectomized Rats," *Planta Medica* 57:420-24, 1991.

Genazzani, E., and Sorrentino, L. "Vascular Action Of Acteina, Active Constituent of *Actaea racemosa* L," *Nature* 194:544-45, 1962.

Jarry, H., et al. "Studies on the Endocrine Effects of the Contents of *Cimicifuga racemosa:* 2. In Vitro Binding of Compounds to Estrogen Receptors," *Planta Medica* 4:316-19, 1985.

Lehmann-Willenbrock, E., and Riedel, H.H. "Clinical and Endocrinologic Studies of the Treatment of Ovarian Insufficiency: Manifestations Following Hysterectomy with Intact Adnexa," *Zentralblatt fur Gynakologie* 110:611-18, 1988.

Black haw

Part of the herbalist's medicine chest for many years, black haw comes from *Viburnum prunifolium*, a deciduous shrub that grows in the eastern United States. The bark of the shrub's roots are used medicinally.

Common dose

Black haw comes as a liquid extract or as the root bark. You can also buy it as capsules or tablets in combination with other herbs and extracts. Some experts recommend the following dose:

- *Tincture* or *bark* taken as tea three times daily.

Side effects

Call your health care practitioner if you experience stomach upset when using black haw.

Interactions

Combining herbs with certain drugs may alter their action or produce unwanted side effects. Don't use black haw if you're taking blood thinners, such as Coumadin.

Why people use this herb

- Chronic diarrhea
- Menstrual pain
- Muscle spasms
- To prevent miscarriage
- To relax the uterus
- Uterine pain

Important points to remember

- Don't take this herb if you're allergic to *V. prunifolium* or related plant species.
- Don't use black haw if you're pregnant or breast-feeding.

Other names for black haw

Other names for black haw include cramp bark, nannyberry, sheepberry, shonny, sloe, stagbush, and sweet haw.

WHAT THE RESEARCH SHOWS

Medical experts caution against using black haw until they know more about its safety and side effects. Most information they have relates to the herb's effects in animals, not humans.

Products containing black haw are sold under such names as Black Haw, PMS Serene, and Utero-Tone.

Selected references

Jarobe, C.H., et al. "Uterine Relaxant Properties of *Viburnum*," *Nature* 5064:837, 1966.

Jarobe, C.H., et al. "1-methyl 2,3-dibutyl hemimellitate: A Novel Component of *Viburnum prunifolium*," *Journal of Organic Chemistry* 34:4202-03, 1969.

Blackroot

With its high tannin content, blackroot has a bitter, nauseating taste. American settlers learned about the herb from Native American Indians. The Delaware Indians called it quitel. The Missouri and Osage Indians referred to it as hini. Early American doctors used blackroot to treat "bilious" fevers.

Blackroot is prepared from the dried roots and rhizome (underground stem) of *Veronicastrum virginicum,* which grows in Canada and the United States.

Common dose

Blackroot comes as dried root or tincture. Some experts recommend the following dose:

- *To induce vomiting* or *to use as a laxative,* 1 gram. To make a tea, mix 1 to 2 teaspoon of dried blackroot in cold water, boil, and simmer for 10 minutes. Drink 1 cup three times a day. When using the tincture, take 1 to 2 milliliters three times a day.

Side effects

Call your health care practitioner if you experience any of these possible side effects of blackroot:

- abdominal pain or cramps
- changes in stool color or odor
- drowsiness
- headache
- nausea
- vomiting.

Why people use this herb

- Constipation
- Jaundice and other symptoms of liver congestion
- To induce vomiting

Ingesting large amounts of dried blackroot tea leaves (½ pound of tea every 3 to 4 days) can cause liver damage.

Interactions

Combining herbs with certain drugs may alter their action or produce unwanted side effects. Don't use blackroot when taking:

- atropine
- Buscopan
- hyoscine

- iron-containing preparations
- Lanoxin
- Transderm-Scōp.

Important points to remember

- Don't use blackroot if you're pregnant or breast-feeding.
- Avoid taking large amounts of blackroot, especially if you have liver disease.
- If you have liver disease, be sure to tell your health care practitioner you're using blackroot. He or she may order periodic liver function tests to check for liver damage.
- Get immediate medical help if you experience symptoms of liver damage, such as jaundice, fever, or pain in the upper right part of your abdomen.

Other names for blackroot

Other names for blackroot include black root, bowman root, brinton root, Culver's physic, Culver's root, high veronica, hini, *Leptandra, Leptandra virginica,* physic root, quitel, tall speed-well, *Veronica,* and *Veronica virginica.*

No known products containing blackroot are available commercially.

WHAT THE RESEARCH SHOWS

Little information is available about blackroot's therapeutic uses or effectiveness. At this time, no evidence supports therapeutic claims for this herb.

Selected references

Galecka, H. "Choleretic and Cholagogic Effects of Certain Hydroxy Acids and Their Derivatives in Guinea Pigs," *Acta Poloniae Pharmaceutica* 26:479-84, 1969.

Haddad, L.M., and Winchester, J.F. *Clinical Management of Poisoning and Drug Overdose,* 2nd ed. Philadelphia: W.B. Saunders Co., 1990.

Lloyd, J.B. *Origin and History of All the Pharmacopeial Vegetable Drugs, Chemicals, and Preparations.* 8th and 9th decennial revisions, Vol. I. Cincinnati: The Caxton Press, 1921.

Millspaugh, C.F. *American Medicinal Plants.* New York: Dover Publications, Inc., 1974. Reprint of 1892 edition.

Blessed thistle

During the Middle Ages, blessed thistle was considered a folk remedy and tonic. It was even used to treat bubonic plague. More recently, the German government has approved blessed thistle as a treatment for heartburn and appetite loss.

An annual plant found mainly in Asia and Europe, blessed thistle (*Cnicus benedictus, Carbenia benedicta, Carduus benedictus)* belongs to the Compositae family. It's related to daisies, asters, and other flowering plants.

Common dose

Blessed thistle comes as:

- capsules (325 or 340 milligrams)
- dried herb (1-ounce packets)
- tincture (1-ounce containers)
- tea.

The dose depends on the intended use and administration method.

Why people use this herb

- Liver disorders
- Menstrual problems
- Poor memory
- Stomach upset
- To stimulate lactation

Side effects

Call your health care practitioner if you experience any of these possible side effects of blessed thistle:

- nausea
- skin irritation from handling the herb
- vomiting.

Interactions

Combining herbs with certain drugs may alter their action or produce unwanted side effects. Don't use blessed thistle when taking other plants from the Compositae family (such as daisies and asters) because cross-sensitivity may occur.

Important points to remember

- Don't use this herb if you're pregnant or breast-feeding.
- Use blessed thistle cautiously if you have a history of skin irritation.

Other names for blessed thistle

Other names for blessed thistle include cardo santo, chardon benit, holy thistle, kardobenediktenkraut, spotted thistle, and St. Benedict thistle.

Products containing blessed thistle are sold under such names as Blessed Thistle Combo and Blessed Thistle Herb.

WHAT THE RESEARCH SHOWS

No animal or human clinical data support claims that blessed thistle has medicinal value.

Selected references

Barrero, A.F., et al. "Biomimetic Cyclization of Cnicin to Malacitanolide, a Cytotoxic Eudesmanolide from *Centaurea malacitana,*" *Journal of Natural Products* 60:1034-35, 1997.

Crellin, J.K., and Philpott, J. *Herbal Medicine Past and Present. A Reference Guide to Medicinal Plants,* Vol. 2. Durham, N.C.: Duke University Press, 1990.

Reynolds, J.E.F., et al., eds. *Martindale, The Extra Pharmacopeia,* 31st ed. London: Royal Pharmaceutical Society of Great Britain, 1996.

Zeller, W., et al. "The Sensitizing Capacity of Compositae plants. VI. Guinea Pig Sensitization Experiments with Ornamental Plants and Weeds Using Different Methods," *Archives of Dermatological Research* 277:28-35, 1985.

Bloodroot

Bloodroot is an ingredient (listed as sanguinarine) in certain toothpastes and oral rinses. Sanguinarine is extracted from the rhizome (underground stem) of *Sanguinaria canadensis*, a perennial plant native to North America. Although bloodroot is used in homeopathic medicine, the Food and Drug Administration considers it unsafe in foods, beverages, and drugs.

Common doses

Bloodroot comes as a tincture and an extract. Some experts recommend the following doses:

- As a *tincture,* 0.3 to 2 milliliters three times a day
- As an *extract* (1:1 in 60% alcohol), 0.06 to 0.3 milliliters three times a day.

Side effects

Call your health care practitioner if you experience any of these possible side effects of bloodroot:

- headache
- irritation of the eye or mucous membranes (from contact with the root dust or components)
- nausea
- vomiting.

Excessive doses of bloodroot can cause:

- low blood pressure
- shock
- coma.

Why people use this herb

- As an expectorant
- Constipation
- Fungal growths
- Nasal polyps
- Ringworm
- Skin cancer
- To induce vomiting
- To stimulate digestion

Interactions

Combining herbs with certain drugs may alter their action or produce unwanted side effects. Don't use bloodroot when taking sanguinarine products containing zinc.

Important points to remember

- This herb's powdered rhizome (underground stem) and juice may destroy the tissues of human and other mammals.
- Don't use bloodroot except under strict supervision and guidance of your dentist or other health care practitioner.

- Don't use this herb if you're pregnant.
- Use bloodroot cautiously and under medical supervision if you have a skin cut, abrasion, or healing tissue.

WHAT THE RESEARCH SHOWS

Most clinical data support the use of bloodroot (as sanguinarine) as an ingredient in toothpaste or oral rinses to control dental plaque. However, one study showed it had no benefit when used in combination with routine periodontal care (such as oral hygiene, scaling, and planing). Besides offering no advantage over routine periodontal care, sanguinarine may be dangerous if ingested orally.

Sanguinarine's effectiveness against skin cancers, fungal infections, and nasal polyps hasn't been proven in controlled clinical trials. Because oral ingestion of this substance has caused tissue destruction, experts don't recommend it.

Other names for bloodroot

Other names for bloodroot include Indian paint, red puccoon, redroot, and tetterwort.

Products containing bloodroot are sold under such names as Lexat and Viadent.

Selected references

Cullinan, M.P., et al. "Efficacy of a Dentrifice and Oral Rinse Containing Sanguinaria Extract in Conjunction with Initial Periodontal Therapy," *Australian Dental Journal* 42:47-51, 1997.

Eisenberg, A.D., et al. "Interactions of Sanguinarine and Zinc on Oral Streptococci and Actinomyces Species," *Caries Research* 25:185-90, 1991.

Kopczyk, R.A., et al. "Clinical and Microbiological Effects of a Sanguinaria-Containing Mouth Rinse and Dentrifice with and without Fluoride During Six Months of Use," *Journal of Periodontology* 62:617-22, 1991.

Blue cohosh

Blue cohosh comes from *Caulophyllum thalictroides*, a plant with bright blue seeds that grows in the eastern United States and Canada. Its active ingredients are extracted from the aerial parts, roots, and rhizomes (underground stems).

Why people use this herb

- Muscle spasms
- Rheumatism
- Scant menstrual flow
- Seizures
- To induce labor

Common doses

Blue cohosh comes as:

- dried powder
- tea
- tablets
- tinctures (1 ounce, 2 ounces)
- capsules (500 milligrams).

Some experts recommend the following doses:

- As *dried rhizome* or *root*, 0.3 to 1 grams three times daily.
- As *liquid extract* (1:1 in 70% alcohol), 0.5 to 1 milliliters three times daily.

Side effects

Call your health care practitioner if you experience any of these possible side effects of blue cohosh:

- chest pain
- mucous membrane irritation from contact with the powdered extract
- severe diarrhea
- stomach cramps or upset
- symptoms of high blood pressure, such as headache, blurred vision, or seizures
- symptoms of high blood sugar, such as extreme thirst, frequent urination, rapid breathing, and a fast, weak pulse.

Children who ingest the seeds may experience poisoning.

Interactions

Combining herbs with certain drugs may alter their action or produce unwanted side effects. Don't use blue cohosh when taking:

- drugs used to lower blood pressure
- drugs used to treat angina (chest pain), such as Adalat, Calan, Cardizem, Inderal, nitroglycerin, Sorbitrate, or Vascor
- nicotine replacement products, such as Nicorette and Nicoderm.

Important points to remember

- Don't use blue cohosh if you're pregnant because it may stimulate the uterus.
- Avoid this herb if you have heart disease.
- Be aware that blue cohosh overdose may cause symptoms resembling those of nicotine poisoning—confusion, muscle twitches, weakness, stomach cramps, seizures, rapid breathing, palpitations, and coma.
- Keep blue cohosh products out of children's reach. Remember that the attractive bright blue seeds are poisonous.

WHAT THE RESEARCH SHOWS

Blue cohosh shows some promise in treating inflammatory diseases and in preventing pregnancy. However, it's potentially toxic and may worsen some conditions. Before experts can recommend it, they must study it thoroughly to assess its risks and benefits.

Other names for blue cohosh

Other names for blue cohosh include blue ginseng, Caulophyllum, squaw root, papoose root, and yellow ginseng.

A product containing blue cohosh is sold as Blue Cohosh Root.

Selected references

Anisimov, M.M., et al. "The Antimicrobial Activity of the Triterpene Glycosides of *Caulophyllum robustum maxim,*" *Antibiotiki I Khimioterapiia* 17:834, 1972.

Benoit, P.S., et al. "Biochemical and Pharmacological Evaluation of Plants. XIV: Antiinflammatory Evaluation of 163 Species of Plants," *Lloydia* 393:160-71, 1976.

Chaudrasekhar, K., and Sarma, G.H.R. "Observations on the Effect of the Low and High Doses of *Caulophyllum* on the Ovaries and the Consequential Changes in the Uterus and Thyroid in Rats," *Journal of Reproduction and Fertility* 38:236-37, 1974.

Scott, C.C., and Chen, K.K. "The Pharmacologic Action of N-methylcytisine," *Therapeutics* 79:334, 1943.

Blue flag

Used by Native Americans to induce vomiting and treat constipation, blue flag comes from *Iris versicolor,* a perennial found abundantly in swamps and low-lying areas in eastern and central North America. When the plant isn't in bloom, many people mistake it for sweet flag (*Acorus calamus*).

The herb's rhizome (underground stem) has a peculiar odor and pungent, acrid taste. The *United States Pharmacopoeia,* a legal compendium of drug standards, lists the rhizome of *Iris versicolor* as an official pharmaceutical ingredient.

Common dose

Blue flag comes as:

- powdered root (20 grains or 1,300 milligrams)
- solid extract (10 to 15 grains, or 650 to 975 milligrams)
- fluid extract (0.5 to 1 fluidrams, or 2.5 to 5 milliliters)
- tincture (1 to 3 fluidrams, or 5 to 15 milliliters).

Some experts recommend the following dose:

- As a *laxative,* 10 to 20 grains of the powdered root or solid extract, or 0.5 to 3 fluidrams of the fluid extract or tincture.

Side effects

Call your health care practitioner if you experience any of these possible side effects of blue flag:

- headache
- mucous membrane irritation
- poisoning symptoms, such as nausea, vomiting, diarrhea, and abdominal pain.

Ingesting fresh root preparations may cause severe nausea and vomiting.

Why people use this herb

- Bruises
- Constipation
- Fluid retention
- Inflammation
- Liver disease
- Sores
- To induce vomiting
- To stimulate the bowel

Interactions

Combining herbs with certain drugs may alter their action or produce unwanted side effects. Tell your health care practitioner about any prescription or nonprescription drugs you're taking.

Important points to remember

- Don't use blue flag if you're pregnant or breast-feeding.
- Avoid taking this herb internally.
- Be aware that blue flag causes severe irritation if it contacts the eyes, nose, or mouth.
- Keep all parts of this plant out of children's reach.

WHAT THE RESEARCH SHOWS

Because blue flag is a known intestinal irritant and may pose a danger in some conditions, medical experts don't recommend it for any disease. In fact, they advise people to avoid this herb until they know more about its risks and benefits.

Other names for blue flag

Other names for blue flag include dagger flower, dragon flower, flag lily, fleur-de-lis, flower-de-luce, liver lily, poison flag, snake lily, water flag, and wild iris.

Products containing blue flag are sold under such names as Iridin and Irisin.

Selected reference

Newall, C.A., et al. *Herbal Medicines: A Guide for Health-Care Professionals,* 1st ed. London: Pharmaceutical Press, 1996.

Bogbean

Bogbean extract comes from the leaves of *Menyanthes trifoliata*, a plant native to European and North American swamps, marshes, and bogs. The fruit of *M. trifoliata* looks like a small bean; hence the name "bogbean." Europeans use bogbean in small amounts as a natural food flavoring.

Common doses

Bogbean comes as dried leaf, liquid extract, and tincture. Some experts recommend the following doses:

- As *dried leaf,* 1 to 2 grams in a tea taken orally three times a day.
- As *extract* (1:1 in 25% alcohol), 1 to 2 milliliters taken orally three times a day at mealtimes with plenty of juice or water.

Side effects

Call your health care practitioner if you experience any of these possible side effects of bogbean:

- bleeding
- nausea
- vomiting.

Bogbean also can cause red blood cell destruction.

Why people use this herb

- Constipation
- Fluid retention
- Fever
- Rheumatism
- Scurvy
- To stimulate the appetite

Interactions

Combining herbs with certain drugs may alter their action or produce unwanted side effects. Don't use bogbean when taking:

- blood thinners, such as heparin and Coumadin
- antiplatelet drugs, such as aspirin, Plavix, or Ticlid.

Important points to remember

- Don't use bogbean if you're pregnant or breast-feeding.
- Call your health care practitioner promptly if you experience unusual bleeding or bruising, abdominal pain, vomiting, or dizziness when using bogbean. Discontinue the herb if these symptoms persist.
- Be aware that ingesting bogbean may cause severe, prolonged nausea and vomiting.
- Keep bogbean fluid extract away from children to avoid poisoning.

WHAT THE RESEARCH SHOWS

Although animal studies indicate a few therapeutic uses for bogbean, results from human studies aren't available to justify its medicinal use. Also, questions about bogbean's safety remain unanswered.

Other names for bogbean

Other names for bogbean include buckbean, marsh trefoil, and water shamrock.

No known products containing bogbean are available commercially.

Selected references

Bishop, C.J., and MacDonald, R.E. "A Survey of Higher Plants for Antibacterial Substances," *Botany* 15:231-59, 1951.

Giaceri, G. "Chromatographic Identification of Coumarin Derivatives in Menyanthes trifoliata," *Fitoterapia* 43:134-38, 1972.

Boldo

Among the most popular medicinal plants in Chile, boldo comes from the leaves and bark of the boldo tree, *Peumus boldus (Boldea boldus)*. Native to Chile and Peru, this small evergreen is naturalized to the Mediterranean region. Boldine—the part of the herb used medicinally—is also found in more than a dozen other trees or shrubs in the laurel, magnolia, and monimia families.

Fossilized boldo leaves more than 13,000 years old with human teeth imprints have been found in Chile. Perhaps they were used medicinally by ancient Chileans or chewed simply for their pleasant, refreshing taste.

More than 60 preparations registered in various countries include boldo as an active ingredient. Chile exports about 800 tons of dried boldo leaves each year, mainly to Argentina, Brazil, France, Germany, and Italy.

Common dose

Boldo comes as a tea, a tincture, and an extract. Some experts recommend the following dose:

- As *dried extract,* 2.5 grams taken orally daily.

Side effects

Call your health care practitioner if you experience any of these possible side effects of boldo:

- exaggerated reflexes
- poor coordination
- seizures.

Large doses of boldo volatile oil may cause poisoning symptoms, including extremely slow breathing.

Interactions

Combining herbs with certain drugs may alter their action or produce unwanted

Why people use this herb

- As a mild hypnotic
- As a sedative
- Common cold
- Constipation
- Digestive disorders
- Earache
- Fluid retention
- Gallbladder disorders
- Gonorrhea
- Gout
- Headache
- Intestinal gas
- Liver disorders
- Menstrual pain
- Nervousness
- Rheumatism
- Stomach upset
- Syphilis
- Tapeworm, pinworm, and other worm infections
- Weakness

side effects. Tell your health care practitioner about any prescription or nonprescription drugs you're taking.

Important points to remember

- Don't use boldo if you have a central nervous system problem or respiratory disorder.
- Don't use this herb if you're pregnant or breast-feeding.
- Keep boldo preparations and plants out of children's reach.
- Avoid ingesting boldo volatile oil because it may be toxic.

WHAT THE RESEARCH SHOWS

Some studies seem to validate claims for boldo's use in digestive disorders. Also, recent findings about the herb's antioxidant and liver-protecting properties warrant additional investigation.

However, more studies must be done to determine its risks and benefits. Until boldo's safety and effectiveness are established, medical experts can't recommend the herb.

Other names for boldo

Other names for boldo include boldine and boldo-do-Chile.

Boldo is a minor ingredient in more than 60 preparations used mainly in South America and Europe.

Selected references

Gotteland, M., et al. "Effect of a Dry Boldo Extract on Oro-cecal Transit in Healthy Volunteers," *Revista Medica de Chile* 123:955-60, 1995.

Kringstein, P., and Cederbaum, A.I. "Boldine Prevents Human Liver Microsomal Lipid Peroxidation and Inactivation of Cytochrome P4502E1," *Free Radical Biology and Medicine* 18:559-63, 1995. Abstract.

Speisky, H., and Cassels, B.K. "Boldo and Boldine: An Emerging Case of Natural Drug Development," *Pharmacological Research* 29:1-12, 1994.

Boneset

Native Americans used boneset to eliminate infection or disease through fever reduction, sweating, and bowel evacuation. They introduced the herb to the colonists, who adopted it to treat malaria and other diseases that cause fever. Boneset became popular during shortages of quinine, the main treatment for malaria at the time.

Boneset comes from the dried leaves and flowering tops of the perennial herb *Eupatorium perfoliatum*, which grows throughout much of the United States and parts of Canada. Some people claim it got its name from its alleged ability to relieve dengue ("breakbone") fever. It was included in the *United States Pharmacopeia*, the legal compendium of drug standards, from 1820 to 1916 and the *National Formulary* from 1926 to 1950. However, the conventional medical community has never advocated its use. More recently, boneset has been included in homeopathic preparations and herbal mixtures sold in Europe and to practicing herbalists.

Common doses

Boneset is available as a tea, an extract, and a topical cream. Some experts recommend the following doses:

- As an *extract,* 10 to 40 drops (2 to 4 grams of plant material) mixed in a liquid taken orally daily.
- As a *tea,* 2 to 6 teaspoons of crushed dried leaves and flowering tops steeped in 1 cup to 1 pint of boiling water.

Why people use this herb

- Acute bronchitis
- As an expectorant
- As a sedative
- Fever
- Flu
- Respiratory congestion

Side effects

Call your health care practitioner if you experience any of these possible side effects of boneset:

- allergic reaction
- diarrhea
- vomiting.

Boneset also can cause liver damage.

Interactions

Combining herbs with certain drugs may alter their action or produce unwanted side effects. Tell your health care practitioner about any prescription or nonprescription drugs you're taking.

Important points to remember

- Don't use boneset if you're pregnant or breast-feeding.
- Tell your health care practitioner you're taking this herb. He or she may order periodic liver function studies to check for liver damage.

WHAT THE RESEARCH SHOWS

Although boneset has been used to reduce fever for more than 200 years, no clinical studies show that it's effective for this purpose. A German study found no difference between aspirin and a homeopathic boneset remedy in relieving discomfort from the common cold.

Medical experts discourage medicinal use of boneset because they don't know enough about its safety and effectiveness. And because proven remedies already exist for many of the herb's claimed therapeutic uses, researchers aren't likely to conduct more boneset studies.

Other names for boneset

Other names for boneset include agueweed, crosswort, eupatorium, feverwort, Indian sage, sweating plant, thoroughwort, and vegetable antimony.

A product containing boneset is sold as Catarrh Mixture.

Selected references

Gassinger, C.A., et al. "A Controlled Clinical Trial for Treating the Efficacy of the Homeopathic Drug *Eupatorium perfoliatum* D2 in the Treatment of the Common Cold," *Arzneimittel-forschung* 31:732-36, 1981.

Smith, L.W., and Culvenor, C.C. "Plant Sources of Hepatotoxic Pyrrolizidine Alkaloids," *Journal of Natural Products* 44:129-52, 1981.

Wagner, H., et al. "Immunostimulating Polysaccharides (Heteroglycans) of Higher Plants," *Arzneimittel-forschung* 35:1069, 1985.

Borage

The borage plant (*Borago officinalis*) is a hardy annual that grows in Europe and the eastern United States. The plant's leaves, stems, flowers, and especially seeds are used medicinally.

Borage leaves have been part of European herbal medicine for centuries. During medieval times, some people steeped the leaves and flowers in wine and drank the concoction to dispel melancholy.

Common dose

Borage comes as softgel capsules (240, 500, and 1,300 milligrams of borage seed oil, which contains 20% to 26% gamma linolenic acid). Some experts recommend the following dose:

- As *borage seed oil,* 1.1 to 1.4 grams taken orally daily.

Why people use this herb

- As an expectorant
- Bronchitis
- Common cold
- Inflammation
- Melancholy
- Rheumatoid arthritis
- To induce sweating

Side effects

Call your health care practitioner if you experience unusual symptoms when using borage.

Ingesting 1 to 2 grams of borage seed oil can cause liver damage.

Interactions

Combining herbs with certain drugs may alter their action or produce unwanted side effects. Tell your health care practitioner about any prescription or nonprescription drugs you're taking.

Important points to remember

- Don't use borage if you're pregnant or breast-feeding.
- Avoid this herb if you have a liver disorder.
- Tell your health care practitioner you're using borage. He or she may recommend periodic liver function studies to check for liver damage.

Other names for borage

Other names for borage include beebread, common borage, common bugloss, cool tankard, ox's tongue, and starflower.

WHAT THE RESEARCH SHOWS

Most claims for borage stem from the fact that it seemed to relieve inflammation in animals and in small, uncontrolled or poorly controlled human studies. However, its exact role in therapy hasn't been resolved and questions about its safety and effectiveness remain. Evidence doesn't substantiate other claims for borage.

Products containing borage are sold under such names as Borage Oil and Borage Power.

Selected references

Karlstad, M. D., et al. "Effect of Intravenous Lipid Emulsions Enriched with Gamma-linolenic Acid on Plasma n-6 Fatty Acids and Prostaglandin Biosynthesis After Burn and Endotoxin Injury in Rats," *Critical Care Medicine* 21:1740-49, 1993.

Leventhal, L. J., et al. "Treatment of Rheumatoid Arthritis with Gamma-linolenic Acid," *Annals of Internal Medicine* 119:867-73, 1993.

Mancuso, P., et al. "Dietary Fish Oil and Fish and Borage Oil Suppress Intrapulmonary Proinflammatory Eicosanoid Biosynthesis and Attenuate Pulmonary Neutrophil Accumulation in Endotoxic Rats," *Critical Care Medicine* 25:1198-1206, 1997.

Pullman-Mooar, S., et al. "Alteration of the Cellular Fatty Acid Profile and the Production of Eicosanoids in Human Monocytes by Gamma-linolenic Acid," *Arthritis and Rheumatism* 33:1526-33, 1990.

Broom

According to folklore and homeopaths, broom relieves irregular heartbeats, rids the body of excess fluid, and causes bowel evacuation or vomiting. Before hops became a standard beer ingredient, broom was added to beer to enhance its taste and boost its intoxicating power.

The crude drug is prepared from the twigs and flowers of *Cytisus scoparius (Sarothamnus scoparius)*, a plant that has been naturalized from Europe to the United States and Canada. Although the Food and Drug Administration has deemed this plant unsafe for human consumption, the German E Commission (which oversees drug use in Germany) considers broom effective in treating certain heart problems.

Common dose

Broom is available as root, cigarettes, teas, and extracts. Experts disagree on what dose to take.

Side effects

Call your health care practitioner if you experience any of these possible side effects of broom:

- headache
- irregular heartbeats
- mind-altering sensations (from smoking the plant parts)
- poisoning symptoms, such as shock, a fast pulse, confusion or other mental changes, vertigo, nausea, and diarrhea (when taken in high doses)
- uterine contractions.

Why people use this herb

- Constipation
- Fluid retention
- Irregular heartbeats
- To induce relaxation and euphoria
- To induce vomiting

Broom also can cause:

- fungal pneumonia (from smoking contaminated broom tops)
- miscarriage.

Interactions

Combining herbs with certain drugs may alter their action or produce unwanted side effects. Don't use broom if you're taking:

- drugs that lower blood pressure
- heart drugs called beta blockers, such as Inderal

- other drugs used to treat heart conditions
- tricyclic antidepressants, such as Sinequan.

Important points to remember

- Don't use broom if you're pregnant because it may cause miscarriage.
- Avoid this herb if you have high blood pressure or a serious heart condition.
- Don't ingest or smoke broom preparations because of potentially dangerous effects on blood vessels.
- Avoid broom if you have a heart pacemaker because it could interfere with pacemaker function.
- Don't confuse this plant with Spanish broom, found in some foods and cosmetics.

Other names for broom

Other names for broom include bannal, broom top, genista, ginsterkraut, hogweed, Irish broom top, sarothamni herb, Scotch broom, and Scotch broom top.

No known products containing broom are available commercially.

WHAT THE RESEARCH SHOWS

A potentially dangerous herb, broom isn't approved for any therapeutic use. Although it may have potential medicinal value, the risk of harm outweighs these purported benefits. Medical experts need more information to analyze the risks and benefits of this herb. Safer and more effective drugs exist for every use that broom's advocates claim.

Selected references

Belpaire, F.M., and Bogaert, M.G. "Cytochrome P450: Genetic Polymorphism and Drug Interactions," *Acta Clinica Belgica* 51:254-60, 1996.

Bird, G.W., and Wingham, J. "Lectins for Polyagglutinable Red Cells: *Cytisus scoparius, Spartium junceum* and *Vicia villosa*," *Clinical and Laboratory Haematology* 2:21-23, 1980.

Leung, A.Y. *Encyclopedia of Common Natural Ingredients Used in Food, Drugs, and Cosmetics.* New York: Wiley-Interscience, 1980.

Young, N.M., et al. "Structural Differences Between Two Lectins from Cytisus scoparius, Both Specific for D-galactose and N-acetyl-D-galactosamine," *Biochemical Journal* 222:41, 1984.

Buchu

Considered a "cooling" diuretic by Ayurvedic medicine, buchu was once listed as a diuretic and antiseptic in the *U.S. National Formulary*. It was also listed in the *British Pharmacopoeia* as a treatment for certain urinary tract disorders. Some Germans use buchu as a diuretic and a treatment for kidney and urinary tract infections. However, German health authorities don't endorse this.

Active components of buchu come from a volatile oil in the leaves of *Barosma betulina (Agathosma betulina)* and the related species *B. serratifolia* and *B. crenulata*, low-lying shrubs in South Africa. The leaves are harvested when the plants flower or bear fruit.

Common doses

Buchu comes as dried leaves (for infusion) and a tincture. Some experts recommend the following doses:

- As an *infusion*, 1 small glass (1 ounce of dried leaves added to 1 pint of boiling water).
- As a *tincture*, 1 to 2 milliliters taken orally three or four times daily.

Why people use this herb

- Fluid retention
- Urinary tract and genital infections

Side effects

Call your health care practitioner if you experience any of these possible side effects of buchu:

- diarrhea, nausea, vomiting (volatile oil)
- increased menstrual flow.

Buchu also can cause miscarriage. Using buchu volatile oil can result in:

- liver damage
- kidney inflammation and dysfunction.

Interactions

Combining herbs with certain drugs may alter their action or produce unwanted side effects. Don't use buchu when taking blood thinners such as Coumadin.

Important points to remember

- Don't use buchu if you're pregnant or breast-feeding.
- Avoid this herb if you have a kidney infection, kidney disease, or a liver disorder because it may worsen these conditions.
- Tell your health care practitioner that you're using buchu. He or she may recommend periodic liver function tests to check for liver damage.
- Avoid ingesting the plant because some components may be toxic.

WHAT THE RESEARCH SHOWS

No studies prove that buchu is effective. Medical experts don't recommend the herb because it may damage the liver.

Other names for buchu

Other names for buchu include agathosma, Barosma betulina, betuline, bocco, and Diosma betulina.

No known products containing buchu are available commercially.

Selected references

Farnsworth, N.R., and Cordell, G.A. "A Review of Some Biologically Active Compounds Isolated from Plants as Reported in the 1974-1975 Literature," *Lloydia* 39:420-55, 1976.

Frawley, D., and Lad, V. *The Yoga of Herbs.* Twin Lakes, Wis.: Lotus Press, 1986.

Buckthorn

Buckthorn comes from the berries of *Rhamnus cathartica,* a thorny shrub or tree native to Europe and naturalized in parts of the United States and Canada. Juice from the berries produces a saffron-colored dye. The bark yields a brilliant yellow. The ripened berries are sometimes mixed with alum, resulting in a sap-green color often used for watercoloring.

Once used mainly as a laxative, buckthorn now serves mainly as a dye. Its laxative action can be severe, and its use in humans was largely discontinued after discovery of *R. purshiana,* a related plant with a gentler action. Until the 19th century, buckthorn was available as a syrup, prepared by boiling buckthorn juice with pimento, ginger, and sugar.

Common dose

Buckthorn comes as a syrup. Experts disagree on what dose to take.

Side effects

Call your health care practitioner if you experience any of these possible side effects of buckthorn:

- abdominal pain
- anxiety
- dehydration symptoms such as thirst
- diarrhea
- nausea
- slow breathing
- trembling
- vomiting.

Why people use this herb

- As a gentle astringent for skin problems
- Constipation

Interactions

Combining herbs with certain drugs may alter their action or produce unwanted side effects. Tell your health care practitioner about any prescription or nonprescription drugs you're taking.

Important points to remember

- Don't use buckthorn if you're pregnant or breast-feeding.
- Use this herb cautiously if you have digestive tract problems, such as irritable bowel syndrome, peptic ulcer disease, ulcerative colitis, or Crohn's disease. Buckthorn may worsen these problems.

- Keep buckthorn berries and preparations out of children's reach.
- Know that gentler and more predictable laxatives than buckthorn are available.

Other names for buckthorn

Other names for buckthorn include common buckthorn, European buckthorn, hartsthorn, purging buckthorn, and waythorn.

Products containing buckthorn are sold under such names as Herbal Laxative, Herbalene, Laxysat Mono Abführ-Tee Nr.2, Neo-Cleanse, and Neo-Lax.

WHAT THE RESEARCH SHOWS

No clinical trials support buckthorn's medicinal use. The herb's violent actions and severe side effects suggest that its risks outweigh its benefits. Medical experts recommend using gentler, more predictable laxatives instead.

Selected references

Lichtensteiger, C.A., et al. "*Rhamnus cathartica* (Buckthorn) Hepatocellular Toxicity in Mice," *Toxicologic Pathology* 25:449-52, 1997.

Millspaugh, C.F. *American Medicinal Plants.* New York: Dover Publications, Inc., 1974. Originally published in 1892.

Bugleweed

Bugleweed comes from the roots, stems, leaves, and flowers of *Lycopus virginicus* and *L. europaeus.* Members of the mint family, these plants are native to Europe and North America.

Common dose

Bugleweed is available as a dried herb and as a liquid extract and tincture. Experts disagree on what dose to take.

Side effects

Call your health care practitioner if you experience unusual symptoms when using bugleweed.

Why people use this herb

- As an astringent
- Fast pulse
- Graves' disease (overactive thyroid)
- Intermittent fever
- Pain relief

Interactions

Combining herbs with certain drugs may alter their action or produce unwanted side effects. Don't use bugleweed when taking:

- heart drugs called beta blockers, such as Inderal (combining these with bugleweed may mask symptoms of an overactive thyroid)
- thyroid hormone replacement drugs.

Important points to remember

- Don't use bugleweed if you're pregnant or breast-feeding.
- Use this herb with extreme caution if you have an underactive pituitary (hypopituitarism), pituitary adenoma, hypogonadism, a thyroid-related tumor, or a similar endocrine disorder.
- Use bugleweed cautiously if you have a heart condition.
- Tell your health care practitioner you're using bugleweed. He or she may want to check for hormone changes caused by bugleweed use.
- Know that this herb hasn't been tested in thyroid conditions other than overactive thyroid.
- If you have a thyroid condition, don't substitute bugleweed for prescribed antithyroid drugs, such as Propyl-Thyracil or Tapazole.
- If you have osteoporosis or take oral contraceptives or fertility drugs, consult your health care practitioner before using bugleweed.

Other names for bugleweed

Other names for bugleweed include carpenter's herb, common bugle, Egyptian's herb, farasyon maiy, gypsy-weed, gypsy-wort, menta de lobo, middle comfrey, Paul's betony, sicklewort, su ferasyunu, water bugle, and water horehound.

No known products containing bugleweed are available commercially.

> **WHAT THE RESEARCH SHOWS**
>
> Information about bugleweed's effects comes solely from animal studies. Results of animal studies don't necessarily apply to people, but they should inspire caution. Bugleweed has been shown to inhibit various hormones, although researchers haven't evaluated the extent of inhibition. The herb may well merit a role in treating Graves' disease, but it must be investigated more thoroughly.

Selected references

Brinker, F. "Inhibition of Endocrine Function by Botanical Agents," *Journal of Naturopathic Medicine* 1:1-14, 1990.

Millspaugh, C.F. *American Medicinal Plants.* New York: Dover Publications, Inc., 1974. Reprint of 1892 edition.

Winterhoff, H., et al. "Endocrine Effects of Lycopus europaeus L. Following Oral Application," *Arzneimittel-forschung* 44:41-45, 1994.

Burdock

Commonly eaten in Asia, burdock is extracted from the dried root of great burdock, *Arctium lappa,* or common burdock, *Arctium minus,* a large biennial grown in China, Europe, and the United States. In the spring, you can identify this herb by the round heads of its purple flowers.

Burdock seeds and leaves have been used in folk medicine for a wide range of ailments. Some Asians eat burdock root.

Common doses

Burdock is available as:

- capsules (425 and 475 milligrams)
- liquid extract
- cream for topical use
- tincture
- dried root
- tea.

Some experts recommend the following doses:

- As a *tea,* 1 cup taken orally three or four times a day.
- As a *compress,* apply externally.

Side effects

Call your health care practitioner if you experience allergic dermatitis (skin inflammation).

Why people use this herb

- Acne
- Arthritis
- Cancer
- Canker sores
- Eczema (a type of skin inflammation)
- Gout
- Hemorrhoids
- HIV
- Kidney stones
- Lower back pain
- Impotence
- Psoriasis (scaly, raised skin patches)
- Rheumatism
- Sciatica
- To purify the blood
- Ulcers

Using a commercial burdock tea contaminated with atropine can cause poisoning symptoms, such as enlarged pupils, blurred vision, and a fast heartbeat.

Interactions

Combining herbs with certain drugs may alter their action or produce unwanted side effects. Don't use burdock when taking insulin or oral drugs for diabetes. Combining burdock with these drugs may decrease your blood sugar too much.

Important points to remember

- Don't use burdock if you're pregnant or breast-feeding.
- Avoid this herb if you're allergic to *Arctium lappa, A. minus,* or related plant species.
- If you have diabetes, be aware that burdock may put you at risk for dangerously low blood sugar. Consult your health care practitioner, who may recommend adjusting your dosage of insulin or other diabetes drugs.
- Be aware that burdock products may be contaminated with atropine, possibly leading to poisoning.

WHAT THE RESEARCH SHOWS

Some studies suggest that burdock might have therapeutic benefits. However, clinical trials haven't been done to verify these benefits. Also, medical experts lack information about the herb's safety and effectiveness.

Other names for burdock

Other names for burdock include bardana, beggar's buttons, clotbur, cockle buttons, cuckold, edible burdock, fox's clote, gobo, great bur, great burdock, happy major, hardock, lappa, love leaves, personata, Philanthropium, thorny burr, and wild gobo.

Products containing burdock are sold under such names as Anthraxiviore and Burdock Root.

Selected references

Bryson, P.D. "Burdock Root Tea Poisoning," *JAMA* 240:1586, 1978.

Bryson, P.D., and Rumack, B.H. "Burdock Root Tea Poisoning," *JAMA* 239:2157, 1978.

Rhoads, P.M., and Anderson, R. "Anticholinergic Poisonings Associated with Commercial Burdock Root Tea," *Clinical Toxicology* 22:581-84, 1985.

Rodriguez, P., et al. "Allergic Contact Dermatitis Due to Burdock *(Arctium lappa),*" *Contact Dermatitis* 33:134-35, 1995.

Butcher's broom

Butchers in Europe and the Mediterranean region once used twigs and leaves from the *Ruscus aculeatus* plant to scrub chopping blocks clean. That's how the herb got its name.

Butcher's broom is extracted from the leaves, rhizomes (underground stems), and roots of *R. aculeatus*, a low-lying evergreen shrub of the Lily family (Liliaceae). Native to the Mediterranean region, it also grows in the southern United States.

Common dose

Butcher's broom comes as:

- capsules (75, 110, 150, 400, 470, and 475 milligrams)
- liquid extract
- tea.

In one study, patients with poor leg circulation and varicose veins received an oral dose of 99 milligrams daily.

Why people use this herb

- Arthritis
- Constipation
- Fluid retention
- Hemorrhoids
- Leg swelling
- Poor leg circulation
- Varicose veins

Side effects

Call your health care practitioner if you experience unusual symptoms when taking butcher's broom.

Interactions

Combining herbs with certain drugs may alter their action or produce unwanted side effects. Don't use butcher's broom when taking:

- drugs called alpha blockers (such as Cardura, Hytrin, and Minipress), used to lower blood pressure or treat benign prostatic hyperplasia (BPH)
- drugs for depression called MAO inhibitors, such as Marplan and Nardil.

Important points to remember

- Don't use butcher's broom if you're pregnant or breast-feeding.
- Use this herb cautiously if you have high blood pressure or BPH or if you're taking an alpha blocker.
- Be aware that scientists don't know the long-term effects of using butcher's broom.

- Keep in mind that if you have poor circulation, this herb may interfere with prescribed drugs you're taking for that condition.

Other names for butcher's broom

Other names for butcher's broom include box holly, knee holly, pettigree, and sweet broom.

Products containing butcher's broom are sold under such names as Butcher's Broom Extract 4:1, Butcher's Broom Root, Hemodren Simple, and Ruscorectal.

WHAT THE RESEARCH SHOWS

Although researchers know that butcher's broom acts on blood vessels, they don't have much information about its effects. One study suggests that the herb is useful in treating chronic poor circulation and varicose veins of the legs. However, this study involved only 40 patients who used butcher's broom in combination with other substances (hesperidin and ascorbic acid).

Butcher's broom may be well tolerated, but more studies are needed to evaluate its effectiveness in treating blood vessel disorders. No evidence supports its use in treating hemorrhoids or arthritis.

Selected references

Bouskela, E., et al. "Effects of *Ruscus* Extract on the Internal Diameter of Arterioles and Venules of the Hamster Cheek Pouch Microcirculation," *Journal of Cardiovascular Pharmacology* 22:221-24, 1993.

Cappelli, R., et al. "Use of Extract of *Ruscus aculeatus* in Venous Disease in the Lower Limb," *Drugs Under Experimental and Clinical Research* 14:277-83, 1988.

Marcelon, G., et al. "Effect of *Ruscus aculeatus* on Isolated Canine Cutaneous Veins," *General Pharmacology* 14:103, 1983.

Rubanyi, G., et al. "Effect of Temperature on the Responsiveness of Cutaneous Veins to the Extract of *Ruscus aculeatus*," *General Pharmacology* 15:431-34, 1984.

Butterbur

Butterbur has been used for thousands of years to treat digestive disorders, asthma, cough, skin diseases, and urinary and genital tract spasms. Active components come from the leaves, flowers, stems, and root stock of *Petasites hybridus, P. officinalis,* or *Tussilago petasites.* Some formulas use extracts from the leaves and roots of *P. frigidus,* also called western coltsfoot. These low-lying perennial herbs of the Composite family (Compositae) are endemic to the United States.

Common doses

Butterbur comes as:

- standardized capsules (25 milligrams)
- *Petasites* extract
- liquid *Petasites* extract (concentration may vary).

Some people smoke *P. frigidus,* drink it as a tea, or use it as a poultice. Experts disagree on what dose to take.

Side effects

Call your health care practitioner if you experience any of these possible side effects of butterbur:

- abdominal pain or pressure
- difficulty breathing
- difficulty swallowing
- difficulty urinating
- eye, skin, or stool discoloration
- prolonged constipation
- severe nausea
- vomiting.

Some experts believe butterbur may cause cancer and liver damage.

Why people use this herb

- Arthritis
- As a sedative
- Asthma
- Cough
- Digestive disorders
- Fluid retention
- Skin disease
- Sores
- Stomach and intestinal pain
- Ulcers
- Urinary and genital tract spasms

Interactions

Combining herbs with certain drugs may alter their action or produce unwanted side effects. Tell your health care practitioner about any prescription or nonprescription drugs you're taking, especially anticholinergics such as atropine.

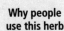

Important points to remember

- Don't use this herb if you're pregnant or breast-feeding.
- Don't use butterbur if you have decreased intestinal or bladder motility because it may worsen symptoms of these disorders.
- If you have asthma, be aware that taking butterbur may make this condition worse if inadequately treated.
- Know that some experts believe this herb may cause cancer or liver damage.

WHAT THE RESEARCH SHOWS

Despite the use of butterbur extract for centuries, scientists don't have enough information to establish its safety and effectiveness in preventing or treating any disease. Animal studies suggest the herb may reduce certain types of muscle spasms and ease inflammation, but no human studies have been done.

Further research may show that the herb's more active components have a beneficial effect, but the extracts would have to be purified and standardized before reliable claims could be made. Active extract components may vary from batch to batch, and potentially hazardous substances have been identified in these plants.

Other names for butterbur

Other names for butterbur include European pestroot, sweet coltsfoot, and Western coltsfoot.

Products containing butterbur are sold under such names as Alzoon, Butterbur Root Extract, Feverfew/Dogwood Supreme, Neurochol, Petaforce, and Wild Cherry Supreme.

Selected references

Brune, K., et al. "Gastroprotective Effects by Extracts of *Petasites hybridus:* The Role of Inhibition of Peptido-leukotriene Synthesis," *Planta Medica* 59:494-96, 1993.

Luthy, J., et al. "Pyrrolizidine Alkaloids in *Petasites hybridus* and *P. albus. Pharmaceutica Acta Helvetiae* 58:98-100, 1983. Abstract.

Moore, M. *Medicinal Plants of the Pacific West.* Santa Fe, N. Mex.: Red Crane Books, 1995.

Weiss, R.F. *Herbal Medicine.* Beaconsfield, England: Beaconsfield Publishers Ltd., 1988.

Cacao tree

Cocoa comes from the seeds of *Theobroma cacao,* the cacao tree. Native to Mexico, this tree now is cultivated in many tropical areas, especially western Africa. *Cacao* refers to the crude material (cacao tree and cacao beans), whereas *cocoa* indicates the processed product.

Many cosmetic, food, and pharmaceutical products contain cacao in one form or another. Chocolate is prepared by mixing cacao powder with sugar, flavoring, and extra cocoa butter fat. Cocoa extract is an ingredient in various beverages. Cocoa powder and cocoa syrup are used to flavor many foods and pharmaceutical products.

Common dose

Cacao comes as cocoa powder, butter, syrup, and extracts. Experts disagree on what dose to take.

Why people use this herb

- As an emollient and skin protectant (in cosmetics)
- As a suppository
- To prevent stretch marks during pregnancy
- To treat wrinkles

Side effects

Call your health care practitioner if you experience any of these possible side effects of cacao:

- acne
- allergic reaction.

Eating 222 grams or more of dark chocolate may cause poisoning symptoms, such as headache, nausea, insomnia, restlessness, excitement, muscle tremors, fast pulse, irregular heartbeats, and mild delirium.

Interactions

Combining herbs with certain drugs may alter their action or produce unwanted side effects. Tell your health care practitioner about any prescription or nonprescription drugs you're taking, especially:

- drugs for depression called MAO inhibitors, such as Nardil and Parnate (don't eat cocoa when taking these drugs)
- Theo-Dur (avoid eating large amounts of cocoa when using this drug).

Important points to remember

- Don't eat cocoa if you're allergic to it.
- Use cocoa cautiously if you're on a low-sodium diet or have irritable bowel syndrome.

- Limit your cocoa intake if you have inflammatory bowel syndrome, heart or blood vessel disease, or irregular heartbeats.
- If you're prone to developing acne, avoid cosmetics that contain cocoa butter.

Other names for cacao

Other names for cacao include chocolate, cocoa, and cocoa butter (theobroma oil).

Many commercial products containing cacao are available as foods, flavorings, or condiments.

> **WHAT THE RESEARCH SHOWS**
>
> Certain antioxidants in cacao may decrease atherosclerosis (plaque buildup in the arteries) and reduce blood clot formation. One study showed that these antioxidants may lower the risk of death from coronary heart disease in elderly men. However, you can also obtain these antioxidants from some fruits and vegetables, which probably have a higher nutritional value than cacao and contain much less fat. Chocolate generally is considered nontoxic.

Selected references

Hertog, M.G.L., et al. "Dietary Antioxidant Flavonoids and Risk of Coronary Heart Disease: The Zutphen Elderly Study," *Lancet* 342:1007-11, 1993.

Mumford, G.K., et al. "Absorption Rate of Methylxanthines Following Capsules, Cola, and Chocolate," *European Journal of Clinical Pharmacology* 51:319-25, 1996.

Sanbongi, C., et al. "Polyphenols in Chocolate, Which Have Antioxidant Activity, Modulate Immune Functions in Humans In Vivo," *Cellular Immunology* 177:129-36, 1997.

Stidworthy, M.F., et al. "Chocolate Poisoning in Dogs," *Veterinary Record* 141:28, 1997.

Calumba

Calumba, from the *Jateorhiza calumba* (*J. palmata*) plant, is native to Mozambique and the forests of eastern Africa, where it's cultivated for use as a dye and flavoring agent. During processing, the plant's root is dried and powdered. As the powder absorbs moisture from the air, it decomposes and changes from green to brownish black.

Common dose

Calumba comes as capsules and an elixir (often prepared without heating as a cold infusion). Experts disagree on what dose to take.

Side effects

Call your health care practitioner if you experience any unusual symptoms when using calumba.

Interactions

Combining herbs with certain drugs may alter their action or produce unwanted side effects. Tell your health care practitioner about any prescription or nonprescription drugs you're taking.

Important points to remember

- Don't use calumba if you're pregnant or breast-feeding.
- If you're using this herb to treat diarrhea, keep in mind that proven drugs for diarrhea exist.

Why people use this herb

- Diarrhea
- Intestinal gas

Other names for calumba

Other names for calumba include *Cocculus palmatus* and columbo root.

Products containing calumba are sold under such names as Amaro Maffioli, Appetiser Mixture, Bitteridina, Ducase, Elixir Spark, Padma-Lax, Richelet, and Travel-Caps.

WHAT THE RESEARCH SHOWS

Medical experts don't recommend this herb because it hasn't been studied in people. With many approved drugs for diarrhea on the market, further investigation and development of calumba for medicinal use isn't likely.

Selected reference

Wada, K., et al. "Columbin Isolated from Calumbae radix Affects the Sleep Time of Anesthetized Mice," *Biological and Pharmaceutical Bulletin* 18:634-36, 1995.

Capsicum

Derived from the dried fruit (pepper) of plants in the Solanaceae family, natural capsicum has been used for centuries—especially the *Capsicum frutescens* and *C. annum* species. Peppers are among the most widely consumed spice in the world. In some Southeast Asian countries, the average person eats nearly 50 milligrams of peppers daily.

Capsaicin, derived from capsicum, is highly potent. Recently, it has gained widespread popularity as an ingredient in nonlethal self-defense sprays. Such sprays have immobilizing effects, such as eyelid spasms, blindness, and incapacitation for up to 30 minutes.

Common dose

Capsicum comes as:

- a cream (0.025%, 0.075%, 0.25%)
- gel (0.025%)
- lotion (0.025%, 0.075%)
- self-defense spray (5%, 10%).

Some experts recommend the following dose:

- As a *topical preparation,* apply three or four times a day.

Why people use this herb

- Bowel disorders
- Chronic laryngitis
- Pain relief
- Poor circulation
- Skin irritation
- Urinary urgency

Side effects

Call your health care practitioner if you experience any of these possible side effects of capsicum:

- back discomfort
- burning pain in the nose, sneezing, or bloody nasal discharge
- closing up of the throat
- cough
- eyelid spasm, extreme burning pain, eye tearing and redness (usually from eye rubbing)
- skin irritation, itching, stinging, or redness
- stomach upset.

Interactions

Combining herbs with certain drugs may alter their action or produce unwanted side effects. Don't use capsicum when taking:

- certain drugs used to lower blood pressure, including Aldomet, Catapres, Tenex, and Wytensin
- drugs for depression called MAO inhibitors, such as Marplan and Nardil.

WHAT THE RESEARCH SHOWS

Topical capsicum preparations have been proven effective in treating pain caused by rheumatoid arthritis, osteoarthritis, diabetes-related nerve problems, postoperative pain, and certain other pain syndromes. These preparations also ease itching, including itching resulting from kidney failure. Long-term use seems to cause no permanent side effects. For some people, the initial burning sensation and delayed onset of action may be the least desirable aspects of capsicum preparations.

One study suggests that inhaling capsicum may ease a runny nose that's not caused by allergy or infection. However, some people can't tolerate taking it this way. Another study explored capsicum as a treatment for urinary urgency, with the preparation administered directly into the bladder. Most patients reported improved symptoms, although they also had side effects, such as a sensation of warmth or burning after urinating. Despite these studies, medical experts caution against ingesting more capsicum than you normally eat in food.

Important points to remember

- Don't use capsicum if you're allergic to it or to chili pepper products.
- Avoid capsicum if you're pregnant because it could stimulate the uterus.
- If you're using capsicum topically for pain relief, remember that it may take up to 28 days to be effective, depending on the condition you're using it for. Apply it at least every 4 to 6 hours. Know that less frequent application may be ineffective.
- Avoid contact with the eyes, mucous membranes, or broken skin. If contact occurs, flush the exposed area with cool, running water as long as necessary.
- To minimize stomach upset, remove the seeds before eating the peppers.

- Be aware that scientists have no evidence that topical use causes permanent injury to the nervous system.
- Don't confuse capsicum peppers with common black peppers or white peppers.

Other names for capsicum

Other names for capsicum include bell pepper, capsaicin, cayenne pepper, chili pepper, hot pepper, paprika, pimiento, red pepper, and tabasco pepper.

Products containing capsicum are sold under such names as Capsin, Cap-Stun, Capzasin, Dolorac, No Pain HP, Pepper Defense, R-Gel, and Zostrix (HP).

Selected references

Bernstein, J.E., et al. "Total Capsaicin Relieves Chronic Post-herpetic Neuralgia," *Journal of the American Academy of Dermatology* 17:93, 1987.

Dasgupta, P., and Fowler, C.J. "Chillies: From Antiquity to Urology," *British Journal of Urology* 80:845-52, 1997.

Robbins, W.R., et al. "Treatment of Intractable Pain with Topical Large-Dose Capsaicin: Preliminary Report," *Anesthesia and Analgesia* 86:579-83, 1998.

Caraway

According to an old superstition, caraway confers the power of retention and prevents theft of items that contain the caraway seed. Traditionally, people gave caraway potions to lovers to keep them from losing interest.

The Arabs, who called the seed *Karawya,* may have been the first of many civilizations to use caraway. The Greek physician Dioscorides (A.D. 40 to 90) advised "pale-faced girls" to take caraway oil, possibly for its reputed stimulant effects.

Now caraway is used mainly as a flavoring agent in foods and pharmaceutical products. An aromatic herb, it comes from *Carum carvi,* a biennial plant that's native to Europe and Asia. Caraway water is produced by soaking 1 ounce of bruised *C. carvi* seeds in 1 pint of cold water for 6 hours. A volatile oil of caraway, distilled from dried, ripened *C. carvi* seeds, is added to such liqueurs as aquavit, Kummel, and L' huile de Venus.

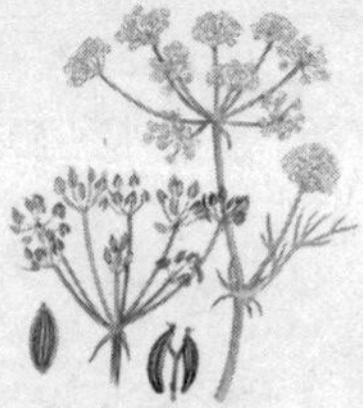

Why people use this herb

- Bronchitis
- Constipation
- Hiatal hernia
- Indigestion
- Intestinal gas
- Laryngitis
- Menstrual cramps
- Sharp intestinal pains
- Stomach ulcers

Common doses

Caraway comes as caraway oil, 5% volatile oil, caraway water, and caraway seed. Some experts recommend the following doses:

- For *adults with intestinal gas,* 1 to 4 drops of the essential oil in 1 teaspoon of water or on a lump of sugar.
- For *infants with sharp intestinal pain,* 1 to 3 teaspoons of caraway water.

Side effects

Call your health care practitioner if you experience any of these possible side effects of caraway:

- diarrhea
- mucous membrane irritation.

Interactions

Combining herbs with certain drugs may alter their action or produce unwanted

side effects. Tell your health care practitioner about any prescription or nonprescription drugs you're taking.

Important points to remember

- Don't use caraway if you're allergic to caraway oil or its components.
- Know that this herb's effectiveness in treating intestinal gas and aiding digestion hasn't been tested. Various approved drugs have been widely tested and may be at least as effective as caraway.
- Check the label carefully before using caraway so that you don't confuse concentrated and plain caraway water.

WHAT THE RESEARCH SHOWS

Clinical trials support only a few of caraway's folklore uses—namely, relieving constipation and easing heartburn not caused by ulcers. For instance, in a small study evaluating the laxative effects of an herbal combination product containing caraway, all patients found relief from constipation within the first 2 days. Also, a combination of caraway and peppermint oil decreased or eliminated pain in patients with heartburn not caused by ulcers. However, these studies aren't definitive.

One study found that caraway oil inhibited certain skin tumors in mice. More studies must be done to evaluate the herb's effect on tumors and explore its potential cancer-fighting properties.

Other names for caraway

Other names for caraway include *Carum carvi,* kummel, kummelol, oleum cari, and oleum carvi.

Products containing caraway are sold under such names as Ajaka, BPC 1973, Cholosum N, Concentrated Caraway Water, Digestozym, Divinal-Bohnen, Euflat 1, Flatulex, Galloselect N, Gastricard N, Globase, Hevert-Carmin, Lomatol, Majocarmin, Metrophyt-V, Neo-Ballistol, Sanvita Magen, Spasmo Claim, and Tirgon.

Selected references

May, B., et al. "Effectiveness of a Fixed Peppermint Oil/Caraway Oil Combination in Non-ulcer Dyspepsia," *Arzneimittel-forschung* 46:1149-53, 1996. Abstract.

Schwaireb, M.H. "Caraway Oil Inhibits Skin Tumors in Female BALB/c Mice," *Nutrition and Cancer* 19:321-25, 1993.

Wattenberg, L.W. "Inhibition of Carcinogenesis by Naturally Occurring and Synthetic Compounds," *Basic Life Sciences* 52:155-66, 1990. Abstract.

Cardamom

A widely used flavoring agent for sweets and coffee, cardamom also is a standard ingredient in curries. Its medicinal use dates back to ancient times. Some people now claim that cardamom sprinkled on cooked cereal can help children with celiac disease who can't tolerate the gluten in grain.

Cardamom seeds are harvested from the fruits of *Elettaria cardamomum*, a large perennial herb native to southern India. When chewed, the seeds have a pleasant taste that may be followed by an increase in saliva and a sensation of warmth in the mouth. The fruits of *E. cardamomum* are gathered before they ripen and split, because seeds from opened fruits are less aromatic.

Why people use this herb

- Bronchitis
- Celiac disease
- Common cold
- Cough
- Indigestion
- Intestinal gas
- To aid digestion
- To stimulate the appetite

Common doses

Cardamom comes as whole or powdered dried seeds, tincture, and fluid extract. Some experts recommend the following doses:

- 15 to 30 grains of powder, 1 fluid dram of tincture, or 5 to 30 drops of fluid extract
- seeds chewed whole
- powder sprinkled on food or mixed in beverages.

Side effects

Call your health care practitioner if you experience allergic skin irritation when using cardamom.

Interactions

Combining herbs with certain drugs may alter their action or produce unwanted side effects. Tell your health care practitioner about any prescription or nonprescription drugs you're taking.

Important points to remember

- Avoid this herb if you're pregnant or breast-feeding.
- Be aware that medical experts don't recommend eating more cardamom than the amounts commonly found in foods.

- If you experience bowel problems even though you've been taking cardamom, consult your health care practitioner.

Other names for cardamom

Other names for cardamom include *Alpinia cardamomum, Amomum cardamon, Amomum repens, Cardamomi semina,* cardamom seeds, *Cardamomum minus,* Malabar cardamom, and *Matonia cardamom.*

No known products containing cardamom are commercially available.

WHAT THE RESEARCH SHOWS

Although herbalists have long claimed that cardamom relieves indigestion and gas, no clinical trials have tested these claims. Thus, the herb's therapeutic benefits remain unproven. Before medical experts can recommend cardamom to treat any medical condition, further studies must be done.

Selected references

Al-Zuhair, H., et al. "Pharmacological Studies of Cardamom Oil in Animals," *Pharmacological Research* 34:79-82, 1996.

Baruah, A.K.S., et al. "Chemical Composition of Alleppey Cardamom Oil by Gas Chromatography," *Analyst* 98:168-71, 1973.

Mobacken, H., and Fregert, S. "Allergic Contact Dermatitis from Cardamom," *Contact Dermatitis* 1:175-76, 1975.

Sukumaran, K., and Kuttan, R. "Inhibition of Tobacco-Induced Mutagenesis by Eugenol and Plant Extracts," *Mutation Research* 343:25-30, 1995.

Carline thistle

Herbalists have used carline thistle to treat everything from the common cold to cancer. The herb's active components come from the seeds, fresh roots, and leaves of the *Carlina acaulis* plant.

Common dose

Carline thistle comes as a liquid and a tea. Experts disagree on what dose to take.

Why people use this herb

- Asthma
- Bronchitis
- Cancer
- Chorea (rapid, involuntary movements)
- Common cold
- Epilepsy
- Fever
- Gallstones
- Gastritis (stomach inflammation and upset)
- Gout
- Headache
- Hysteria
- Inflammation
- Itchy skin
- Kidney stones
- Nervousness
- Painful menstruation
- Rheumatism
- Rickets
- Skin inflammation from allergies
- To promote labor and childbirth
- Tuberculosis
- Worms
- Wounds

Side effects

Call your health care practitioner if you experience any of these possible side effects of carline thistle:

- muscle spasms
- pain.

An overdose of carline thistle may cause seizures.

Interactions

Combining herbs with certain drugs may alter their action or produce unwanted side effects. Tell your health care practitioner about any prescription or nonprescription drugs you're taking.

Important point to remember

- Avoid this herb if you're pregnant or breast-feeding.

Other names for carline thistle

Other names for carline thistle include *Artemisia vulgaris, Carlina vulgaris,* felon herb, mugwort, and *Radix cardopatiae*.

No known products containing carline thistle are available commercially.

WHAT THE RESEARCH SHOWS

Some studies indicate carline thistle might be an effective bladder irrigant. Researchers who used the herb to flush patients' bladders after a certain type of surgery reported that the patients lost less blood and had fewer blood infections and inflammations.

Other research suggests carline thistle may ease skin itching and allergic skin inflammation. However, scientists know little about the herb's safety. Until well-designed, controlled human trials are done, medical experts can't recommend the herb for any use.

Selected references

Davidov, M.I., et al. "Postadenectomy Phytoperfusion of the Bladder," *Urologiia Nefrologiia* 5:19-20, 1995.

Tamuki, A., and Muratsu, M. "Clinical Trial of SY Skin Care Series Containing Mugwort Extract," *Skin Research* 36:369-78, 1994. Abstract.

Tezhka, T., et al. "The Clinical Effects of Mugwort Extract on Pruritic Skin Lesions," *Skin Research* 35:303-11, 1992. Abstract.

Cascara sagrada

The dried bark of *Rhamnus purshiana,* a plant found along the Pacific Northwest, cascara sagrada was used as a laxative by Native Americans. The bark should be aged for at least 1 year. Three-year-old bark is preferred for its milder laxative effect.

To prepare the herb, people collect it in the summer by peeling off sections of bark and rolling them into large quills. Then they carefully sun-dry the bark to avoid exposing its inner surface to the sun and thus make sure it retains its yellow color. Then they process the drug into its final form.

Common doses

Cascara sagrada comes as capsules, bitter and sweet fluid extracts, and dried bark for teas. (The tea has an extremely bitter taste.) Some experts recommend the following doses:

- As an *aromatic fluid extract (sweet cascara),* 5 milliliters taken orally.
- As *extract capsules,* 300 milligrams taken orally.
- As *liquid extract (bitter cascara),* 1 to 5 milliliters taken orally.

Side effects

Call your health care practitioner if you experience any of these possible side effects of cascara sagrada:

- abdominal pain
- diarrhea
- discolored urine
- stomach cramps
- vomiting.

Cascara sagrada also can cause body water and salt imbalances, fatty stools, and laxative dependency.

Why people use this herb

- Chronic constipation

Interactions

Combining herbs with certain drugs may alter their action or produce unwanted side effects. Tell your health care practitioner about any prescription or nonprescription drugs you're taking.

Important points to remember

- Use this herb cautiously if you're pregnant. Be aware that other laxatives, such as Metamucil or Colace, may be preferred during pregnancy.
- Avoid cascara sagrada if you're breast-feeding. The herb enters the breast milk and may cause diarrhea in a breast-fed infant.
- To help prevent constipation, drink lots of fluids, consume more fiber, eat regular meals, and get regular exercise.
- If you have chronic constipation (lasting more than 1 week), see your health care practitioner. You may have something more serious than simple constipation.
- Keep in mind that the fresher the bark used to make the preparation, the greater the risk of side effects.
- Avoid long-term use of this herb because it can lead to laxative dependency or abuse.

WHAT THE RESEARCH SHOWS

The Food and Drug Administration has approved cascara sagrada as a safe and effective laxative. Nonetheless, experts warn people who take it for chronic constipation to use it cautiously to avoid laxative abuse. Most health care practitioners recommend standardized laxative drugs over cascara sagrada tea because these drugs can be taken in the correct dosage and cause fewer side effects.

Other names for cascara sagrada

Other names for cascara sagrada include Californian buckthorn and sacred bark.

Products containing cascara sagrada are sold under such names as Bassoran with Cascara, Bicholax, Cas-Evac, Casvlium, and Kondremul with Cascara.

Selected references

Covington, T.R., et al., eds. *Handbook of Nonprescription Drugs,* 11th ed. Washington, D.C.: American Pharmaceutical Association, 1996.

Morton, J.F. *Major Medicinal Plants: Botany, Culture and Uses.* Springfield, Ill: Charles C. Thomas Pub., Ltd., 1977.

Castor bean

Castor oil, made from the castor bean, is an official product used as a laxative, as a protectant in hair conditioners, and in skin creams intended to treat rash. It's obtained by cold-pressing the seeds of *Ricinus communis,* a perennial herb believed to be native to Africa and India.

Castor oil flowers develop into spiny capsules containing three seeds (also called "beans"). As they dry, the capsules explode, scattering the seeds.

Why people use this herb

- Cysts
- Eye irritation
- Preoperative bowel evacuation
- To soften bunions and corns
- Warts
- Worms

Common dose

Castor oil comes as:

- an emulsion (Alphamul 60% [90 or 3,780 milliliters], Emulsoil 95% [63 milliliters], Fleet Flavored Castor Oil 67% [45 or 90 milliliters], Neoloid 36.4% [118 milliliters])
- a liquid (100% [60, 120, or 480 milliliters])
- a purge (95% [30 or 60 milliliters]).

Some experts recommend the following dose:

- For *constipation,* 15 to 60 milliliters of castor oil taken orally every day.

Side effects

Call your health care practitioner if you experience abdominal pain or cramping when using castor oil. Large oral doses can cause:

- acute intestinal pain
- nausea
- severe bowel evacuation
- vomiting.

Chronic use of castor oil may lead to:

- allergic reactions (from handling the seeds)
- symptoms of body water and salt loss, such as dehydration, thirst, and weakness.

Chewing the leaves or seeds can cause poisoning, which may lead to such symptoms as abdominal pain, nausea and vomiting, liver and kidney injury, mouth and esophageal irritation, seizures, and even death.

Interactions

Combining herbs with certain drugs may alter their action or produce unwanted side effects. Tell your health care practitioner about any prescription or nonprescription drugs you're taking.

Important points to remember

- Don't use this herb if you're pregnant or breast-feeding.
- Use castor oil cautiously if you think you may have appendicitis, rectal bleeding, or bowel obstruction. Also use it cautiously if you're sensitive to castor oil.
- Keep in mind that refrigerating castor oil improves its taste.
- Drink plenty of fluids (6 to 8 glasses) daily to help avoid constipation.
- Don't use castor oil for more than a few days at a time.

WHAT THE RESEARCH SHOWS

Although castor oil is an approved laxative, other laxatives are gentler and taste better. If you want to use it, buy a standardized form rather than a nonstandardized herbal preparation. Other purported uses for castor oil have little or no supporting clinical evidence.

Other names for castor oil

Other names for castor oil include African coffee tree, bofareira, castor oil plant, Mexico weed, palma Christi, tangantangan oil plant, wonder tree, and wunderbaum.

Products containing castor oil are sold under such names as Alphamul, Aromatic Castor Oil USP 23, Castor Oil Caps USP 23, Emulsoil, Fleet Castor Oil Emulsion, Neoloid, Purge, Ricino Koki, and Unisoil.

Selected reference

Kinamore, P.A., et al. "Abrus and Ricinus Ingestion: Management of Three Cases," *Clinical Toxicology* 17:401-05, 1980.

Catnip

Catnip comes from *Nepeta cataria,* a minty-scented perennial common in Europe and cultivated in the United States. Many cat owners buy catnip for their pets. If catnip causes euphoria and sexual stimulation in cats, as some people believe, these effects most likely stem from the herb's scent, not its consumption.

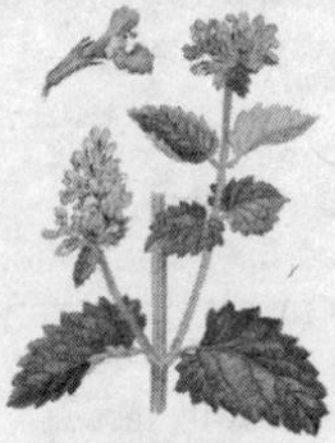

Why people use this herb

- Anemia
- As a stimulant
- Bronchitis
- Cancer
- Colic in infants
- Common cold
- Diarrhea
- Fever
- For mind-altering effects (when smoked)
- Headache
- Hiccups
- Hives
- Indigestion
- Insomnia
- Intestinal gas
- Lack of menstruation
- Muscle spasms
- Painful menstruation
- Restlessness
- Toothache
- To induce sweating

Common doses

Catnip comes as:

- capsule (380 milligrams)
- liquid
- elixir
- tincture
- tea.

Some experts recommend the following doses:

- As a *tea,* pour boiling water on 2 teaspoons of the dried leaves, brew for 10 to 15 minutes, and drink.
- As a *tincture,* 2 to 4 milliliters taken orally three times a day.

Side effects

Call your health care practitioner if you experience any of these possible side effects of catnip:

- an overall ill feeling
- headache
- nausea and vomiting (with large doses).

Interactions

Combining herbs with certain drugs may alter their action or produce unwanted side effects. Tell your health care practitioner about any prescription or nonprescription drugs you're taking.

Important points to remember

- Don't use this herb if you're pregnant or breast-feeding.
- Before using catnip as a sleep aid, be aware that no scientific evidence supports this use. See your health care practitioner, who may refer you to a sleep disorder specialist.

Other names for catnip

Other names for catnip include cataria, catmint, catnep, catrup, cat's-play, catwort, field balm, and nip.

Products containing catnip are sold under such names as Catnip, Catnip & Fennel, Catnip & Fennel Extract, Catnip Herb, and Catnip Mist.

> **WHAT THE RESEARCH SHOWS**
>
> Catnip may have sedative effects, but scientists don't have evidence to back this claim. According to one case report, though, catnip altered the mental status of a toddler after he'd eaten many raisins soaked in catnip tea. More studies are needed to evaluate the herb's safety and effectiveness for its purported therapeutic uses.

Selected references

Hatch, R.C. "Effects of Other Drugs on Catnip-Induced Pleasure Behavior in Cats," *American Journal of Veterinary Research* 33:143-55, 1972.

Osterhoudt, K.C., et al. "Catnip and the Alteration of Human Consciousness," *Veterinary and Human Toxicology* 39:373-75, 1997.

Sherry, C.J., and Hunter, P.S. "The Effect of an Ethanolic Extract of Catnip on the Behavior of the Young Chick," *Experientia* 35:237-38, 1979.

Cat's-claw

Cat's-claw gets its name from the small thorns at the base of the plant's leaf, which look like feline claws. Plant components are extracted from the roots, stem bark, and leaves of *Uncaria tomentosa, U. guianensis,* and other species of the woody vine belonging to the Rubiaceae family. These plants are native to the Amazon. Peru boasts about 20 different plants called cat's-claw. Because some species are toxic, the plant must be verified botanically.

In the 1970s, preliminary research at Peru's National Institute of Health showed promising results in children who received cat's-claw as a leukemia treatment.

Why people use this herb

- Arthritis
- Birth control
- Inflammatory digestive tract disorders, such as diverticulitis, gastritis, Crohn's disease, dysentery, and ulcers
- Rheumatism

Common dose

Cat's-claw comes as:

- tablets and capsules (25, 150, 175, 300, and 350 milligrams of the standard extract; 400, 500, and 800 milligrams, 1 gram, and 5 grams of the raw herb)
- teas
- tinctures
- cut, dried, or powdered bark, roots, and leaves.

Some experts recommend the following dose:

- 500 to 1,000 milligrams taken orally three times a day.

Side effects

Call your health care practitioner if you experience symptoms of low blood pressure, such as dizziness or weakness, when using cat's-claw.

Interactions

Combining herbs with certain drugs may alter their action or produce unwanted side effects. Don't use cat's-claw when taking:

- drugs to lower blood pressure
- blood thinners such as Coumadin.

Important points to remember

- Don't use this herb if you're scheduled for a skin graft or organ transplant, if you have a blood clotting disorder, or if you're taking a blood thinner.
- Avoid cat's-claw if you're pregnant or breast-feeding.
- Consult your health care practitioner if you develop unusual bleeding, tiny purple or red spots on your skin, bleeding gums, or unexplained bruising.
- Rise slowly from a sitting or lying position to avoid dizziness caused by low blood pressure.
- If you're taking cat's-claw for birth control, use a second form of contraception for added safety.

WHAT THE RESEARCH SHOWS

Cat's-claw may have benefits in treating certain diseases, although it must be studied further. Current research focuses on the herb's potential use in treating AIDS, leukemia and other cancers, viral infections, allergic respiratory diseases, stomach and digestive disorders, and osteoarthritis. Clinical trials also are investigating whether cat's-claw can help combat such viruses as herpes simplex, herpes zoster, and HIV.

Other names for cat's-claw

Other names for cat's-claw include life-giving vine of Peru, samento, and una de gato.

Products containing cat's-claw are sold under such names as Cat's Claw Inner Bark Extract and Vegicaps.

Selected references

Chen, C.X., et al. "Inhibitory Effect of Rhynchophylline on Platelet Aggregation and Thrombosis," *Chung-Kuo Yao Li Hsueh Pao* 13:126-30, 1992.

Harada, M., and Ozaki, Y. "Effect of Indole Alkaloids from *Gardneria* Genus and *Uncaria* Genus on Neuromuscular Transmission in the Rat Limb In Situ," *Chemical and Pharmaceutical Bulletin* 24:211, 1976.

Hemingway, S.R., and Philipson, J.D. "Alkaloids from South American Species of *Uncaria* (Rubiaceae)," *Journal of Pharmacy and Pharmacology* 26(suppl): 113, 1974.

Zhang, W., et al. "Effect of Rhyncophylline on the Contraction of Rabbit Aorta," *Chung-Kuo Yao Li Hsueh Pao* 8:425-29, 1987.

Celandine

Celandine comes from the roots and flowering tops of *Chelidonium majus*, a member of the poppy family (Papaveraceae) common to North America, Europe, and Asia. Some people use the milky, orange juice from the stems and other *C. majus* parts for medicinal purposes.

Celandine is an ingredient in an antiretroviral drug that may act against the Epstein-Barr and herpes viruses. Ukrain, derived from celandine, is available by prescription in Europe but not approved for use in the United States. Celandine products available in the United States (manufactured as herbal nutritional supplements or topical herbal treatments) haven't been tested by the Food and Drug Administration (FDA).

Why people use this herb

- Biliary tract blockages
- Cancer
- Colonic polyps
- Digestive disorders
- Eye irritation
- Gallstones
- Hepatitis
- Jaundice
- Liver disease
- To loosen bad teeth
- To remove nodules, warts, and similar growths
- To soften calluses and corns

Common doses

Celandine comes as extract, tincture, and tea. (In Eastern Europe, it's also available as a prescribed injection.) The dose depends on the product used and the intended purpose.

The dose of Ukrain (used in Europe to treat tumors) depends on the person's immune status. The drug is given by intravenous injection, with single doses ranging from 5 to 20 milligrams depending on tumor mass, speed of tumor growth, extent of the disease, and the person's immune status. In several studies, people received Ukrain injections every other day.

Side effects

Call your health care practitioner if you experience any of these possible side effects of celandine:

- dizziness
- drowsiness
- fatigue
- frequent urination
- insomnia

- nausea
- restlessness
- thirst
- tingling, itching, and stabbing pains in the tumor area.

Celandine also can cause:
- damage to an embryo
- low blood pressure
- possible liver damage.

Interactions
Combining herbs with certain drugs may alter their action or produce unwanted side effects. If you're using Ukrain, don't take:
- digitalis drugs, used to treat heart failure
- morphine and related drugs
- oral drugs used to lower blood sugar
- sulfa drugs such as Bactrim.

Important points to remember
- Don't use celandine if you're pregnant or breast-feeding.
- Don't give this herb to children.
- Don't use celandine for more than 2 weeks at a time.
- If you have, or suspect you may have, a serious liver or stomach disorder, don't use this or any other herbal supplement or fresh herb.
- Know that the *C. majus* plant is highly toxic. Contact with the sap causes skin inflammation. Oral consumption can cause abdominal pain, vomiting, diarrhea, fainting, severe stomach inflammation, other serious stomach problems, coma, and even death.
- Be aware that oral ingestion of celandine has led to poisoning and death.
- Don't use herbal extracts in your eyes or on your skin unless the FDA has approved them for such use. Eye or skin contact may lead to blindness, infection, or skin sores.
- Don't take celandine instead of prescribed drugs for diagnosed ailments.
- Be aware that greater celandine isn't related to lesser celandine *(Ranunculus ficaria)*.

Other names for celandine
Other names for celandine include celandine poppy, common celandine, felonwort, garden celandine, greater celandine, rock poppy, swallow wort, tetter wort, and wart wort.

WHAT THE RESEARCH SHOWS

Research indicates that Ukrain (derived from celandine) has been effective against cancers of the esophagus, breast, cervix, testes, urethra, and ovaries; colorectal cancer; malignant melanoma; optic nerve tumors; and, in AIDS patients, Kaposi's sarcoma. Scientists believe Ukrain might one day play an important role in treating cancer and other diseases, but they must conduct more research before the Food and Drug Administration can approve such use.

Because of the serious risk of complications from self-treatment of liver, digestive, and eye diseases and skin inflammation, medical experts don't recommend celandine supplements or topical agents. They also caution against using this herb to self-treat or prevent diseases and against ingesting *Chelidonium majus*, the plant that celandine comes from.

Products containing celandine are sold under such names as Bloodroot/Celandine Supreme, Cacau, Celandine Extract, Celandine Tops and Roots, Cytopure, Fennel/Wild Yam Supreme, No. 2040 Headache Remedy, No. 2090 Indigestion Remedy, and Venancapsan. Ukrain is available only in Europe.

Selected references

Anonymous. "UKRAIN Information for Physicians." Nowicky Pharma. Ukrainian Anticancer Institute, Vienna, Austria. Sept. 1, 1997.

Brzosko, W.J., et al. "Influence of Ukrain on Breast Cancer," *Drugs under Experimental and Clinical Research* 22:127-33, 1996. Abstract.

Vavreckova, C., et al., "Benzophenanthridine Alkaloids of *Chelidonium majus.* II. Potent Inhibitory Action Against the Growth of Human Keratinocytes," *Planta Medica* 62:491-94, 1996.

Celery

Around 450 B.C., the ancient Greeks made wine from celery and served it as an award at athletic games. Celery tonics and elixirs have been used since the late 19th century. Today, of course, we use celery to flavor food, soap, and gum. High in fiber, this vegetable is popular with dieters.

Celery comes from *Apium graveolens*, a widely cultivated biennial herb. Steam distillation of the seeds yields oil of celery.

Common dose

Celery comes in capsules (450 and 505 milligrams). Experts disagree on what dose to take.

Side effects

Call your health care practitioner if you experience any of these possible side effects of celery:

- allergic reactions, such as throat closure, facial swelling, and hives
- blisters
- skin inflammation.

Large doses can cause slowing of the nervous system, resulting in such symptoms as drowsiness.

Interactions

Combining herbs with certain drugs may alter their action or produce unwanted side effects. Tell your health care practitioner about any prescription or nonprescription drugs you're taking.

Important point to remember

- Avoid celery capsules if you're pregnant or breast-feeding.

Why people use this herb

- Arthritis
- As a digestive aid
- As a sedative
- As an aphrodisiac
- Asthma
- Bronchitis
- Cough
- Fever
- Fluid retention
- Headache
- Heartburn
- Hiccups
- Hives
- Intestinal gas
- Lack of menstruation
- Liver disorders
- Muscle spasms
- Nervousness or hysteria
- Rheumatism
- Spleen disorders
- Tension headache
- Toothache
- To sterilize the urinary tract
- Urine retention
- Vomiting

Other names for celery

Other names for celery include apium, celery seed, celery seed oil, marsh parsley, smallage, and wild celery.

Products containing celery are sold under such names as Cachets Lesourd, Dr. Brown's Cel-Ray, Guaiacum Complex, Herbal Diuretic Complex, Rheumatic Pain, and Vegetex.

WHAT THE RESEARCH SHOWS

Several therapeutic claims for celery have been verified. For instance, celery lowered blood pressure in a small study of patients with high blood pressure. Nonetheless, medical experts don't recommend using it in amounts greater than those normally found in food.

Selected references

Birmingham, D.J., et al. "Phytotoxic Bullae Among Celery Harvesters," *Archives of Dermatology* 83:73, 1961.

Hashim, S., et al. "Modulatory Effects of Essential Oils From Spices on the Formation of DNA Adduct by Aflatoxin B1 In Vitro," *Nutrition and Cancer* 21:169-71, 1994.

Centaury

Herbalists' claims for centaury stem from its traditional use as a bitter tonic to stimulate the appetite. Active components are extracted from the leaves, stems, and flowers of *Centaurium erythraea, C. umbellatum,* and *C. minus*. These annual or biennial herbs belong to the Gentian family (Gentianaceae). Vermouth and some nonalcoholic beverages contain trace amounts of centaury.

Common doses

Centaury is available as the crude herb. For most uses, experts recommend the following dose:

- 2 to 4 milliliters of a liquid extract (1:1 in 25% alcohol) or infusion taken three times a day.

Why people use this herb

- As an astringent in cosmetics
- Kidney stones

Some German experts suggest 1 to 2 grams of the crude herb daily.

Side effects

Call your health care practitioner if you experience unusual symptoms when using centaury.

Interactions

Combining herbs with certain drugs may alter their action or produce unwanted side effects. Tell your health care practitioner about any prescription or nonprescription drugs you're taking.

Important points to remember

- Avoid centaury if you're pregnant or breast-feeding.
- Be aware that medical experts know little about this herb's effectiveness.
- Avoid chronic centaury use because long-term effects aren't known.
- Know that some people refer to *C. erythraea* as *Erythraea centaurium.*

Other names for centaury

Other names for centaury include bitter herb, Centaurea, common centaury, European centaury, lesser centaury, and minor centaury.

No known products containing centaury are available commercially.

WHAT THE RESEARCH SHOWS

Medical experts caution against using centaury for any medical condition because they know nothing about its safety or effectiveness. No information from human clinical trials is available.

Selected references

Berkan, T., et al. "Anti-inflammatory, Analgesic and Antipyretic Effects of an Aqueous Extract of *Erythraea centaurium,*" *Planta Medica* 57:34-37, 1991.

Schimmer, O., and Mauthner, H. "Polymethoxylated Xanthones from the Herb of *Centaurium erythraea* with Strong Antimutagenic Properties in *Salmonella typhimurium,*" *Planta Medica* 62:561-64, 1996.

Chamomile

Chamomile comes in several varieties. The German or Hungarian version, called *Matricaria recutita (M. chamomilla)*, is known as "true" chamomile. Roman or English chamomile comes from *Chamaemelum nobile (Anthemis nobile)*.

Common dose

Chamomile comes as capsules (354 and 360 milligrams), a liquid, and a tea. It's also found in many cosmetic products. Most experts recommend the following dose:

- As a *tea*, add 1 tablespoon of the flower head to hot water for 10 to 15 minutes, and take up to four times a day.

Why people use this herb

- Eczema (skin inflammation)
- Eye irritation
- Hemorrhoids
- Insomnia
- Menstrual disorders
- Migraine
- Skin blisters and loosening
- Stomach disorders
- Throat discomfort
- To clean the skin

Side effects

Call your health care practitioner if you experience any of these possible side effects of chamomile:

- allergic conjunctivitis (eye inflammation)
- skin irritation
- severe allergic reaction (chest tightness, wheezing, hives, itching, and rash)
- vomiting.

Interactions

Combining herbs with certain drugs may alter their action or produce unwanted side effects. Tell your health care practitioner about any prescription or nonprescription drugs you're taking, especially:

- blood thinners such as Coumadin (don't use chamomile when taking these drugs)
- any other drugs, because chamomile may make them less effective.

Important points to remember

- Don't use chamomile if you're pregnant or breast-feeding because the herb may trigger miscarriage. Also, be aware that some chamomile components have caused damage to animal embryos and fetuses.

- Use chamomile cautiously if you're allergic to components of the herb's volatile oil or if you have a history of skin irritation.
- Avoid chamomile if you have a history of asthma or allergic dermatitis.
- Be aware that long-term consumption of chamomile tea may have a cumulative therapeutic effect.

WHAT THE RESEARCH SHOWS

Researchers found that oral chamomile induced a deep sleep in patients undergoing cardiac catheterization. Scientists don't have enough information to verify claims that chamomile eases muscle spasms and inflammation and is effective in treating digestive disorders.

Other names for chamomile

Other names for chamomile include common chamomile, English chamomile, German chamomile, Hungarian chamomile, Roman chamomile, sweet false chamomile, true chamomile, and wild chamomile.

Products containing chamomile are sold under such names as Chamomile Flowers, Chamomile Tea, Chamomile Organic, Chamomilla, and Classic Chamomile.

Selected references

Fidler, P., et al. "Prospective Evaluations of a Chamomile Mouthwash for Prevention of 5-FU-Induced Oral Mucositis," *Cancer* 77:522-24, 1996.

Habersang, S., et al. "Pharmacological Studies with Compounds of Chamomile. IV. Studies on Toxicity of Alpha-Bisabolol," *Planta Medica* 37:115-23, 1979.

Mann, C., and Staba, E.J. "The Chemistry, Pharmacology, and Commercial Formulations of Chamomile," in *Herbs, Spices and Medicinal Plants: Recent Advances in Botany, Horticulture and Pharmacology,* Vol 1. Arizona: Oryx Press, 235-80, 1986.

Chaparral

Native Americans traditionally used chaparral for medicinal purposes. The herb's active components come from the leaves of *Larrea tridentata* or *L. divaricata,* a desert-dwelling evergreen shrub native to the southwestern United States and Mexico.

From the late 1950s to the 1970s, some people drank chaparral tea to fight cancer. In 1970, the Food and Drug Administration removed the herb from its "generally recognized as safe" list.

Common dose

Chaparral comes as tablets, capsules, and teas. Experts disagree on what dose to take. For daily consumption, some recommend the tea.

Side effects

Call your health care practitioner if you experience skin irritation when using chaparral.

Chaparral can also cause kidney cancer, kidney cysts, and liver damage.

Why people use this herb

- Bronchitis
- Common cold
- Pain
- Skin disorders

Interactions

Combining herbs with certain drugs may alter their action or produce unwanted side effects. Tell your health care practitioner about any prescription or nonprescription drugs you're taking.

Important point to remember

- Know that this herb can cause serious liver damage. The damage usually resolves once the person stops using chaparral. However, some people have experienced severe irreversible liver damage and acute liver failure and required liver transplants. Call your health care practitioner promptly if you experience possible symptoms of liver damage, such as jaundice and fatigue.

Other names for chaparral

Other names for chaparral include creosote bush, greasewood, and *Hediondilla.*

No known products containing chaparral are commercially available.

WHAT THE RESEARCH SHOWS

Studies investigating chaparral's active component in treating cancer, AIDS, and Alzheimer's disease have shown conflicting results. Further research is needed. In the meantime, medical experts don't recommend this herb because it has been linked to liver damage.

Selected references

Cunningham, D.C., et al. "Proliferative Responses of Normal Human Mammary and MCF-7 Breast Cancer Cells to Linoleic, Conjugated Linoleic Acid and Eicosanoid Synthesis Inhibitors in Culture," *Anticancer Research* 17:197-203, 1997.

Goodman, Y., et al. "Nordihydroguaiaretic Acid Protects Hippocampal Neurons Against Amyloid Beta-Peptide Toxicity, and Attenuated Free Radical and Calcium Accumulation," *Brain Research* 654:171-76, 1994.

Pavani, M., et al. "Inhibition of Tumoral Cell Respiration and Growth by Nordihydroguaiaretic Acid," *Biochemical Pharmacology* 48:1935-42, 1994.

Sheikh, N.M., et al. "Chaparral-Associated Hepatotoxicity," *Archives of Internal Medicine* 157:913-19, 1997.

Chaste tree

According to legend, monks chewed chaste-tree leaves to maintain their celibacy vows. The herb comes from the dried fruits and root bark of *Vitex agnus-castus*. A German formula[illegible] chaste tree is used for certain menstrual disorders, premenstrual syndrome, breast pain, inadequate lactation, and menopause symptoms.

Common dose

Chaste tree is available as capsules, tinctures, and teas. A German study used a dose of a 20 milligram capsule taken orally twice a day.

Side effects

Call your health care practitioner if you experience any of these possible side effects of chaste tree:

- abdominal pain
- cramping
- diarrhea
- headache
- increased menstrual flow
- itching
- rash.

Why people use this herb

- Acne
- Inadequate lactation
- Ovarian insufficiency
- To regulate the menstrual cycle
- Uterine bleeding

Interactions

Combining herbs with certain drugs may alter their action or produce unwanted side effects. Tell your health care practitioner about any prescription or nonprescription drugs you're taking.

Important points to remember

- Avoid this herb if you're pregnant or breast-feeding or if you're trying to get pregnant.
- Be aware that most information on chaste tree comes from foreign studies whose results are hard to interpret.

names for chaste tree

ther names for chaste tree include agneau chaste, chasteberry, gatillier, hemp tree, keuschbaum, and monk's pepper.

No known products containing chaste tree are commercially available.

> **WHAT THE RESEARCH SHOWS**
>
> A German study showed that chaste tree had value in treating women with certain reproductive hormone imbalances. However, another report argued against using this herb in women with multiple follicular development because of the alterations in hormone levels that resulted.
>
> Medical experts believe the herb may be worth investigating in disorders specific to women but don't yet have enough data on its long-term safety and effectiveness to recommend it.

Selected references

Cahill, D., et al. "Multiple Follicular Development Associated with Herbal Medicine," *Human Reproduction* 9:1469-70, 1994.

Hirobe, C., et al. "Cytotoxic Flavonoids from Vitex agnus-castus," *Phytochemistry* 46:521-24, 1997.

Milewicz, A., et al. "Vitex agnus-castus Extract in the Treatment of Luteal Phase Defects Due to Latent Hyperprolactinemia. Results of a Randomized Placebo-Controlled Double-Blind Study," *Arzneimittel-forschung* 43:752-56, 1993.

Sliutz, G., et al. "Agnus castus Extracts Inhibit Prolactin Secretion of Rat Pituitary Cells," *Hormone and Metabolic Research* 25:253-55, 1993.

Chaulmoogra oil

Modern leprosy drugs wouldn't exist without chaulmoogra oil, which comes from the seeds of *Hydnocarpus wightiana, H. anthelmintica,* and *Taraktogenos kurzii*. This herb was discovered in the 1920s by Joseph Rock, a botanist who'd heard that a certain plant he'd never seen could cure leprosy. While searching for the plant throughout the Far East and India, he obtained some seeds in an Indian market. Rock learned that they came from a tall local tree with leathery leaves and large, white flowers. He collected the seeds and naturalized the plant in Hawaii. About 20 years later, active components from the seeds provided the basic materials for the first leprosy drugs.

Common dose

Chaulmoogra oil is available as a topical oil. Some people inject a salt form of the oil under the skin. Experts disagree on what dose to take.

Why people use this herb

- Leprosy

Side effects

Call your health care practitioner if you experience stomach irritation after injecting chaulmoogra oil under the skin. Also be aware that such injections may cause calcium deposits to form under the skin.

Interactions

Combining herbs with certain drugs may alter their action or produce unwanted side effects. Tell your health care practitioner about any prescription or nonprescription drugs you're taking.

Important points to remember

- Don't use this herb if you're pregnant or breast-feeding.
- If you suspect you may have leprosy, seek medical advice from a health care practitioner who has experience in leprosy treatment. He or she may recommend more conventional treatment.
- Don't try to self-inject this herb except under close supervision of a health care practitioner who has experience in leprosy treatment.

Other names for chaulmoogra oil

Other names for chaulmoogra oil include chaulmogra oil, gynocardia oil, and hydnocarpus oil.

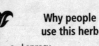

WHAT THE RESEARCH SHOWS

Medical experts caution people not to use chaulmoogra oil because safer leprosy treatments exist. The herb's role in treating leprosy and other disorders hasn't been determined.

No known products containing chaulmoogra oil are available commercially.

Selected references

Noordeen, S.K. "A Look at World Leprosy," *Leprosy Review* 62:72-86, 1991.

Ohtaka, K. "Patients with Calcinosis Cutis: National Leprosarium Matsuoka Hoyo-En' Aomori' Japan," *Nippon Rai Gakkai Zasshi* 61:98-101, 1992.

Chickweed

Components of chickweed, a widely occurring "weed," are extracted from the leaves, stems, and flowers of *Stellaria media*. A member of the Caryophyllaceae family, this plant is native to Europe.

Common doses

Chickweed comes as:

- capsules
- crude herb
- liquid extract (alcohol-free available)
- oils
- ointments
- tea bags (caffeine-free)
- tinctures.

Some experts recommend the following doses:

- As *capsules,* 3 capsules taken orally three times daily.
- As *liquid extract,* 15 to 30 drops (diluted) taken orally up to three times daily.
- As an *ointment,* apply liberally to affected areas as needed up to four times daily.
- As a *tea,* several times daily as needed.

Why people use this herb

- As an expectorant
- Burns
- Cough
- Dry, chapped skin
- Fever
- Inflammatory conditions such as rheumatism, eczema, and psoriasis
- Insect stings and bites
- Itching
- Rashes
- Skin irritation
- Sore throat
- Stomach ulcers
- To "cleanse" the blood
- To drain abscesses and boils
- To lose weight
- Wounds

Side effects

Call your health care practitioner if you experience symptoms of nitrate poisoning, such as dizziness, weakness, headache, and fainting spells, when using chickweed.

Interactions

Combining herbs with certain drugs may alter their action or produce unwanted side effects. Tell your health care practitioner about any prescription or nonprescription drugs you're taking.

Important points to remember

- Don't use this herb if you're pregnant or breast-feeding.

- Be aware that chickweed may cause nitrate poisoning because it contains nitrate. One person who ingested excessive amounts experienced paralysis.

Other names for chickweed

Other names for chickweed include mouse-ear, satinflower, star chickweed, starweed, stitchwort, tongue grass, white bird's-eye, and winterweed.

A product containing chickweed is sold as Chickweed.

WHAT THE RESEARCH SHOWS

Clinical evidence doesn't support herbalists' claims that chickweed is effective in treating a wide range of ailments.

Selected reference

Budzianowski, J., et al. "Studies on Antioxidative Activity of Some C-glycosylflavones," *Polish Journal of Pharmacology* 43:395-401, 1991.

Chicory

Some people use chicory as a coffee substitute because of the herb's coffeelike flavor and aroma. Unlike coffee, it may have a sedative effect. In fact, some people add it to coffee to offset the stimulation caused by caffeine.

Active chicory components come from the dried roots of *Cichorium intybus*, a European biennial or perennial herb. Some people use the leaves of young plants as potherbs, blanching older plants' leaves and eating them like celery. The roots can be boiled and eaten with butter. More commonly, they're roasted and added to coffee or tea for a bitter taste. The roasted, dried root serves as a coffee substitute.

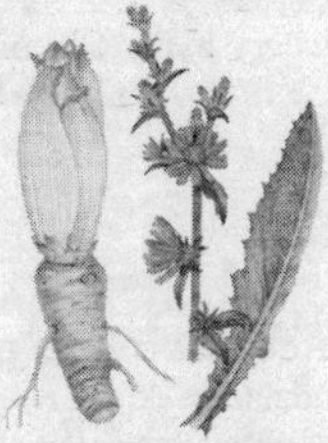

Common dose

Chicory comes as the crude herb, root (roasted and unroasted), and extracts. Some experts recommend the following dose:

- As the *crude herb*, 3 grams taken orally daily.

Why people use this herb

- As a coffee or tea additive (to counteract caffeine's stimulant effect)
- As a coffee substitute
- Constipation
- Fluid retention

Side effects

Call your health care practitioner if you experience skin irritation when using chicory.

Interactions

Combining herbs with certain drugs may alter their action or produce unwanted side effects. Tell your health care practitioner about any prescription or nonprescription drugs you're taking.

Important point to remember

- Use chicory with caution or avoid it entirely if you have heart disease. The herb may act on the heart.

Other names for chicory

Other names for chicory include blue sailors, garden endive, succory, and wild succory.

A product containing chicory is sold as Chicory.

WHAT THE RESEARCH SHOWS

Claims that chicory combats the stimulant effects of coffee and tea remain unproven. The herb may have some use in treating irregular heartbeats, but more research is needed. Chicory's laxative properties also remain unproven. Medical experts advise against using chicory until studies are completed.

Selected references

Benoit, P.S., et al. "Biological and Phytochemical Evaluation of Plants. XIV. Anti-inflammatory Evaluation of 163 Species of Plants," *Lloydia* 39:160-71, 1976.

Malten, K.E. "Chicory Dermatitis from September to April," *Contact Dermatitis* 9:232, 1983.

Chinese rhubarb

One of the oldest and best known Chinese herbal medicines, rhubarb is used to manufacture liqueurs and aperitifs. Active components of Chinese rhubarb come from the dried root bark of *Rheum palmatum*, a large perennial plant that's native to Tibet and northwest China. Chinese rhubarb is more potent than the European and North American rhubarb species used for food and medicinal purposes.

Why people use this herb

- As an astringent
- Bleeding
- Burns
- Constipation
- Diarrhea
- Digestive tract bleeding
- Eye inflammation
- Indigestion
- Injuries
- Jaundice
- Menstrual disorders
- Sores

Common doses

Chinese rhubarb comes as:

- tablets
- tincture (water- or alcohol-based)
- syrup
- extract.

Some experts recommend the following doses:

- For *diarrhea,* 1 teaspoon of tincture or decoction taken orally daily.
- For *constipation,* ½ to 1 teaspoon of tincture or 1 to 2 teaspoons of decoction taken orally daily.
- For *bleeding from the upper digestive tract*, 3-gram tablets or powder taken two or four times daily.

Side effects

Call your health care practitioner if you experience any of these possible side effects of Chinese rhubarb:

- skin irritation (from handling the leaves)
- bright yellow or red urine.

Eating Chinese rhubarb leaves can cause poisoning symptoms such as abdominal pain, nausea, and vomiting. Ingesting large amounts may cause seizures and death.

Interactions

Combining herbs with certain drugs may alter their action or produce unwanted side effects. Tell your health care practitioner about any prescription or nonprescription drugs you're taking.

Important points to remember

- Don't use Chinese rhubarb if you're pregnant or breast-feeding, if you think you may be pregnant, or if you're planning to become pregnant.
- Avoid this herb if you have intestinal problems such as ulcers or sharp intestinal pains.
- Don't give this herb to children under age 2. In older children, give only a lower-strength preparation.
- Don't use Chinese rhubarb for more than 2 weeks because it may cause intestinal problems or laxative dependence.
- Keep in mind that this herb may turn your urine bright yellow or red.
- Don't prepare Chinese rhubarb formulations at home because of the risk of oxalic acid poisoning.
- Keep this plant out of the reach of children and pets.
- Use a lower-strength preparation if you're over age 65.
- Remember that Chinese rhubarb isn't the same as rhubarb found in the United States.

WHAT THE RESEARCH SHOWS

Most studies on Chinese rhubarb come from Asia and their results are hard to interpret. However, in patients with digestive tract bleeding, rhubarb helped to control bleeding, decrease blood loss, reduce the need for blood-clotting drugs, resolve fever, and increase colon activity. What's more, the herb didn't affect the stomach or duodenum (the first portion of the small intestine).

Another Chinese study showed that giving Chinese rhubarb in combination with two prescribed drugs slowed the progression of kidney failure better than did either drug when used alone. (The prescribed drugs were an ACE inhibitor, which lowers blood pressure, and Capoten, used to lower blood pressure, manage heart failure, or treat kidney problems in diabetics who use insulin.) Chinese researchers suggest that patients with chronic kidney disease receive this combination before more radical treatment.

Western scientists are intrigued with Chinese rhubarb's potential for treating kidney failure and digestive tract bleeding. Future studies should focus on these aspects of the herb. But with little information about the herb's safety and effectiveness, medical experts can't recommend it for these uses at this time.

Other names for Chinese rhubarb

Other names for Chinese rhubarb include Himalayan rhubarb, medicinal rhubarb, rhei radix, rhei rhizoma, rubarbo, and Turkish rhubarb.

Products containing Chinese rhubarb are sold under such names as Dahuang Liujingao and Extractum Rhei Liquidum.

Selected references

Dong-hai, J., et al. "Resume of 400 Cases of Acute Upper Digestive Tract Bleeding Treated by Rhubarb Alone," *Pharmacology* 20:128-30, 1980.

Kang, Z., et al. "Observation of Therapeutic Effect in 50 Cases of Chronic Renal Failure Treated with Rhubarb and Adjuvant Drugs," *Journal of Traditional Chinese Medicine* 13:249-52, 1993. Abstract.

Zhang, G., and El Nahas, A.M. "The Effect of Rhubarb Extract on Experimental Renal Fibrosis," *Nephrology, Dialysis, Transplantation* 11:186-90, 1996.

Zhang, J.H., et al. "Clinical Effects of Rheum and Captopril on Preventing Progression of Chronic Renal Failure," *Chinese Medical Journal* 103:788-93, 1990. Abstract.

Cinnamon

A popular spice used in cooking, cinnamon also is found in small amounts in many toothpastes, mouthwashes, gargles, lotions, liniments, soaps, detergents, and other products. Active components come from the dried bark, leaves, and twigs of various species of *Cinnamomum*—Ceylon cinnamon *(C. zeylandicum)*, Saigon cinnamon (*C. loureirii)*, and others. *C. zeylanium* grows in Sri Lanka, southeastern India, Indonesia, South America, and the West Indies. The essential oils are removed by steam-distilling the dried bark and leaves.

Why people use this herb

- Abdominal pain
- Chest pain
- Common cold
- Diarrhea
- Fungal infections
- Gynecologic disorders
- High blood pressure
- Kidney problems
- Pain
- Rheumatism

Common dose

Cinnamon comes as dried bark, dried leaves, powder, and cinnamon oil. Experts disagree on what dose to take.

Side effects

Call your health care practitioner if you experience any of these possible side effects of cinnamon:

- allergic reactions, including skin irritation, second-degree burns, fast breathing, increased perspiration, and unusual excitement followed by drowsiness
- facial flushing
- gingivitis (gum inflammation)
- inflamed, cracked lips
- inflammation in or around the mouth
- fast pulse
- shortness of breath
- tongue inflammation.

Cinnamon also can cause increased intestinal activity.

Interactions

Combining herbs with certain drugs may alter their action or produce unwanted side effects. Tell your health care practitioner about any prescription or nonprescription drugs you're taking.

Important points to remember

- If you're pregnant or breast-feeding, don't use cinnamon in amounts greater than those normally found in foods.
- Be aware that cinnamon and its components can cause allergic reactions, such as skin irritation (including second-degree burns) and mucous membrane reactions.
- Know that some children use cinnamon products as recreational drugs.

WHAT THE RESEARCH SHOWS

Few studies have evaluated claims for cinnamon's proposed uses. More research must be done to determine whether it's safe and effective. In the meantime, medical experts caution against using cinnamon except as a spice.

Other names for cinnamon

Other names for cinnamon include *Batavia cassia, Batavia cinnamon, Cassia, Cassia lignea,* Ceylon cinnamon, Chinese cinnamon, cinnamomom, false cinnamon, Padang cassia, Panang cinnamon, Saigon cassia, and Saigon cinnamon.

Various manufacturers produce cinnamon for use as a spice.

Selected references

Pilapil, V.R. "Toxic Manifestations of Cinnamon Oil Ingestion In a Child," *Clinical Pediatrics* 28:276, 1989.

Viollon, C., and Chaumont, J.P. "Antifungal Properties of Essential Oils and Their Main Components upon *Cryptococcus neoformans*," *Mycopathologia* 128:151-53, 1994.

Clary

In the 16th century, Rhine Valley winemakers added clary to their wines to make them more potent. Clary also has purported medicinal and aromatherapy uses.

Clary comes from *Salvia sclarea,* a perennial herb native to southern Europe. Some people use the seeds of this plant to remove dust particles from the eyes. To obtain the highly aromatic essential oil, herbalists steam-distill the plant's flowering tops.

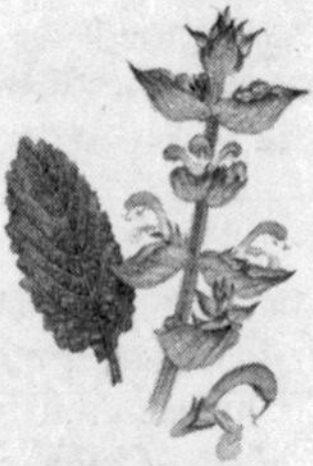

Why people use this herb

- Anxiety
- As a sedative
- Depression
- Digestive problems
- Inflammation
- Irregular menstrual periods
- Kidney problems
- Menopausal symptoms
- Menstrual pain
- Mental fatigue
- Muscle spasms
- Poor libido
- Premenstrual syndrome
- Sore throat
- To improve sex drive
- To cause euphoria

Common doses

Clary comes as an essential oil (5 or 10 milliliters, or clear liquid). Some experts recommend the following doses:

- For *mental fatigue, anxiety, depression,* or *poor libido,* apply 2 drops of essential oil to a piece of cloth and inhale.
- For *massage,* apply 2 to 4 drops of essential oil to 2 teaspoons of carrier oil or lotion.
- For *baths,* add 2 to 10 drops of essential oil to bath water.
- For *menstrual pain,* apply 4 drops of essential oil to a piece of cloth and use as a warm compress.
- For *sore throat, hoarseness,* or *laryngitis,* add 3 drops of essential oil to a glass of water, rinse mouth, and gargle.

Side effects

Call your health care practitioner if you experience any of these possible side effects of clary:

- drowsiness
- euphoria
- headache
- increased menstrual bleeding.

Interactions

Combining herbs with certain drugs may alter their action or produce unwanted side effects. Don't use clary when drinking alcohol because it may increase the effects of alcohol.

Important points to remember

- Don't use clary if you've ever had an estrogen-sensitive cancer. (Ask your health care practitioner if you're not sure.)
- Avoid this herb if you're pregnant or breast-feeding.
- Call your health care practitioner if you experience increased menstrual bleeding or a change in your menstrual cycle.
- When using clary, avoid hazardous activities, such as driving a car, until you know how this herb affects you.
- Avoid using clary with alcohol and other drugs that slow the nervous system because the combination may cause excessive sedation.
- Report unusual symptoms to your health care practitioner.
- Be aware that clary's benefits and risks are poorly documented.

WHAT THE RESEARCH SHOWS

Despite herbalists' many claims for clary, controlled studies haven't shown that the herb is clinically effective. For this reason, medical experts don't recommend it.

Other names for clary

Other names for clary include clary oil, clary sage, clear eye, eyebright, muscatel sage, orvale, see bright, and toute-bonne.

No known products containing clary are available commercially.

Selected references

Lis-Balchin, M., and Hart, S. "A Preliminary Study of the Effect of Essential Oils on Skeletal and Smooth Muscle In Vitro," *Journal of Ethnopharmacology* 58:183-87, 1997.

Ulubelen, A., et al. "Terpenoids from *Salvia sclarea*," *Phytochemistry* 36: 971-74, 1994.

Clove

A well-known spice, clove comes from *Syzgium aromaticum* (also called *Eugenia caryophyllata* or *Caryophyllus aromaticus),* an evergreen tree native to Southeast Asia. Active components are extracted by steam distillation from the dried flower buds.

Although Germany has approved clove as a local anesthetic and an antiseptic, the American Dental Association (ADA) sanctions it only for professional use by dentists.

Why people use this herb

- As a mouthwash
- Toothache

Common doses

Clove is available as drops (85% eugenol), mouthwash, and fluid or oil extract. It's also found in some cigarettes. The dose depends on the product used. Some experts recommend the following doses:

- As *fluid extract,* 5 to 30 drops.
- As *oil extract,* 1 to 5 drops.
- As *mouthwash,* ½ to 1 ounces of clove oil.

Side effects

Call your health care practitioner if you cough up blood when using clove.

Clove also can cause:

- local tissue irritation
- mouth sensitivity
- pulmonary edema
- sudden lower airway closure.

Smoking clove cigarettes can damage soft tissues and injure the airway linings.

Interactions

Combining herbs with certain drugs may alter their action or produce unwanted side effects. Tell your health care practitioner about any prescription or nonprescription drugs you're taking.

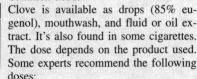

Important points to remember

- Avoid topical clove oil because it may damage the dental pulp and related tissues.
- Know that the ADA doesn't consider clove oil and eugenol, its component, to be safe and effective nonprescription drugs for toothache.
- Keep in mind that toothache or dental pain may signal a more serious problem. Seek professional dental advice if you experience such pain.
- Be aware that applying clove oil or products containing eugenol may damage the dental pulp or soft tissue of the mouth.

WHAT THE RESEARCH SHOWS

Some studies suggest clove may help reduce inflammation and fight infection. However, no well-controlled human studies have evaluated whether clove oil or eugenol is effective in relieving pain or combating infection. According to the Food and Drug Administration, insufficient data on eugenol exist.

Other names for clove

Other names for clove include caryophyllum, *Eugenia aromatica,* oil of clove, and oleum caryophylli.

Products containing clove are sold under such names as Dent-Zel-Ite Toothache Relief Drops and Red Cross Toothache Medication.

Selected references

Briozzo, J., et al. "Antimicrobial Activity of Clove Oil Dispersed in a Concentrated Sugar Solution," *Journal of Applied Bacteriology* 66:69-75, 1989.

Hackett, P.H., et al. "Clove Cigarettes and High Altitude Pulmonary Edema," *JAMA* 253:3551-52, 1985. Letter.

Rasheed, A., et al. "Eugenol and Prostaglandin Biosynthesis," *New England Journal of Medicine* 310:50-51, 1984. Letter.

Coffee

Coffee comes from the fruits of the *Coffea arabica* bush. Grown in semitropical regions, this bush commonly is cultivated for its seeds (called beans after roasting). Freshly picked berries are sun-dried ("natural" or dry process) or subjected to depulping machines and then dried ("washed" or wet process). Before green (unripened) beans are roasted, caffeine is extracted from them with organic solvents. Roasting and blending of other beans gives each coffee its characteristic flavor.

The best known coffee-growing areas are Central and South America, Africa, Jamaica, and Hawaii. Americans seem to prefer Colombian and Central American coffee over Brazilian and African varieties.

Why people use this herb

- To improve exercise tolerance
- To increase alertness
- To relax or expand the airways

Common dose

Coffee comes as whole dried or ground beans, or as freeze-dried or spray-dried crystals (instant coffee). Many pain-relievers, stimulants, allergy medicines, cold products, and dietary aids contain caffeine.

Experts disagree on what dose to take. The lethal caffeine dose is 10 grams.

Side effects

Call your health care practitioner if you experience any of these possible side effects of coffee:

- fast pulse
- headache, possibly from increased blood pressure
- increased urination
- insomnia
- mild delirium and excitation
- muscle twitches and tremors
- nausea
- restlessness.

Coffee also may cause:

- gastroesophageal reflux disease (GERD, a condition in which stomach contents flow backward into the esophagus)

- glaucoma
- increased risk of seizures (in people receiving electroconvulsive therapy)
- peptic ulcer disease
- worsening of heart and blood vessel disease.

Interactions

Combining herbs with certain drugs may alter their action or produce unwanted side effects. Tell your health care practitioner about any prescription or nonprescription drugs you're taking.

Important points to remember

- Avoid coffee if you're pregnant or breast-feeding.
- Be aware that you may have caffeine withdrawal symptoms (such as headache) if you abruptly stop drinking coffee after chronic consumption.
- Know that most medical experts no longer believe caffeine can worsen an irregular heartbeat or cause a lasting blood pressure increase.
- If you have high cholesterol or triglyceride levels, consult a health care practitioner about the benefits of minimizing your coffee intake.
- Don't drink coffee if you have GERD. It may worsen the condition.

WHAT THE RESEARCH SHOWS

Coffee is relatively harmless and may even have certain benefits. In studies, caffeine helped cold sufferers feel more alert and less ill. In elderly people, caffeine helped prevent after-meal blood pressure decreases, which may reduce the risk of accidental falls.

However, coffee can cause problems in some people. Taking a conservative view, some medical experts recommend that pregnant and breast-feeding women and people with high cholesterol, high blood pressure, or stomach disease limit their coffee intake.

Other names for coffee

Other names for coffee include bean juice, *Coffea arabica,* café, espresso, java, robusta coffee, and santos coffee.

Many manufacturers sell coffee. Product names include Maxwell House, Eight O'clock, Bean Company, and Folgers.

Selected references

Graboys, T.B., et al. "The Effect of Caffeine on Ventricular Ectopic Activity in Patients with Malignant Ventricular Arrhythmia," *Archives of Internal Medicine* 149:637-39, 1989.

Van Dusseldorp, M., et al. "Effect of Decaffeinated Versus Regular Coffee on Blood Pressure," *Hypertension* 14(5):563-69, 1989.

Cola tree

Cola tree is the main source of caffeine in carbonated soft drinks. Its extract is a common flavoring in these drinks.

The herb comes from the evergreens *Cola nitida* and *C. acuminata*. Native to western Africa, Sri Lanka, and Indonesia, these trees belong to the same family as cacao (chocolate). Active herbal components are extracted from the seeds.

Why people use this herb

- As an aphrodisiac
- Depression
- Diarrhea
- Fluid retention
- Heartburn
- Heart disease
- Mood and personality disorders
- To clean the teeth and freshen the breath
- To increase alertness
- To stimulate the heart
- Wounds

Common doses

Cola tree is available as nuts or seeds. Seed extracts are available as capsules, tablets, and fluid extracts. Some experts recommend the following doses:

- As *fluid extract,* 5 to 40 drops (¼ to 2 teaspoons) orally up to three times a day, taken at meals with juice or water.
- As *solid extract,* 2 to 8 grains (130 to 520 milligrams) orally per dose.
- As a *decoction,* 1 to 2 teaspoons of the unextracted powder boiled in 1 cup of water for 10 to 15 minutes.

Side effects

Call your health care practitioner if you experience any of these possible side effects of cola tree:

- allergic reactions
- an excited or nervous feeling
- anxiety
- bright yellow staining of the inside of the mouth (from chewing cola nuts)
- palpitations
- stomach pain.

Cola tree also can cause:

- changes in brain, kidney, liver, and testicular enzyme activity
- decreases in certain hormones
- fast pulse
- high blood pressure

- low blood pressure
- slow pulse.

Interactions

Combining herbs with certain drugs may alter their action or produce unwanted side effects. Don't use cola tree when taking drugs that relieve pain and reduce fever, such as aspirin.

Important points to remember

- Don't use cola nut or its extract if you're pregnant or breast-feeding.
- Avoid this herb if you have high blood pressure, irregular heartbeats, or a stomach ulcer. Also avoid it if you're at increased risk for stroke.
- If you're allergic to chocolate, avoid cola tree because of possible cross-sensitivity.
- If you smoke cigarettes and also chew cola nuts, be aware that you're at increased risk for mouth cancer.
- If you experience mood changes while using cola nut, consult your health care practitioner.

WHAT THE RESEARCH SHOWS

The German Commission E (Germany's counterpart to the U.S. Food and Drug Administration) considers cola nut useful in treating mental and physical fatigue. Small amounts of cola nut extract probably are harmless–equivalent to a strong cup of coffee or the standard dose of a nonprescription caffeine product. Other components of cola nut haven't been studied.

Although caffeine and theobromine in cola nuts have potential value in treating certain nervous and respiratory disorders, medical experts instead recommend taking a single-ingredient drug with a standardized dose and known side effects. Studies have explored caffeine's effects on animals' nervous systems and hearts, but the implications for people aren't known. More studies must be done to identify all side effects and toxic effects of cola nut.

Other names for cola tree

Other names for cola tree include kola nut and kolanut.

Products containing cola tree are sold under such names as Colloidal Energy Formula, Kola Nut, Starter, and Ultra Diet Pep. (Most commercial preparations are standardized to approximately 10% caffeine content.)

Selected references

Atawodi, S.E., et al. "Nitrosatable Amines and Nitrosamide Formation in Natural Stimulants: *Cola acuminata, C. nitida,* and *Garcinia cola,*" *Food and Chemical Toxicology* 33:625-30, 1995.

Ebana, R.U., et al. "Microbiological Exploitation of Cardiac Glycosides and Alkaloids from *Garcinia kola, Borreria ocymoides, Kola nitida,* and *Citrus aurantifolia,*" *Journal of Applied Bacteriology* 71:398-401, 1991.

Gaye, F., et al. "Experimental Study of Variations of Salivary pH Affected by Chewing Cola," *Dakar Medical* 35:148-55, 1990.

Ibu, J.O., et al. "The Effect of *Cola acuminata* and *Cola nitida* on Gastric Acid Secretion," *Scandinavian Journal of Gastroenterology* 124 (Suppl):39-45, 1986.

Coltsfoot

Asians and Europeans first used coltsfoot 2,000 years ago to treat asthma, bronchitis, and cough. More recently, the herb has served as a candy flavoring. Although some people recommend smoking coltsfoot for respiratory relief, heat destroys the herb's soothing effect.

Why people use this herb

- Asthma
- Bronchitis
- Cough

Active components of coltsfoot are extracted from the dried leaves, flowers, and, sometimes, the roots of *Tussilago farfara*. This low-growing perennial herb is found in Europe, England, Canada, and the northern United States.

Common doses

Coltsfoot is available as extract, tincture, syrup, and tea. Some experts recommend the following doses:

- As a *decoction* (prepared by boiling the dried herb), 0.6 to 2.9 grams taken orally.
- As a *liquid extract* (1:1 in 25% alcohol), 0.6 to 2 milliliters taken orally three times daily.
- As a *tincture* (1:5 in 45% alcohol), 2 to 8 milliliters taken orally three times daily.
- As a *syrup* (liquid extract 1:4 in syrup), 2 to 8 milliliters taken orally three times daily.
- As a *tea,* 1 to 3 teaspoons of dried flowers or leaves in 1 cup of boiling water taken orally three times daily.

Side effects

Call your health care practitioner if you experience any of these possible side effects of coltsfoot:

- appetite loss
- diarrhea
- fever
- jaundice (yellowish skin discoloration)
- nausea
- vomiting.

Coltsfoot also can cause:

- increased blood pressure
- upper respiratory tract infection.

Interactions

Combining herbs with certain drugs may alter their action or produce unwanted side effects. Don't use coltsfoot if you're taking drugs used to lower blood pressure.

Important points to remember

- Avoid coltsfoot if you're pregnant or breast-feeding.
- Use this herb cautiously if you have high blood pressure.
- Use coltsfoot cautiously if you're allergic to chamomile or ragweed because cross-sensitivity may occur.
- Report unusual symptoms while taking this or any other herb.

Other names for coltsfoot

Other names for coltsfoot include ass's-foot, bullsfoot, coughwort, farfara, fieldhove, filius ante patrem, foalswort, hallfoot, horse-hoof, kuandong hua, and pas díane.

No known products containing coltsfoot are commercially available.

WHAT THE RESEARCH SHOWS

Coltsfoot's safety and effectiveness haven't been well studied. The little information available comes from animal research.

Medical experts advise anyone who's considering using coltsfoot to take into account its possible effects on the heart and blood vessels, its cancer-causing potential, and the risk of an allergic reaction. According to the Food and Drug Administration, its safety is undefined. Canada has banned the herb.

Selected references

Hirono, J., et al. "Carcinogenic Activity of Coltsfoot, *Tussilago farfara*," *Japanese Journal of Cancer Research* 67:125-29, 1976.

Hwang, S., et al. "L-652,469 as a Dual Receptor Antagonist of Platelet Activating Factor and Dihydropyridines from *Tussilago farfara*," *European Journal of Pharmacology* 141:269-81, 1987.

Li, Y.P., et al. "Evaluation of Tussilagone: A Cardiovascular-Respiratory Stimulant Isolated from Chinese Herbal Medicine," *General Pharmacology* 19:261-63, 1988.

Comfrey

Comfrey is extracted from the leaves and roots of *Symphytum officinale,* a perennial herb of the Borage family (Boraginaceae). The plant grows in temperate regions such as North America, western Asia, and Australia.

Common doses

Comfrey is available as a tea (dried leaf and whole root), a blended plant extract (also called "green drink"), and a cream. Oil from the leaves and root may be incorporated in ointments or used as a compress.

Although comfrey has been used as a tea, medical experts in the United States and Canada don't recommend internal use because the herb may be toxic. Limit external application to a maximum of 10 days.

Why people use this herb

- Ulcers of the bowel, stomach, liver, and gallbladder
- Wounds

Side effects

Call your health care practitioner if you experience unusual symptoms when using comfrey.

Comfrey can cause liver damage. In animals, the herb has been linked to liver and bladder tumors.

Interactions

Combining herbs with certain drugs may alter their action or produce unwanted side effects. Tell your health care practitioner about any prescription or nonprescription drugs you're taking.

Important points to remember

- Don't take comfrey internally.
- Avoid this herb if you're pregnant or breast-feeding.
- Don't give comfrey to young children.
- Don't use comfrey root for medicinal purposes. Limit external application of the mature leaves to intact skin to 10 days.
- Try commercially available antiseptic ointments and creams before using comfrey on wounds. If you do use comfrey on a wound, monitor wound appearance and size.

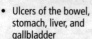

WHAT THE RESEARCH SHOWS

Despite the long history of therapeutic claims for several ailments, comfrey can cause liver damage and shouldn't be consumed. Although animal studies suggest comfrey may promote wound healing, commercially available topical antiseptic agents are more likely to be safe and effective.

Other names for comfrey

Other names for comfrey include blackwort, bruisewort, knitbone, and slippery root.

No known products containing comfrey are available commercially.

Selected references

Hirono, I., et al. "Carcinogenic Activity of *Symphytum officinale*," *Journal of the National Cancer Institute* 61(3):865-69, 1978.

Mattocks, A.R. "Toxic Pyrrolizidine Alkaloids in Comfrey," *Lancet* 11:1136-37, 1980.

Condurango

Condurango is the dried bark of *Marsedenia condurango,* a member of the milkweed family (Asclepiedaceae) that's native to Ecuador and other parts of South America. In the late 1800s, some people considered condurango a cure for early stages of lymphoma and cancer of the breast, esophagus, face, lips, neck, skin, stomach, and tongue.

Why people use this herb

- Bleeding
- Cancer
- Chronic syphilis
- Fluid retention
- Indigestion caused by tension or anxiety
- Pain
- To stimulate the appetite

Common doses

Condurango comes as dried or powdered bark, liquid extract, and tincture. Some experts recommend the following doses:

- As *dried bark,* 1 to 4 grams taken orally.
- As *powdered bark,* 1 to 2 teaspoons mixed with 1 cup of boiling water and left to stand for 10 to 15 minutes before consuming.
- As a *tincture,* 1 to 2 milliliters taken orally three times a day.

Side effects

Call your health care practitioner if you experience any of these possible side effects of condurango:

- nervous system stimulation (stiff neck and facial muscles, restlessness, excitable reflexes, or seizures)
- vision problems, vertigo, sweating, and increased urine output (from ingesting 12 grams or more of the bark).

Ingesting the bark may cause:

- poisoning
- seizures ending in paralysis (with overdose).

Interactions

Combining herbs with certain drugs may alter their action or produce unwanted side effects. Don't use condurango when taking:

- atropine
- Epitol
- iron-containing products

- Lanoxin
- Norvir
- Paxil
- scopolamine
- Zoloft.

Important points to remember

- Don't use condurango if you have a liver disorder or a history of seizures or other nervous system problems.
- Avoid condurango if you're pregnant or breast-feeding.
- Tell your health care practitioner you're using this herb. He or she may recommend periodic liver function studies to check for liver damage.
- Immediately report symptoms of liver damage, such as fever, jaundice (yellow skin discoloration), and pain in the upper right area of the abdomen.
- Immediately discontinue the herb if you experience stiff or rigid muscles, excitable reflexes, or seizures.
- Avoid hazardous activities, such as driving, until your tolerance to the herb is known.

WHAT THE RESEARCH SHOWS

Although condurango reduced tumors in rats, human studies are lacking. Medical experts caution against taking excessive amounts of this herb because of the risk of liver damage, nervous system stimulation, and drug interactions.

Other names for condurango

Other names for condurango include condor-vine bark, condurango bark, condurango blanco, eagle-vine bark, gonolobus condurango triana, and marsedenia condurango.

Products containing condurango are sold under such names as Conduran, Condurango, and Condurango Bark.

Selected references

Hayashi, K., et al. "Antitumor Active Glycosides from Condurango Cortex," *Chemical and Pharmaceutical Bulletin* 28:1954-58, 1980.

Klaassen, C.D. *Casarett and Doull's Toxicology: The Basic Science of Poisons,* 5th ed. New York: McGraw-Hill Book Co., 1996.

Coriander

A flavoring agent typically used with other ingredients, coriander is known as Chinese parsley in Asian cuisines and as cilantro in Spanish cuisines. Fruits, meat products, and alcoholic beverages contain the highest coriander levels.

An essential oil from the dried, ripe fruits of *Coriandrum sativum* is distilled to obtain the active components of the herb. The two plant varieties commonly used are *C. sativum* var. *vulgare* and *C. sativum* var. *microcarpum*. Some people incorrectly refer to coriander fruits as seeds.

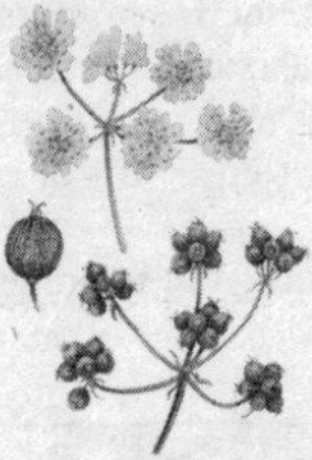

Why people use this herb

- Arthritis
- As an ingredient in some creams, lotions, and perfumes
- Pinworms, tapeworms, and other worm infections

Common dose

Coriander comes as a crude extract of the fruits. Experts disagree on what dose to take.

Side effects

Call your health care practitioner if you experience an allergic reaction to the essential oil. Coriander also may cause fatty liver, a condition that leads to appetite loss, an enlarged liver, and abdominal discomfort.

Interactions

Combining herbs with certain drugs may alter their action or produce unwanted side effects. Tell your health care practitioner about any prescription or nonprescription drugs you're taking, especially drugs that lower blood sugar.

Important points to remember

- Avoid coriander if you're pregnant or breast-feeding.
- Be aware that evidence doesn't support medicinal use of coriander.
- Don't ingest this herb in amounts greater than those commonly found in foods.

Other names for coriander

Other names for coriander include Chinese parsley, cilantro, and oriander.

No known products containing coriander are available commercially.

> **WHAT THE RESEARCH SHOWS**
>
> No human data support medicinal claims for coriander. Therefore, medical experts recommend using it only as a flavoring agent.

Selected references

Al-Said, M.S., et al. "Post-coital Antifertility Activity of the Seeds of *Coriandrum sativum* in Rats," *Journal of Ethnopharmacology* 21:165-73, 1987.

Hashim, S., et al. "Modulatory Effects of Essential Oils from Spices on the Formation of DNA Adduct by Aflatoxin B1 In Vitro," *Nutrition and Cancer* 21:169-75, 1994.

Corkwood

Corkwood comes from the leaves, stems, and root bark of *Duboisia myoporoides*, a member of the Solanaceae family. Native to Australia, this tree was the main source of the anticholinergic drugs scopolamine and atropine before other commercial sources became available. Some people chew the leaves for their stimulant effect.

Why people use this herb

- As an atropine substitute
- As a stimulant
- To stun animals during hunting

Common dose

Corkwood comes as an extract of the corkwood tree (leaves and stems) in tablets and liquid. Experts disagree on what dose to take.

Side effects

Call your health care practitioner if you experience any of these possible side effects of corkwood:

- blurred vision
- constipation
- disorientation
- drowsiness
- dry mouth or skin
- euphoria
- fatigue
- urine retention.

Corkwood also may cause:

- euphoria
- excitation (in high doses)
- hallucinations (in high doses)
- paralyzed eye muscles
- pulse rate changes.

Interactions

Combining herbs with certain drugs may alter their action or produce unwanted side effects. Don't use corkwood while taking:

- anticholinergic drugs, such as atropine
- heart drugs called beta blockers, such as Inderal
- Lanoxin

- Symmetrel
- tricyclic antidepressants.

Important points to remember

- Don't use corkwood if you're allergic to atropine or if you have glaucoma, heart or blood vessel disease, intestinal or urinary tract obstruction, myasthenia gravis, or kidney disease.
- Avoid corkwood if you're pregnant or breast-feeding.

Other names for corkwood

Other names for corkwood include corkwood tree and pituri.

No known products containing corkwood are available commercially.

WHAT THE RESEARCH SHOWS

Although corkwood leaves and stems have been used medicinally (mainly as an atropine substitute), no clinical studies have been done. Some people have experienced toxic effects from occupational or accidental exposure, after absorbing the herb through the mucous membranes and upper respiratory tract. Medical experts caution against using the plant medicinally.

Selected references

Coulsen, J.F., and Griffin, W.J. "The Alkaloids of *Duboisia myoporoides*. I. Aerial Parts," *Planta Medica* 15:459-466, 1967.

Coulsen J.F. and Griffin W.J. "The Alkaloids of *Duboisia myoporoides*. II. Roots," *Planta Medica* 16:174-81, 1968.

Pearn, J. "Corked Up: Clinical Hyoscine Poisoning with Alkaloids of the Native Corkwood, *Duboisia*," *Medical Journal of Australia* 2:422-23, 1981.

Couchgrass

Common in Europe, couchgrass has been introduced to the United States. Most medicinal couchgrass products use the roots of the *Agropyron repens* plant.

Why people use this herb

- Arthritis
- Bladder inflammation
- Fluid retention
- Premenstrual syndrome
- Urinary tract infection

Common dose

Couchgrass comes as capsules (380 milligrams) and tablets (60 milligrams). The manufacturer of Diuplex, a product containing couchgrass, suggests a dose of 2 to 3 tablets taken orally once or twice daily.

Side effects

Call your health care practitioner if you experience skin irritation when using couchgrass. Couchgrass also can cause depletion of body salts.

Interactions

Combining herbs with certain drugs may alter their action or produce unwanted side effects. Tell your health care practitioner about any prescription or nonprescription drugs you're taking.

Important points to remember

- Avoid this herb if you're pregnant or breast-feeding.
- Be aware that couchgrass may cause ergot poisoning (ergotism) if the herb's grain is infected with a fungus-containing ergot. Symptoms of ergot poisoning include burning and freezing sensations, numbness, painful muscle cramps, and poor circulation in the hands and feet. With prolonged ergot ingestion, gangrene may occur. *Convulsive* ergotism may cause seizures, extreme hunger, retching, tongue biting, or unusual breathing patterns. *Hallucinogenic* ergotism may cause vivid hallucinations along with symptoms of one of the other ergotism forms.
- If you're using unprocessed couchgrass, discard portions with black spores.

Other names for couchgrass

Other names for couchgrass include dog grass, quack grass, *Triticum,* twitchgrass, and wheat grass.

WHAT THE RESEARCH SHOWS

Scientists have little information about the safety and effectiveness of couchgrass. No clinical trials or published case reports are available.

Products containing couchgrass are sold under such names as Aqua-Rid, Arcocaps and Diuplex.

Selected reference

Reynolds, J., ed. *Martindale: The Extra Pharmacopoeia,* 21st ed. London: Royal Pharmaceutical Society of Great Britain, 1996.

Cowslip

Active components of cowslip come from the flowers of *Primula veris*, a plant that's native to the mountains of western North America.

Why people use this herb

- Anxiety
- Hysteria
- Insomnia
- Irritability
- Restlessness

Common doses

Cowslip comes as dried flowers and liquid extract. Some experts recommend the following doses:

- As *dried flowers*, 1 to 2 grams taken orally as an infusion three times daily.
- As *liquid extract* (1:1 solution in 25% alcohol), 1 to 2 milliliters taken orally three times daily.

Side effects

Call your health care practitioner if you experience any of these possible side effects of cowslip:

- diarrhea
- nausea
- skin irritation
- vomiting.

Cowslip also can cause:

- heart dysfunction
- liver damage
- red blood cell destruction
- severe digestive tract irritation (from raw cowslip leaves).

Interactions

Combining herbs with certain drugs may alter their action or produce unwanted side effects. Don't use cowslip while taking:

- diuretics
- drugs that lower blood pressure
- sedatives.

Important points to remember

- Don't use cowslip if you're pregnant or breast-feeding.
- Call your health care practitioner if you experience an allergic re-

action, stomach or intestinal problems, or symptoms of liver damage (such as jaundice).

Other names for cowslip

Other names for cowslip include American cowslip, artetyke, arthritica, buckles, crewel, drelip, fairy cup, herb Peter, key of heaven, keyflower, may blob, mayflower, Our Lady's keys, paigle, palsywort, password, peagle, petty mulleins, and plumrocks.

No known products containing cowslip are available commercially.

WHAT THE RESEARCH SHOWS

Scientists know little about cowslip's chemical properties. Until the herb's safety has been established, medical experts caution against taking it for long periods or using large doses.

Selected reference

Cebo, B., et al. "Pharmacologic Properties of Saponin Fraction from Polish Crude Drugs," *Herba Polonica* 22:154-62, 1976.

Cranberry

A trailing evergreen shrub *(Vaccinium macrocarpon, V. oxycoccus,* or *V. erythrocarpum),* cranberry grows in various climates—most notably, acidic bogs from Tennessee to Alaska. A juice or powdered concentrate is made from whole berries (fruit); the skins and seeds are then screened out.

For more than a century, people have been drinking cranberry juice to help prevent urinary tract infections. Two chemical components in the juice reduce the ability of bacteria to adhere to the lining of urinary tract cells.

Common doses

Cranberry comes as:

- capsules (475 and 500 milligrams)
- juices (usually 10% to 20% pure)
- powdered concentrates of varying strengths.

Some experts recommend the following doses:

- As a *juice,* 10 to 16 ounces taken orally every day.
- As *concentrate,* 1 to 2 capsules of concentrate taken orally every day.

Why people use this herb

- Cancer
- Skin irritation caused by contact with urine (in people with urostomies)
- To prevent urinary tract infections
- To treat certain drug overdoses

Side effects

Call your health care practitioner if you experience diarrhea when using cranberry.

Interactions

Combining herbs with certain drugs may alter their action or produce unwanted side effects. Tell your health care practitioner about any prescription or nonprescription drugs you're taking.

Important points to remember

- Use cranberry cautiously if you have benign prostatic hypertrophy or urinary tract obstruction.
- If you have diabetes, keep in mind that you're prone to urinary tract infections. If you're using cranberry juice to help prevent such in-

fections, use only the sugar-free variety to reduce your carbohydrate intake.

- To help prevent urinary tract infections, drink sufficient fluids to ensure adequate urine flow.
- Notify your health care practitioner if you continue to have symptoms of urinary tract infection (such as painful urination or urinary bleeding) after the infection has been treated.

WHAT THE RESEARCH SHOWS

For acute urinary tract infection, medical experts recommend prescribed antibiotics. However, cranberry juice may help prevent such infections, especially in diabetics and other people prone to them. Cranberry juice seems to be a safe, inexpensive, and reasonably effective alternative to long-term preventive antibiotic use (which can be costly, cause side effects, and increase the risk of bacterial resistance). Future studies might find cranberry juice useful in treating conditions linked to urine retention, such as an enlarged prostate, spina bifida, and diabetes.

Other names for cranberry

Other names for cranberry include bog cranberry, isokarpalo (in Finland), marsh apple, mountain cranberry, pikkukarpalo (in Finland), and small cranberry.

Products containing cranberry are sold under such names as Cranberry Power, Cranberry Whole Fruit, Cran Relief, Cran-Tastic.

Selected references

Avorn, J., et al. "Reduction of Bacteriuria and Pyuria After Ingestion of Cranberry Juice," *JAMA* 271:751-54, 1994.

Ofek, I., et al. "Anti-Escherichia coli Adhesion Activity of Cranberry and Blueberry Juices," *Advances in Experimental Medicine and Biology* 408:179-83, 1996.

Sobota, A.E. "Inhibition of Bacterial Adherence by Cranberry Juice: Potential Use for the Treatment of Urinary Tract Infections," *Journal of Urology* 131:1013-16, 1984.

Cucumber

A low-growing annual vegetable, cucumber originated in northern India, where it was domesticated more than 3,000 years ago. History records a few noteworthy cucumber fanatics, including the Roman emperor Tiberius, who ate some cucumber daily and ordered his gardeners to find ways to grow cucumbers out of season. Columbus included cucumbers in his experimental gardens on Hispaniola (Haiti) during his second voyage in 1494.

Why people use this herb

- Fluid retention
- Facial cleansing
- High blood pressure
- Low blood pressure
- Skin irritation

Common doses

Cucumber comes as seeds and juice and is found in many cosmetics. Some experts recommend the following doses:

- As a *diuretic,* steep 1 to 2 ounces of the ground seed in water and drink.
- As a *cosmetic,* apply the extracted juice topically.

Side effects

Call your health care practitioner if you experience symptoms of body water and salt loss (such as dehydration, increased thirst, lightheadedness, or dizziness) when using cucumber medicinally.

Interactions

Combining herbs with certain drugs may alter their action or produce unwanted side effects. Tell your health care practitioner about any prescription or nonprescription drugs you're taking, especially diuretics.

Other names for cucumber

Cucumber is also called wild cowcumber.

No known products containing cucumber are available commercially.

Selected reference

Liener, I.E. *Toxic Components of Plant Foodstuffs.* London: Academic Press, 1980.

WHAT THE RESEARCH SHOWS

Medicinal and therapeutic claims for cucumber have little evidence to support them. With many safe and effective prescription diuretics available, there's little reason to use cucumber to treat fluid retention.

Daffodil

Traditionally, preparations made from boiled daffodil bulbs were used to induce vomiting. Today, some people use daffodil in the form of powdered flowers or extract from *Narcissus pseudonarcissus*, in the Narcissus family (Amaryllidaceae). These plants are common in Europe and the United States.

Why people use this herb

- Burns
- Joint pain
- Muscle strain
- Respiratory congestion
- To induce vomiting
- Wounds

Common dose

Daffodil comes as powdered flowers and extract. Some experts recommend the following dose:

- *To induce vomiting,* 20 grains to 2 drams of powdered flowers or 2 to 3 grains of extract taken orally.

Side effects

Call your health care practitioner if you experience any of these possible side effects of daffodil:

- excessive salivation
- nausea
- skin irritation
- unusually small pupils
- vomiting.

Daffodil also can cause:

- collapse of the respiratory system, heart, and blood vessels
- death (by paralyzing the central nervous system).

Interactions

Combining herbs with certain drugs may alter their action or produce unwanted side effects. Tell your health care practitioner about any prescription or nonprescription drugs you're taking.

Important points to remember

- Avoid this herb if you're pregnant or breast-feeding.
- Don't consume any part of the daffodil plant. The flowers and bulbs are poisonous, and ingesting even small quantities can lead to rapid death. Accidental poisoning by daffodil bulbs has been reported in the United States, Britain, Switzerland, Germany, Finland, Sweden, and the Netherlands.

- Keep plant parts out of reach of children and pets.

Other names for daffodil

Other names for daffodil include daffydown-dilly, fleur de coucou, Lent lily, *Narcissus,* and porillon.

No known products containing daffodil are available commercially.

WHAT THE RESEARCH SHOWS

In studies, a substance derived from daffodil inhibited HIV and cytomegalovirus infections. This leads scientists to believe the herb has potential for biochemical research and may contribute to the development of new laboratory tests for these viruses.

However, little evidence supports medicinal uses of daffodil. Therapeutic claims aren't based on controlled studies in people. What's more, daffodil plants are toxic and must not be taken internally.

Selected references

Balzarini, J., et al. "Alpha-(1,3)- and Alpha-(1-6)-mannose Specific Plant Lectins are Markedly Inhibitory to Human Immunodeficiency Virus and Cytomegalovirus Infections In Vitro," *Antimicrobial Agents and Chemotherapy* 35:410-16, 1991.

Gude, M., et al. "An Investigation of the Irritant and Allergenic Properties of Daffodils *(Narcissus pseudonarcissus* L., Amaryllidaceae). A Review of Daffodil Dermatitis," *Contact Dermatitis* 19:1-10, 1988.

Daisy

The Iroquois Indians used the daisy to aid digestion. Several chemical compounds come from the fresh or dried flowers and leaves of *Bellis perennis*, a common perennial herb.

Why people use this herb

- Arthritis
- As an expectorant
- Bruises
- Cough
- Diarrhea
- Kidney disorders
- Liver disorders
- Muscle spasms
- Nasal inflammation
- Pain
- Rheumatism
- Skin disorders
- To aid digestion
- To "purify" the blood
- Wounds

Common doses

Daisy comes as a dried herb and a tincture. Some experts recommend the following doses:

- As a *tincture,* 2 to 4 milliliters taken three times daily.
- As an *infusion,* 1 teaspoon of dried herb steeped in boiling water for 10 minutes, taken three times daily.

Side effects

Call your health care practitioner if you experience unusual symptoms when using daisy for medicinal purposes.

Interactions

Combining herbs with certain drugs may alter their action or produce unwanted side effects. Tell your health care practitioner about any prescription or nonprescription drugs you're taking.

Important points to remember

- Don't use daisy medicinally if you're pregnant or breast-feeding.
- Although daisies have been eaten in some parts of the world, their effects haven't been documented. Use caution when ingesting.

Other names for daisy

Other names for daisy include bairnwort, bruisewort, common daisy, and day's eye.

WHAT THE RESEARCH SHOWS

Although the daisy has a long history of safety, this history is based on verbal reports, not clinical data. The herb's chemical components haven't been thoroughly evaluated.

No known products containing daisy are available commercially.

Selected reference

Launert, E. *The Hamlyn Guide to Edible and Medicinal Plants of Britain and Northern Europe.* London: Hamlyn Publishing Group Ltd., 1981.

Damiana

Damiana comes from the leaves of *Turnera diffusa,* a shrub found in Mexico, South America, and the southwestern United States. Some herbalists believe damiana can "improve the sexual ability of the enfeebled and aged." The herb has an aromatic scent and a pleasing taste.

Common doses

Damiana is available as a tincture, capsule, powder, or tea. Some experts recommend the following doses:

- As a *tincture,* up to 2.5 milliliters taken orally three times daily.
- As a *powdered herb,* 18 grams in a 500-milliliter decoction, taken as a tea three times a day.

Side effects

Call your health care practitioner if you experience hallucinations when using damiana. Damiana also can cause irritation of the urethra, which might explain why some people believe the herb has aphrodisiac effects. Taking excessive amounts may result in liver injury.

Why people use this herb

- As an aphrodisiac
- Constipation
- Depression
- Fluid retention
- To induce euphoria and relaxation

Interactions

Combining herbs with certain drugs may alter their action or produce unwanted side effects. Tell your health care practitioner about any prescription or nonprescription drugs you're taking.

Important points to remember

- Don't use damiana if you're pregnant or breast-feeding.
- Avoid hazardous activities, such as driving, until you know how this herb affects you.

Other names for damiana

Other names for damiana include herba de la pastora, Mexican damiana, old woman's broom, and rosemary.

Products containing damiana are sold under such names as Damiania and Damiana Root.

WHAT THE RESEARCH SHOWS

Although some herbalists believe damiana has aphrodisiac and hallucinogenic effects, no evidence supports these claims. A detailed review of damiana's history indicates such claims stem from a hoax.

Selected reference

Lowry, T.P. "Damiana," *Journal of Psychoactive Drugs* 16:267-68, 1984.

Dandelion

A well-known herbal remedy and natural food item, dandelion is one of nine herbal ingredients in a British product used to treat viral hepatitis. Some people roast dandelion root and use it as a coffee substitute. Others make wine and schnapps from dandelion flowers or add the herb to soups and salads. Dandelion contains more vitamin A than carrots.

Active herbal components come from the leaves and roots of *Taraxacum officinale* or *T. laevigatum*. These common, low-growing weeds are native to Europe and Asia and naturalized worldwide.

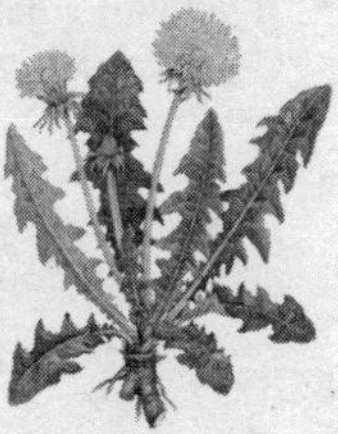

Common doses

Dandelion comes as capsules, extracts, and teas. Some experts recommend the following doses:

- As *dried root,* 2 to 8 grams taken orally by infusion or decoction three times daily.
- As *dried leaf,* 4 to 10 grams taken orally by infusion three times daily.
- As *fluid extract* (1:1 in 25% alcohol), 4 to 8 milliliters (1 to 2 teaspoons) taken orally three times daily.
- As *tincture of root* (1:5 in 45% alcohol), 5 to 10 milliliters taken orally three times daily.
- As *juice of root,* 4 to 8 milliliters taken orally three times daily.

Why people use this herb

- Constipation
- Digestive complaints
- Fluid retention from premenstrual syndrome, heart failure, or high blood pressure
- Gallbladder problems
- Liver disorders
- Rheumatism
- To aid weight reduction
- To help remove corns, calluses, and warts
- To stimulate bile production

Side effects

Call your health care practitioner if you experience skin irritation when using dandelion.

Dandelion can also cause:

- blockage of the digestive or biliary tract
- gallbladder inflammation
- gallstones.

Interactions

Combining herbs with certain drugs may alter their action or produce unwanted side effects. Don't use dandelion while taking:

- diuretics
- drugs that lower blood pressure
- drugs that lower blood sugar.

Important points to remember

- Don't use dandelion if you're pregnant or breast-feeding.
- If you have diabetes, check your blood sugar level carefully when using dandelion. The herb may make your blood sugar level drop too low.
- If you're taking dandelion along with a drug used to lower blood pressure, be aware that you may feel dizzy or lose consciousness briefly when rising from a sitting or lying position.

WHAT THE RESEARCH SHOWS

In a small group of patients, dandelion root successfully treated chronic nonspecific colitis (inflammation of the colon). In these patients, the herb relieved abdominal pain, constipation, and diarrhea.

Nonetheless, scientists have little information to justify dandelion's reported therapeutic uses. Although the plant has been used in foods without side effects, medical experts caution against ingesting large amounts.

Other names for dandelion

Other names for dandelion include lion's tooth, priest's crown, and wild endive.

A product containing dandelion is sold as Dandelion.

Selected references

Mascolo, N., et al. "Biological Screening of Italian Medicinal Plants for Anti-Inflammatory Activity," *Phytotherapy Research* 1:28-9, 1987.

Racz-Kotilla, E., et al. "The Action of *Taraxacum officinale* Extracts on the Body Weight and Diuresis of Laboratory Animals," *Planta Medica* 26(3):212-17, 1974.

Devil's claw

The hooks that cover the fruit of *Harpagophytum procumbens,* the source of devil's claw, account for the herb's odd name. The hooks promote the plant's spread by animals. The drug is extracted from the roots and secondary tubers of *H. procumbens,* a member of the Pedalia family (Pedaliaceae).

Common dose

Devil's claw comes as:

- capsules (200, 420, 499, 510, and 750 milligrams)
- tinctures
- teas.

In one study, people received 2,000 milligrams orally daily.

Why people use this herb

- Allergies
- Arteriosclerosis (hardening of the arteries)
- Arthritis
- Boils
- Digestive tract problems
- Headache
- Heartburn
- Kidney disorders
- Liver disorders
- Lumbago
- Malaria
- Menopause symptoms
- Menstrual pain
- Nicotine poisoning
- Rheumatism
- Severe stabbing pains
- Skin cancer
- To stimulate the appetite

Side effects

Call your health care practitioner if you experience unusual symptoms when using devil's claw.

Interactions

Combining herbs with certain drugs may alter their action or produce unwanted side effects. Tell your health care practitioner about any prescription or nonprescription drugs you're taking, especially drugs for irregular heartbeats.

Important points to remember

- Avoid devil's claw if you have gastric or duodenal ulcers or if you're breast-feeding.
- Don't use this herb if you're pregnant, think you may be pregnant, or plan to become pregnant. Devil's claw may stimulate uterine contractions and cause miscarriage.
- If you're using devil's claw to ease inflammation, keep in mind that you may get better results by taking one of the many prescription or nonprescription drugs with known risks and benefits.

Other names for devil's claw

Other names for devil's claw include grapple plant and wood spider.

Products containing devil's claw are sold under such names as Devil's Claw, Devil's Claw Capsule, Devil's Claw Secondary Root, and Devil's Claw Vegicaps.

> **WHAT THE RESEARCH SHOWS**
>
> Except for a single study, scientists have no evidence that devil's claw eases inflammation or has therapeutic value in treating any other disorder. Larger and well-designed clinical studies must be done to evaluate its safety and effectiveness in treating arthritis.

Selected references

Moussard, C., et al. "A Drug in Traditional Medicine, *Harpagophytum procumbens:* No Evidence for NSAID-Like Effect on Whole Blood Eicosanoid Production in Humans," *Prostaglandins Leukotrienes and Essential Fatty Acids* 46:283-86, 1992.

Whitehouse, L.W., et al. "Devil's Claw *(Harpagophytum procumbens):* No Evidence for Anti-inflammatory Activity in the Treatment of Arthritic Disease," *Canadian Medical Association Journal* 129:249-51, 1983.

DHEA

DHEA has been touted as an immune booster, an anti-aging miracle drug, and a treatment for many disorders ranging from depression to tumors. DHEA is made from steroid precursors found in the yam. Europe and China produce most of the commercially available DHEA.

Common dose

DHEA is available as:

- capsules (5, 25, or 50 milligrams)
- timed-release tablets (15 milligrams)
- cream (4 ounces, combined with other vitamins and herbs).

In most studies, people received a dose of 50 milligrams orally daily.

Why people use this herb

- Atherosclerosis (plaque buildup in the arteries)
- Certain autoimmune disorders
- Diabetes
- Depression
- To enhance the immune system
- To prevent osteoporosis
- To slow the effects of aging
- Tumors

Side effects

Call your health care practitioner if you experience any of these possible side effects of DHEA:

- excessive body hair growth
- increased aggressiveness
- insomnia
- irritability.

Interactions

Combining herbs with certain drugs may alter their action or produce unwanted side effects. Tell your health care practitioner about any prescription or nonprescription drugs you're taking, especially other androgen or estrogen hormones.

Important points to remember

- Don't use DHEA if you have prostate cancer, benign prostatic hypertrophy, or a breast or uterine tumor. DHEA may promote growth of these tumors.
- Avoid this herb if you're pregnant or breast-feeding.
- If you're over age 40, don't take DHEA unless you've been screened aggressively for hormonally sensitive cancers.
- Report mood or behavior changes to your health care practitioner.

WHAT THE RESEARCH SHOWS

Most claims for DHEA are based on laboratory and nonprimate studies. Although decreasing DHEA levels in humans may indicate aging and degenerative diseases, scientists lack conclusive evidence that DHEA can prevent or treat these diseases. They also know little about the safety of long-term DHEA use. Larger and more comprehensive trials are needed to determine an appropriate role for DHEA in medicine.

Other names for DHEA

DHEA is also called dehydroepiandrosterone.

Products containing DHEA are sold under such names as Born Again's DHEA Eyelift Serum, DHEA Men's Formula, DHEA with Antioxidants 25 milligrams, and DHEA with Bioperine 50 milligrams.

Selected reference

Wolkowitz, O.M., et al. "Dehydroepiandrosterone Treatment of Depression," *Biological Psychiatry* 41:311-18, 1997.

Dill

Dill may have gotten its name from its sedative and antigas properties: The old Norse word *dilla* means "to lull." In the Middle Ages, magicians used dill in potions and magic spells, and people grew the herb in their gardens to ward off witchcraft and enchantments.

All parts of the dill plant are used, but most dill products come from the dried ripe fruit, seeds, or flowers of *Anethum graveolens,* a member of the carrot family (Umbelliferae). Some people put dill in "gripe water," which they give to infants to relieve gas and sharp intestinal pains. Dill also promotes milk flow in breastfeeding women and cattle.

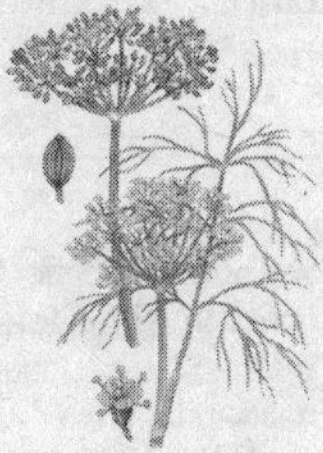

Common doses

Dill comes as dried fruit, distilled or concentrated dill water, and dill oil. Some experts recommend the following doses:

- As *dried fruit,* 1 to 4 grams taken orally three times daily.
- As *distilled dill water,* 2 to 4 milliliters taken orally three times daily.
- As *concentrated dill water,* 0.2 milliliters taken orally three times daily.
- As *dill oil,* 0.05 to 2 milliliters taken orally three times daily.

Side effects

Call your health care practitioner if you experience unusual symptoms while using dill.

Why people use this herb

- Bad breath
- Hiccups
- Insomnia
- Intestinal gas
- Muscle spasms
- Stomach pain
- To aid digestion
- To improve the appetite
- To stimulate lactation
- To strengthen nails

Interactions

Combining herbs with certain drugs may alter their action or produce unwanted side effects. Tell your health care practitioner about any prescription or nonprescription drugs you're taking.

Important points to remember

- Don't use dill if you're on a low-salt (low-sodium) diet because of its high sodium content.
- Use dill cautiously if you're allergic to other spices. Cross-sensitivity may occur.
- Seek advice from your health care practitioner before taking dill.

Other names for dill

Other names for dill include dill seed and dillweed.

Products containing dill are sold under such names as Atkinson & Barker's Gripe Mixture, Concentrated Dill Water BPC 1973, Neo, Neo Baby Mixture, Nurse Harvey's Gripe Mixture, and Woodwards Gripe Water.

WHAT THE RESEARCH SHOWS

The potential benefits of dill remain unproven. Most clinical data on this herb come from foreign sources or animal studies. No human data from the United States support the use of dill for intestinal gas or sharp intestinal pains in infants or as a milk flow stimulant. More studies must be done to determine if dill is safe or effective.

Selected reference

Morton, J.F. *Atlas of Medicinal Plants of Middle America: Bahamas to Yucatan.* Springfield, Ill: Charles C. Thomas Publisher, 1981.

Dong quai

Dong quai comes from the roots of *Angelica polymorpha* var. *sinensis*, a fragrant perennial herb native to China, Korea, and Japan.

Common dose

Dong quai comes as tablets (fluid extract, 0.5 grams) and raw root (4.5 to 30 grams to be boiled or soaked in wine). In some countries, it also comes in injectable forms. In one study, people received a dose of 1 gram of the root.

Side effects

Call your health care practitioner if you experience any of these possible side effects of dong quai:

- bleeding
- diarrhea
- fever
- skin sensitivity to sunlight.

Interactions

Combining herbs with certain drugs may alter their action or produce unwanted side effects. Don't use dong quai while taking blood thinners.

Important points to remember

- Don't ingest volatile oil of dong quai because one of its components can cause cancer.
- Don't use this herb if you're pregnant or breast-feeding because it may harm the fetus. Report planned or suspected pregnancy.
- Report unusual bleeding or bruising.
- Know that some of the herb's components increase the risk of certain cancers.

Why people use this herb

- Abscess
- Buerger's disease (a condition of obstruction, inflammation, and blood clotting in a blood vessel)
- Chronic runny nose
- Constipation
- Excessive fetal movement
- Gynecologic disorders, such as irregular menstruation, painful menstruation, premenstrual syndrome, and chronic pelvic infection
- Headache
- Hepatitis
- High blood pressure
- Infections, including those producing pus
- Liver cirrhosis
- Malaria
- Raynaud's disease (a condition of intermittent slowing of blood flow to the fingers, toes, ears or nose)
- Severe stabbing pains
- Shingles
- Toothache
- Ulcers

- To help prevent skin sensitivity to sunlight, use sunblock and wear adequate clothing and sunglasses.
- Don't use this herb for its estrogen-like effects because these effects haven't been proven.

Other names for dong quai

Other names for dong quai include Chinese angelica, dry-kuei, FP3340010/FP334015/FT334010, tang-kuei, and women's ginseng.

Products containing dong quai are sold under such names as Dong Kwai, Dong Quai Capsules, and Dong Quai Fluid Extract.

WHAT THE RESEARCH SHOWS

Only a few animal studies support the many therapeutic claims for dong quai. The herb seems to have more than 18 active chemical components, which exert widely divergent effects. Some components can cause cancer and others have unknown side effects. Extensive testing of individual components must be done before dong quai can be deemed safe or effective.

Selected reference

Hirata, J.D., et al. "Does Donq Quai Have Estrogenic Effects in Postmenopausal Women? A Double-Blind Placebo-Controlled Trial," *Fertility and Sterility* 68:981-86, 1997.

Echinacea

Echinacea dietary supplements are extracted from the dried roots and rhizomes (underground stems) of *Echinacea angustifolia* or *E. pallida* and from the fresh juice of the roots or above-ground parts of *E. purpurea*. Native to North America, these plants flower from May through October in fields from Saskatchewan south to Tennessee and Texas.

Why people use this herb

- Abscesses
- Burns
- Colon cancer
- Eczema (a type of skin inflammation)
- Liver cancer
- Upper respiratory tract infection
- Urinary tract infection
- Varicose leg ulcers
- Skin wounds

Common doses

Echinacea comes as:

- capsules (125 milligrams, 355 milligrams [85 milligrams of herbal extract powder], or 500 milligrams)
- tablets (335 milligrams)
- hydroalcoholic extracts
- fresh-pressed juice
- glycerite (dissolved in glycerin)
- lozenges
- tinctures.

Some experts recommend the following doses:

- As an *expressed juice,* 6 to 9 milliliters taken orally daily.
- As a *powdered herb,* 900 milligrams to 1 gram taken orally three times daily.
- As a *tincture,* 0.75 to 1.5 milliliter (15 to 30 drops) taken orally two to five times daily, or 60 drops taken orally three times daily.
- As a *tea,* 2 teaspoons (4 grams) of coarsely powdered herb simmered in 1 cup of boiling water for 10 minutes. However, tea isn't recommended because some of echinacea's useful active compounds don't dissolve in water.

Side effects

Call your health care practitioner if you experience an allergic reaction when using echinacea. Such reactions are most likely to occur in people sensitive to plants in the daisy family.

Interactions

Combining herbs with certain drugs may alter their action or produce unwanted side effects. Tell your health care practitioner about any prescription or nonprescription drugs you're taking.

Important points to remember

- Don't take echinacea if your immune system is suppressed (for instance, if you have tuberculosis, HIV infection, or AIDS) or if you have an autoimmune disease such as collagen disease or multiple sclerosis.
- Avoid this herb if you're pregnant or breast-feeding.
- Don't give an alcohol-based tincture to children and don't use these tinctures if you are an alcoholic, have liver disease, or are taking Antabuse or Flagyl.
- Know that your immune system may become overstimulated and then suppressed if you take echinacea for a long time. Don't use this herb longer than 8 weeks. Some experts believe 10 to 14 days probably is long enough.

Other names for echinacea

Other names for echinacea include American cone flower, black sampson, black susans, cock-up-hat, comb flower, coneflower, echinacea care liquid, hedgehog, Indian head, Kansas snakeroot, Missouri snakeroot, narrow-leaved purple coneflower, purple coneflower, purple Kansas coneflower, red sunflower, scurvy root, and snakeroot.

WHAT THE RESEARCH SHOWS

According to a 1999 study, people who use echinacea continuously for a long time have more upper respiratory infections than those who don't take the herb. The study also found that echinacea was ineffective in treating upper respiratory infections. However, it involved only one echinacea form. Other herb forms may produce different results.

All told, scientists need more information before they can define echinacea's role in treating or preventing disease. Until then, medical experts caution against delaying medical treatment of an illness that continues or worsens despite taking echinacea for 1 week or longer. As for toxicity, no animal studies using large doses have found toxic effects.

Products containing echinacea are sold under such names as Coneflower Extract, Echinacea, Echinacea Angustifolia Herb, Echinacea Fresh Freeze-Dried, Echinacea Glycerite, Echinacea Herb, Echinacea Herbal Comfort Lozenges, Echinacea Plus, and Echinacea Purpurea.

Selected references

Combest, W.L., and Nemecz, G. "Echinacea," *U.S. Pharmacist* October:126-32, 1997.

Jacobson, M. "The Structure of Echinacein, the Insecticidal Component of American Coneflower Roots," *Journal of Organic Chemistry* 32:1646-47, 1967.

Lersch, C., et al. "Stimulation of the Immune Response in Outpatients with Hepatocellular Carcinomas by Low Doses of Cyclophosphamide (LDCY), *Echinacea purpurea* Extracts (Echinacein), and Thymostimulin," *Arch Gescwulstforsch* 60:379-83, 1990.

Lersch, C., et al. "Nonspecific Immunostimulation with Low Doses of Cyclophosphamide (LDCY), Thymostimulin, and *Echinacea purpurea* Extract (Echinacein) in Patients with Far Advanced Colorectal Cancers. Preliminary Results," *Cancer Investigation* 10:343-48, 1992.

Elderberry

People once used elderberry as an insect repellent, placing sprays of the flower in horses' bridles or adding powdered flowers to water and dabbing it on the skin. Some people mix elderberry with sage, lemon juice, vinegar, and honey to use as a gargle. Elderberry juice has been used in hair dye and scented ointments. Children sometimes make pipes or pea-shooters from the hollowed stems of the elder—sometimes suffering cyanide poisoning as a result.

Several trees and shrubs of the *Sambucus* species, such as *S. nigra* and *S. canadensis,* produce elderberries. Herbalists typically use the flowers and berries, probably because the inner bark and leaves contain most of the potentially poisonous substances.

Why people use this herb

- Asthma
- Burns
- Cancer
- Chafed skin
- Common cold
- Epilepsy
- Gout
- Headache
- Liver disease
- Measles
- Psoriasis (scaly, raised skin patches)
- Sharp stabbing pains
- Swelling
- Syphilis
- Toothache
- To repel insects
- Wounds

Common dose

Elderberry comes as:

- ointments and aqueous solutions of the bark and leaves
- oils
- solutions
- wine.

Experts disagree on what dose to take.

Side effects

Call your health care practitioner if you experience any of these possible side effects of elderberry:

- diarrhea (from *S. ebulus* berries or leaves of any *Sambucus* species)
- vomiting (from eating a lot of *S. racemosa* berries).

Ingesting the bark, roots, leaves, or unripe berries of the elderberry plant can cause cyanide poisoning.

Interactions

Combining herbs with certain drugs may alter their action or produce unwanted side effects. Tell your health care practitioner about any prescription or nonprescription drugs you're taking.

Important points to remember

- Use elderberry products with caution because of the risk of cyanide poisoning.
- Never eat the plant's leaves, stems, or green parts. They're poisonous.
- Don't use this herb if you're pregnant or breast-feeding.
- Avoid anything made with berries of the dwarf elder (*S. ebulus*), thought to be especially poisonous. Large doses can cause vertigo, vomiting, and diarrhea (symptoms of cyanide poisoning).
- Never eat uncooked elderberries because of the risk of cyanide poisoning.
- Know that eating 60 milligrams of cyanide has caused death. Keep the elderberry plant away from children and pets, and have the telephone number for the nearest poison control center handy.

WHAT THE RESEARCH SHOWS

Medical experts don't recommend using elderberry products as laxatives because of the risk of cyanide poisoning. Besides, many safe, effective laxatives and cathartics are available. The same is true for the other conditions for which elderberries have been used. For instance, many proven anti-inflammatory products are available to treat rheumatism symptoms.

Other names for elderberry

Other names for elderberry include antelope brush (*Sambucus tridentata*), black elder (*S. nigra*), blue elderberry (*S. caerulea*), boretree, common elder (*S. canadensis*), danewort (*S. ebulus*), dwarf elder, elder, European elder, pipe tree, red elderberry, red-fruited elder (S. *pubens, S. racemosa*), *Sambucus*, and sweet elder.

Products containing elderberry are sold under such names as Elderberry Power and Elder Flowers.

Selected references

Swanston-Flatt, S.K., et al. "Glycaemic Effects of Traditional European Plant Treatments for Diabetes. Studies in Normal and Streptozotocin Diabetic Mice," *Diabetes Research* 10:69-73, 1989.

Yesilada, E., et al. "Inhibitory Effects of Turkish Folk Remedies on Inflammatory Cytokines: Interleukin-1^{alpha}, Interleukin-1^{beta} and Tumor Necrosis Factor Alpha," *Journal of Ethnopharmacology* 58:59-73, 1997.

Elecampane

In France and Switzerland, elecampane root was used to prepare absinthe, a potent cordial popular at the turn of the century. In Europe and Asia, the herb has been used as a remedy for centuries.

Elecampane comes from the dried roots and rhizomes (underground stems) of 2- to 3-year-old *Inula helenium* plants. This perennial herb, native to the temperate regions of Europe, Asia, and Africa, has yellow flowers with large heads.

Why people use this herb

- Asthma
- Bronchitis
- Cough
- Fluid retention
- Indigestion
- Lung disease
- *Mycobacterium tuberculosis* (a type of tuberculosis)
- Snakebite
- To stimulate the appetite

Common doses

Elecampane comes as powdered root preparations, fluid extracts, and lotions. Some experts recommend the following doses:

- As *fresh root,* 1 to 2 tablespoons taken orally three times daily.
- As *dried root,* 2 to 3 grams taken orally three times daily.
- As *extract,* 3 grams of dried root in 20 milliliters of alcohol and 10 milliliters water taken orally three times daily.

Side effects

Call your health care practitioner if you experience a skin reaction after coming in contact with elecampane.

Interactions

Combining herbs with certain drugs may alter their action or produce unwanted side effects. Tell your health care practitioner about any prescription or nonprescription drugs you're taking.

Important points to remember

- Watch for skin inflammation after contact with elecampane.
- If you have allergies, wear long sleeves and gloves when handling the herb.

Other names for elecampane

Other names for elecampane include aunee, elf dock, elfwort, horseheal, scabwort, velvet dock, and wild sunflower.

WHAT THE RESEARCH SHOWS

Researchers believe elecampane may have value as an expectorant, an antiseptic, and a mild digestive stimulant. However, well-designed human studies haven't been done. The herb seems to be safe and well tolerated, but medical supervision is still recommended.

No known products containing elecampane are available commercially.

Selected references

Fokina, G.I., et al. "Experimental Phytotherapy of Tick-Borne Encephalitis," *Voprosy Virusologii* 36:18-21, 1991. Abstract.

Reiter, M., and Brandt, W. "Relaxant Effects on Tracheal and Ileal Smooth Muscles of the Guinea Pig," *Arzneimittel-forschung* 35:408-14, 1985. Abstract.

Rhee, J.K., et al. "Alterations of *Clonorchis sinensis* EPG by Administration of Herbs in Rabbits," *American Journal of Chinese Medicine* 13:65-69, 1985. Abstract.

Ephedra

Chinese practitioners have been using ephedra for several years. In the United States, the herb has street names of "natural ecstasy" as a stimulant and "natural fen-phen" as a diet aid. The Food and Drug Administration (FDA) warns against using the diet aid and has banned the stimulant version.

This herb comes from the ephedra species—an evergreen with a pinelike odor that grows in certain desert regions of Asia and the United States. Of the many ephedra species, the most common are *Ephedra sinica* and *E. nevadensis*. Herbalists use parts of the plant's seeds and stems.

Why people use this herb

- Bronchial asthma
- Chills
- Common cold
- Cough
- Fever
- Flu
- Fluid retention
- Headache
- Joint pain
- Nasal congestion
- To stimulate the nervous system
- To suppress the appetite

Common dose

Ephedra comes as unprocessed extracts of root and above-ground parts, tablets (approximately 7 milligrams), and teas. Some experts recommend the following dose:

- As a *tea,* place ½ ounce of dried branches in a pint of boiling water and steep for 10 to 20 minutes.

Be aware that the FDA prohibits the sale of ephedra in quantities of 8 milligrams or more per dose and cautions against taking more than 8 milligrams every 6 hours or more than 24 milligrams daily. The FDA also warns not to use ephedra products for more than 7 days in a row.

Side effects

Call your health care practitioner if you experience any of these possible side effects of ephedra:

- anxiety
- confusion
- constipation
- dizziness
- headache
- insomnia

- irregular heartbeats
- nervousness
- psychosis
- restlessness
- skin inflammation
- urine retention.

This herb also can cause heart attacks, psychosis, and uterine contractions.

Interactions

Combining herbs with certain drugs may alter their action or produce unwanted side effects. Don't use this herb with:

- drugs to relieve depression called MAO inhibitors (such as Marplan and Nardil)
- ephedrine
- heart drugs called beta blockers (such as Inderal)
- phenothiazines such as Thorazine, used for anxiety, nausea, vomiting, or psychosis
- Sudafed
- Theo-Dur.

Important points to remember

- Don't take ephedra if you're pregnant because it can stimulate the uterus.
- Be aware that many of the heart attacks, seizures, and strokes reported to the FDA occurred in previously healthy young adults using ephedra.
- Know that the FDA has linked 17 deaths and hundreds of serious side effects to ephedra products containing the alkaloid ephedrine.
- Avoid ephedra if you have heart disease, high blood pressure, diabetes, or an enlarged prostate.
- Watch for side effects—especially chest pain, shortness of breath, palpitations, dizziness, or fainting—when using ephedra. Seek medical help immediately if you experience any of these.
- Take less than 8 milligrams every 6 hours and never more than 24 milligrams daily. Also, don't use ephedra for more than 7 consecutive days.

Other names for ephedra

Other names for ephedra include brigham tea, cao ma huang (Chinese ephedra), desert tea, epitonin, herba ephedrae, herbal, joint fir, ma huang, mahuuanggen (root), Mexican tea, Mormon tea, muzei mu huang (Mongolian ephedra), natural ecstasy, popotillo, sea grape, squaw tea, teamster's tea, yellow astringent, yellow horse, and zhong ma huang (intermediate ephedra).

Products containing ephedra are sold under such names as Herbal Fen-Phen, Power Trim, and Up Your Gas.

WHAT THE RESEARCH SHOWS

Scientists believe the main components in some *Ephedra* species may be valuable in treating certain conditions, especially fluid retention. However, standardized formulations of ephedra's active chemicals are available over the counter, so medical experts don't recommend taking the herbal product.

Selected reference

Wang, G.Z., and Hikokichi, O. "Experimental Study in Treating Chronic Renal Failure with Dry Extract and Tannins of Herbal Ephedra," *Chinese Journal of Stomatology* 14:485, 1994.

Eucalyptus

Herbal eucalyptus products come from the leaves of the eucalyptus globulus labill plant. The herb was first used more than 100 years ago to relieve stuffy nose.

Common doses

Eucalyptus is available as an oil and a lotion. Some experts recommend the following doses:

- For *various uses,* 0.05 to 0.2 milliliters of eucalyptol, 0.05 to 0.2 milliliter of eucalyptus oil, or 2 to 4 grams of fluid extract taken orally.
- For *topical use,* mix 30 milliliters of oil with 500 milliliters of water.

Side effects

Call your health care practitioner if you experience any of these possible side effects of eucalyptus:

- bluish gray skin
- burning sensation in the stomach
- delirium
- dizziness
- muscle weakness
- nausea
- small pupils
- vomiting.

Why people use this herb

- Nasal congestion

Eucalyptus also can cause seizures.

Interactions

Combining herbs with certain drugs may alter their action or produce unwanted side effects. Tell your health care practitioner about any prescription or nonprescription drugs you're taking.

Important points to remember

- Avoid eucalyptus products if you're pregnant or breast-feeding.
- Don't use eucalyptus oil if you're taking drugs or other treatments to lower your blood sugar.
- Dilute the herb before you swallow it or apply it to your skin.
- Keep eucalyptus oil away from children and pets.

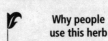

Other names for eucalyptus

Other names for eucalyptus include fevertree, gum tree, and Tasmanian blue gum.

Products containing eucalyptus are sold under such names as Eucalyptamint and Eucalyptus Oil.

> **WHAT THE RESEARCH SHOWS**
>
> Although many people take eucalyptus, scientists have little information to support claims for its medicinal use. Until researchers test the herb's ability to combat infections, medical experts recommend using established drugs, not eucalyptus, to treat infections.

Selected references

Egawa, H., et al. "Antifungal Substances Found in Leaves of Eucalyptus Species," *Specialia* 15:889-90, 1977.

Hong, C., et al. "Effects of a Topically Applied Counterirritant (Eucalyptamint) on Cutaneous Blood Flow and on the Skin and Muscle Temperature," *American Journal of Physical Medicine and Rehabilitation* 70:29-33, 1991.

Santos, F., et al. "Mast Cell Involvement in the Rat Paw Oedema Response to 1,8-cineole, the Main Constituent of Eucalyptus and Rosemary Oils," *European Journal of Pharmacology* 331:253-58, 1997.

Eyebright

Euphrasia officinalis, the plant that eyebright comes from, has been used since the Middle Ages to treat bloodshot or irritated eyes—a practice that evolved because the spotted and striped flowers resemble bloodshot eyes. An annual, _E. officinalis_ grows to roughly 1 foot tall.

Common doses

Eyebright comes as a lotion or an infusion to drink. Some experts recommend the following doses:

- As an *eye compress,* soak a pad in an infusion of eyebright and apply it to your eyes.
- As an *eyewash,* use 5 to 10 drops of tincture in water.
- As an *infusion,* steep eyebright in boiling water and take orally.

Why people use this herb

- Blepharitis (inflammation of the eyelids and eyelash follicles)
- Conjunctivitis (inflammation of the eye's mucous membrane lining)
- Eye fatigue
- Stye (infection of an eyelid gland)

Side effects

Call your health care practitioner if you experience any of these possible side effects of eyebright:

- confusion
- headache
- itching
- red, swollen eyelid rims
- severe pressure in the eyes with tearing
- sneezing
- stuffy nose
- unusual eye sensitivity to light
- vision problems
- weakness.

Interactions

Combining herbs with certain drugs may alter their action or produce unwanted side effects. Tell your health care practitioner about any prescription or nonprescription drugs you're taking.

Important points to remember

- Don't use this herb to treat an eye condition because it may lead to eye infection.
- Medical experts caution against using eyebright because it may cause cell damage.
- Report vision changes or eye swelling, redness, or discharge to your health care practitioner.
- Wear sunglasses and avoid bright light when using this herb.

WHAT THE RESEARCH SHOWS

Scientific studies don't support the use of eyebright for eye problems. Medical experts caution that herbal preparations generally carry a high risk of infection because they may not be sterile.

Other names for eyebright

Other names for eyebright include meadow eyebright and red eyebright.

No known products containing eyebright are available commercially.

Selected reference

Trovato, A., et al. "In Vitro Cytotoxic Effect of Some Medicinal Plants Containing Flavonoids." *Bollettino Chimico Farmaceutico* 135:263-66, 1996.

False unicorn root

False unicorn root is extracted from the root system of *Chamaelirium luteum* in autumn. Native to North America, the plant usually is harvested from the wild. From 1916 to 1947, false unicorn root was listed as a "uterine tonic" and diuretic in the *U.S. National Formulary*, a list of drugs and their formulas.

Common dose

False unicorn root comes as dried root, chopped root for decoction, tincture, and a component of tablets used for menopause symptoms. Some experts recommend the following dose:

- For *menopause symptoms,* 5 to 10 drops of tincture taken orally four to six times daily. Or, if using a decoction, drink ½ cup twice daily.

Why people use this herb

- Liver disorders
- Menstrual problems
- Uterine problems
- "Weakness" of the genital and urinary tracts

Side effects

Call your health care practitioner if you experience unusual symptoms when using false unicorn root.

Interactions

Combining herbs with certain drugs may alter their action or produce unwanted side effects. Tell your health care practitioner about any prescription or nonprescription drugs you're taking.

Important points to remember

- Don't use false unicorn root if you're pregnant or breast-feeding.
- Be aware that the herb's purported benefits may take months to appear.

WHAT THE RESEARCH SHOWS

Scientific studies don't support the use of false unicorn root for conditions of the uterus and ovaries. The herb hasn't been studied in people.

Other names for false unicorn root

Other names for false unicorn root include blazing star, fairywand, helonias dioica, and starwort.

No known products containing false unicorn root are available commercially.

Selected reference

Grieve, M. *A Modern Herbal*. New York: Barnes & Noble, Inc., 1996.

Fennel

Fennel usually is obtained from the seeds of *Foeniculum vulgare*, from which the essential oil is extracted. Some people also use the plant's root for cooking or other purposes.

Common dose

Fennel comes as volatile oil in water—2% (Sweet Fennel) and 4% (Bitter Fennel). Some experts recommend the following dose:

- For *digestive problems,* 0.1 to 0.6 milliliter of the oil taken daily or 5 to 7 grams of the fruit taken daily.

Side effects

Call your health care practitioner if you experience any of these possible side effects of fennel:

- nausea
- skin irritation from sunlight exposure
- vomiting.

Fennel also may cause:

- pulmonary edema
- seizures
- tumors.

Why people use this herb

- To enhance sex drive
- To increase lactation in breast-feeding women
- To promote childbirth and delivery
- To stimulate menstruation

Interactions

Combining herbs with certain drugs may alter their action or produce unwanted side effects. Tell your health care practitioner about any prescription or nonprescription drugs you're taking.

Important points to remember

- Know that you could be allergic to fennel if you're allergic to members of the same plant family, such as celery, carrots, or mugwort.
- Don't use fennel medicinally if you're pregnant or breast-feeding.
- Stay out of the sun if you experience skin irritation.
- If you grow fennel, don't confuse it with hemlock, which may cause death if eaten.

Other names for fennel

Other names for fennel include aneth fenouil, bitter fennel, carosella, common fennel, fenchel, fenouil, fenouille, finocchio, Florence fennel, funcho, garden fennel, hinojo, large fennel, sweet fennel, and wild fennel.

Products containing fennel are sold under such names as Bitter Fennel and Sweet Fennel.

WHAT THE RESEARCH SHOWS

Because fennel hasn't been studied scientifically, medical experts don't recommend using the herb to treat any medical condition.

Selected references

Fyfe, L., et al. "Inhibition of *Listeria monocytogenes* and *Salmonella enteriditis* by Combinations of Plant Oils and Derivatives of Benzoic Acid: The Development of Synergistic Antimicrobial Combinations," *International Journal of Antimicrobial Agents* 9:195-99, 1997.

Lis-Balchin, M., and Hart, S. "A Preliminary Study of the Effect of Essential Oils on Skeletal and Smooth Muscle In Vitro," *Journal of Ethnopharmacology* 58:183-87, 1997.

Malini, T., et al. "The Effects of *Foeniculum vulgare* Mill Seed Extract on the Genital Organs of Male and Female Rats," *Indian Journal of Physiology and Pharmacology* 29:21, 1985.

Fenugreek

Fenugreek, or *Trigonella foenum-graecum,* is native to countries along the Mediterranean's eastern shore. The plant is cultivated in India, Egypt, Morocco, and, occasionally, England. Herbalists use only the seeds, which grow in sickle-like pods. Each pod contains about 10 to 20 brownish seeds.

Fenugreek smells and tastes like maple syrup. In fact, drinking fenugreek tea may cause the urine to smell like maple syrup. People used to add the herb to liquid medicines to mask the taste.

Common doses

Fenugreek is available as unprocessed seeds, extracts in liquid and spray, seeds in a dried powder or capsules, and a poultice. Some experts recommend the following doses:

- As *seeds,* 1 to 6 grams taken orally three times daily.
- As a *powdered drug,* dissolve 50 grams in ¼ liter of water and apply topically.

Why people use this herb

- Constipation
- Diabetes
- Digestive tract irritation
- Gout
- Indigestion
- Inflamed lymph glands
- Inflamed tissue
- Leg ulcers
- Muscle pain
- Poor appetite
- Tuberculosis
- Wounds

Side effects

Call your health care practitioner if you experience any of these possible side effects of fenugreek:

- bleeding
- bruising
- headache
- low blood sugar symptoms, such as dizziness, hunger, trembling, profuse sweating, and a fast pulse.

Interactions

Combining herbs with certain drugs may alter their action or produce unwanted side effects. Tell your health care practitioner about any prescription or nonprescription drugs you're taking, especially drugs that lower blood sugar.

Don't use fenugreek while taking:

- blood thinners such as Coumadin
- other oral drugs.

Important points to remember

- Don't use fenugreek if you're pregnant because it may stimulate uterine contractions.
- Tell your health care practitioner if you experience unusual bleeding or bruising or if other drugs you're taking seem less effective while using fenugreek.
- If you're diabetic, check your blood sugar carefully until you know how fenugreek affects it.
- Learn about low blood sugar symptoms and management of it.
- If you're using fenugreek to lower your blood sugar or cholesterol level, remember that effective and tested drugs are available.
- Be aware that the Food and Drug Administration says fenugreek is "generally recommended as safe" at concentrations below 0.05%.

WHAT THE RESEARCH SHOWS

Although fenugreek may hold promise in treating diabetes and high cholesterol, researchers haven't tested the herb on people. What's more, existing drugs have proven benefits in these conditions.

Other names for fenugreek

Other names for fenugreek include bird's-foot, Greek hayseed, and trigonella.

Products containing fenugreek are sold under such names as Fenugreek Seed and Fenu-Thyme.

Selected references

Ahsan, S.K., et al. "Effect of *Trigonella foenum-graecum* and *Ammi majus* on Calcium Oxalate Urolithiasis in Rats," *Journal of Ethnopharmacology* 26:249, 1989.

Newall, C.A., et al. *Herbal Medicines. A Guide for Health-Care Professionals.* London: The Pharmaceutical Press, 1996.

Feverfew

A European plant now cultivated in the United States and Canada, feverfew bears yellow flowers and yellow-green leaves from July to October. Usually, the leaves are dried or used fresh in teas and extracts. The most common botanical name for feverfew is *Chrysanthemum parthenium*.

The chemical parthenolide has the highest concentration in the leaves and flowering tops during the summer, before the seeds are set. The parthenolide level drops rapidly thereafter. This may explain the difference in parthenolide levels between brands of feverfew capsules and tablets.

Common doses

Feverfew is available as:

- capsules (pure leaf—380 milligrams; leaf extract—250 milligrams)
- liquid
- tablets (commonly used to make infusions or teas).

Some experts recommend the following doses:

- To *treat migraine,* 543 micrograms of parthenolide taken orally daily.
- To *prevent migraine,* 25 milligrams of freeze-dried leaf extract taken orally daily; 50 milligrams of leaf taken orally daily with food; or 50 to 200 milligrams of above-ground plant parts taken orally daily.

Why people use this herb

- Asthma
- Fever
- Insect bites
- Menstrual problems
- Psoriasis (scaly, raised skin patches)
- Rheumatism
- Stomachache
- Threatened miscarriage
- Toothache
- To prevent migraines

Side effects

Call your health care practitioner if you experience any of these possible side effects of feverfew:

- allergic reaction
- mouth sores
- post-feverfew syndrome—moderate to severe pain with stiff joints and muscles after discontinuing the herb.

Interactions

Combining herbs with certain drugs may alter their action or produce unwanted side effects. Tell your health care practitioner about any prescription or nonprescription drugs you're taking.

Important points to remember

- Don't use feverfew if you're pregnant or breast-feeding.
- Stay alert for an allergic reaction, mouth sores, and skin sores.
- To avoid the discomfort of post-feverfew syndrome, discontinue the herb gradually, not abruptly.

Other names for feverfew

Other names for feverfew include altamisa, bachelors' button, chamomile grande, featherfew, featherfoil, febrifuge plant, midsummer daisy, mutterkraut, nosebleed, Santa Maria, wild chamomile, and wild quinine.

Products containing feverfew are sold under such names as Feverfew, Feverfew Glyc, and Feverfew Power.

Selected references

Groenewegen, W.A., and Heptinstall, S. "A Comparison of the Effects of an Extract of Feverfew and Parthenolide, a Component of Feverfew, on Human Platelet Activity In Vitro," *Journal of Pharmacy and Pharmacology* 43:553-57, 1990.

Heptinstall, S., et al. "Parthenolide Content and Bioactivity of Feverfew (*Tenacetum parthenium* [L.] Schultz-Bip.). Estimation of Commercial and Authenticated Feverfew Products," *Journal of Pharmacy and Pharmacology* 44:391-95, 1992.

Johnson, E.S., et al. "Efficacy of Feverfew as Prophylactic Treatment of Migraine," *BMJ* 291:569-73, 1985.

Murphy, J.J., et al. "Randomised, Double-Blind, Placebo-Controlled Trial of Feverfew in Migraine Prevention," *Lancet* 2:189-92, 1988.

WHAT THE RESEARCH SHOWS

A few studies found feverfew effective in preventing migraines. However, researchers must conduct more studies to establish better dosage guidelines and identify specific drug interactions.

Feverfew may be the only treatment that can prevent migraines in people who don't benefit from standard drug therapy. Although experts disagree on what dose to take, standardized feverfew preparations with doses based on parthenolide content have brought the best results in experiments.

Figwort

A tall, snapdragon-like plant, figwort goes by the botanical names *Scrophularia nodosa* and *S. ningpoensis*. Usually, herbalists use the dried leaves and flowers, although the Chinese also use the root.

Common doses

Figwort comes as a tincture, compress, soak, and wash. Some experts recommend the following doses, although they disagree on how often to take the herb:

- As an *infusion,* 2 to 8 grams of dried herb taken orally.
- As *liquid extract,* 2 to 8 milliliters taken orally.
- As *tincture*, 2 to 4 milliliters taken orally.

Side effects

Call your health care practitioner if you experience any of these possible side effects of figwort:

- diarrhea
- irregular heartbeats
- nausea
- slow pulse
- vomiting.

Figwort also can cause a type of irregular heartbeat called heart block.

Why people use this herb

- Chronic skin conditions
- Digestive disorders
- Eczema (a type of skin inflammation)
- Inflammation
- Itching
- Psoriasis (scaly, raised skin patches)
- To stimulate the heart

Interactions

Combining herbs with certain drugs may alter their action or produce unwanted side effects. Don't use figwort while taking:

- digitalis drugs used to treat heart failure or certain irregular heartbeats
- heart drugs called beta blockers (such as Inderal)
- heart drugs called calcium channel blockers (such as Calan and Procardia).

Important points to remember

- Don't use figwort if you have heart disease.
- Avoid this herb if you're pregnant or breast-feeding.
- Call your health care practitioner if you experience light-headedness, weakness, shortness of breath, or pulse rate changes.

WHAT THE RESEARCH SHOWS

Researchers haven't studied figwort to identify possible benefits and safety risks. However, medical experts warn people—especially those with heart disease—not to use it.

Other names for figwort

Other names for figwort include carpenter's-square, common figwort, rose-noble, scrofula plant, square stalk, stinking christopher, and throatwort.

No known products containing figwort are available commercially.

Selected reference

Inouye, H., et al. "Purgative Activities of Iridoid Glucosides," *Planta Medica* 25:285-88, 1974.

Flax

Herbalists today use soluble fiber made from mature flax seeds *(Linum usitatissimum)* for cures and poultices. The plant has a more varied history, though. Archeologists have traced flax seeds and fibers back 10,000 years, when prehistoric people wove it into clothing. American settlers used flax to make fabrics called linsey-woolsey and linen. Linseed oil, expressed from flaxseeds, is used in paints and varnishes. Researchers currently are looking for more uses for flax.

Flaxseed cakes are used as cattle feed. Flax also has been a source of waxes and waterproofing products. Folklore about the slimy residue of flaxseeds includes tales of people falling into large vats of seeds and drowning.

Why people use this herb

- Atherosclerosis (plaque buildup in the arteries)
- Colon problems caused by laxative abuse
- Constipation
- Diverticulitis (inflammatory disease of the intestine)
- High cholesterol
- Irritable bowel syndrome
- Skin inflammation

Common doses

Flax is available as:

- powder
- capsules
- softgel capsules (1,000 milligrams)
- oil.

Some experts recommend the following doses:

- For *all internal uses,* 1 to 2 tablespoons of oil or mature seeds taken orally in two or three equal daily doses.
- For *topical use,* 30 to 50 grams of flax meal applied as a hot, moist poultice or compress, as needed.

Side effects

Call your health care practitioner if you experience any of these possible side effects of flax:

- diarrhea
- intestinal gas
- nausea.

All plant parts contain harmful substances. Stay alert for overdose symptoms—shortness of breath, rapid breathing, weakness, and poor muscle coordination progressing to paralysis and seizures.

Interactions

Combining herbs with certain drugs may alter their action or produce unwanted side effects. Don't use flax when taking:

- laxatives
- oral drugs
- stool softeners.

Important points to remember

- Don't use flax if you're pregnant or breast-feeding because it may harm the fetus or cause miscarriage.
- Don't use flax if you have prostate cancer or constipation.
- Never eat immature flaxseeds.
- Keep flax away from children and pets.
- If you use flax, drink plenty of fluids to minimize intestinal gas.
- Tell your health care practitioner if other drugs you're taking seem less effective.
- Refrigerate flaxseed oil to prevent its breakdown.
- Remember that proven cholesterol-lowering treatments are available. Flax, on the other hand, is unproven.

Other names for flax

Other names for flax include flaxseed, linseed, lint bells, and linum.

Products containing flax are sold under such names as Barlean's Flax Oil, Barlean's Vita-Flax, and Flaxseed.

WHAT THE RESEARCH SHOWS

Use of flax as a source of omega-3 fatty acids and to treat inflammatory diseases deserves more investigation. But most of the herb's uses aren't proven. Also, researchers haven't analyzed the herb's potentially harmful chemicals for long-term effects.

Selected references

Bierenbaum, M.L., et al. "Reducing Atherogenic Risk in Hyperlipidemic Humans with Flax Seed Supplementation: A Preliminary Report," *Journal of the American College of Nutrition* 12:501, 1993.

Dobelis, I.N., ed. *Magic and Medicine of Plants*. Pleasantville, N.Y.: The Reader's Digest Association, Inc., 1986.

Suttman, U., et al. "Weight Gain and Increased Concentrations of Receptor Proteins for Tumor Necrosis Factor After Patients with Symptomatic HIV Infection Received Fortified Nutrition Support," *Journal of the American Dietetic Association* 96:565-69, 1996.

Thompson, L.U., et al. "Variability in Anticancer Lignan Levels in Flaxseed," *Nutrition and Cancer* 27:26-30, 1997.

Fumitory

Fumitory comes from *Fumaria officinalis,* a plant that's native to Europe and North Africa and also grows in Asia, North America, and Australia. The leaves and flowers are used to produce herbal preparations.

Why people use this herb

- Constipation
- Fluid retention
- Heart problems related to coronary blood flow disorders
- Gallbladder and liver diseases
- Skin eruptions

Common doses

Fumitory comes as dried herb, a liquid extract, and a tincture. Some experts recommend the following doses:

- As *dried herb,* 2 to 4 grams taken orally three times daily.
- As a *tea,* 2 to 4 grams of the dried herb steeped in hot water and taken orally three times daily.
- As *liquid extract* (1:1 in 25% alcohol), 2 to 4 milliliters taken orally three times daily.
- As a *tincture* (1:5 in 45% alcohol), 1 to 4 milliliters taken orally three times daily.

Side effects

Call your health care practitioner if you experience any of these possible side effects of fumitory:

- low blood pressure symptoms, such as dizziness and weakness
- sedation
- slow pulse.

At high or toxic doses, fumitory can cause seizures. The herb also can increase pressure within the eye, causing glaucoma (which may lead to vision loss).

Interactions

Combining herbs with certain drugs may alter their action or produce unwanted side effects. Don't use fumitory while taking:

- drugs used to lower blood pressure
- heart drugs called beta blockers (such as Inderal)

- heart drugs called calcium channel blockers (such as Calan and Procardia)
- Lanoxin and other drugs that slow the heart rate.

Important points to remember

- Don't take fumitory if you're pregnant or breast-feeding.
- Avoid this herb if you have glaucoma or an illness that makes you prone to seizures.
- If you use fumitory, report light-headedness, weakness, shortness of breath, or pulse rate changes to your health care practitioner.

> **WHAT THE RESEARCH SHOWS**
>
> Researchers haven't tested fumitory on people, so its safety and usefulness remain unproven.

Other names for fumitory

Other names for fumitory include earth smoke, hedge fumitory, and wax dolls.

No known products containing fumitory are available commercially.

Selected references

Gorbunov, N.P., et al. "Pharmacological Correction of Myocardial Ischemia and Arrhythmias in Reversible Coronary Blood Flow Disorders and Experimental Myocardial Infarct in Dogs," *Kardiologiia* 20:84-87, 1980.

Hentschel, C., et al. "*Fumaria officinalis* (fumitory)—Clinical Applications," *Fortschritte der Medizin* 113:291-92, 1995.

Preininger, V. "The Pharmacology and Toxicology of the Papaveraceae Alkaloids," in *The Alkaloids XV*. Edited by Manske, R.H.F. London: Academic Press, 1975.

Galangal

Galangal is the dried root of *Alpinia officinarum,* a native plant of eastern and southeastern Asia. The herb is botanically and chemically related to ginger.

Why people use this herb

- Fungal infections
- Rheumatism (painful joints and muscles)

Common dose

Galangal comes as a dried root. Some experts recommend the following dose:

- 1 gram taken orally.

Side effects

Call your health care practitioner if you experience diarrhea, nausea, or vomiting when using galangal.

Interactions

Combining herbs with certain drugs may alter their action or produce unwanted side effects. Tell your health care practitioner about any prescription or nonprescription drugs you're taking.

Important points to remember

- Don't take galangal if you are pregnant, suspect you're pregnant, or are planning to become pregnant.
- Avoid this herb if you have a chronic digestive tract disease.
- Consult your health care practitioner before taking this herb.

Other names for galangal

Other names for galangal include *Alpinia officinarum*, China root, Chinese ginger, colic root, East Indian root, galanga, kaempferia galanga, and rhizoma galangae.

No known products containing galangal are available commercially.

WHAT THE RESEARCH SHOWS

Galangal hasn't been thoroughly tested as a treatment for rheumatic disorders or fungal infections. Until more research is done on its benefits and potential risks, medical experts won't recommend it.

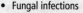

Selected references

Janssen, A., and Scheffer, J.J. "Acetoxychavicol Acetate, an Antifungal Component of *Alpinia galanga*," *Planta Medica* 51:507, 1985.

Morita, H., and Itokawa, H. "Cytotoxic and Antifungal Diterpenes from the Seeds of *Alpinia galanga*," *Planta Medica* 54:117, 1988.

Qureshi, S., et al. "Toxicity Studies on *Alpinia galanga* and *Curucuma longa*," *Planta Medica* 58:124, 1992.

Galanthamine

Galanthamine comes from the bulbs of a spring flower called common snowdrop *(Galanthus nivalis)*. The herb also is available as a chemical synthetic. A 1983 journal report suggested that Odysseus used the common snowdrop as an antidote to Circe's poisonous drugs in Homer's epic poem *The Odyssey*. If true, this would have been the first recorded use of galanthamine to reverse drug intoxication.

Common dose

Galanthamine comes as:

- coated tablets (5 and 10 milligrams)
- ampules (5 milligrams).

Some experts recommend the following dose:

- For *Alzheimer's disease,* initially 5 milligrams taken three times daily, then increased to 30 to 40 milligrams daily.

Why people use this herb

- Alzheimer's disease
- Myasthenia gravis
- Post-polio paralysis
- To reverse neuromuscular blockade (in which drugs are given to stop unwanted muscle movement)

Side effects

Call your health care practitioner if you experience any of these possible side effects of galanthamine:

- abdominal pain
- agitation
- diarrhea
- dizziness
- light-headedness
- nausea
- sleep disturbances
- vomiting.

Interactions

Combining herbs with certain drugs may alter their action or produce unwanted side effects. Don't use galanthamine while taking drugs to relieve depression called MAO inhibitors (such as Marplan and Nardil) or if you've been exposed to organophosphate fertilizers (used in gardens and on farms).

Important points to remember

- Don't use this herb if you have a slow pulse, extremely poor muscle tone, recent heart attack, epilepsy, unusually increased muscle activity, Parkinson's disease, diabetic crisis, or a blockage of the respiratory, digestive, or urinary tract.

- Consult your health care practitioner before taking galanthamine.
- Remember that established treatments are available for the conditions for which galanthamine is used.
- Avoid hazardous activities until you know how the herb affects you.

WHAT THE RESEARCH SHOWS

Some research supports galanthamine's use in Alzheimer's disease, and scientists can predict its effects and safety. More studies are needed to define its exact role in treating this condition. Meanwhile, medical experts emphasize that proven drugs are available, so using galanthamine is questionable.

Other names for galanthamine

Other names for galanthamine include galanthamine hydrobromide.

A product containing galanthamine is sold as Nivalin.

Selected references

Bores, G.M., et al. "Pharmacological Evaluation of Novel Alzheimer's Disease Therapeutics: Acetylcholinesterase Inhibitors Related to Galanthamine," *Journal of Pharmacology and Experimental Therapeutics* 277:728-38, 1996.

Dal-Bianco, P., et al. "Galanthamine Treatment in Alzheimer's Disease," *Journal of Neural Transmission Supplementum* 33:59-63, 1991.

Kewitz, H., et al. "Galanthamine, a Selective Nontoxic Acetylcholinesterase Inhibitor Is Significantly Superior Over Placebo in the Treatment of SDAT," *Neuropsychopharmacology* 10 (Suppl Part 2):130, 1994.

Plaitakis, A., and Duvoisin, R.C. "Homerís Moly Identified as *Galanthus nivalis* L.: Physiologic Antidote to Stramonium Poisoning," *Clinical Neuropharmacology* 6:1-5, 1983.

Garlic

Garlic, or *Allium sativum*, is among the most extensively researched and described medicinal plants. Usually, the fresh garlic bulb is dried, crushed into a powder, and compressed to produce a tablet. However, raw whole cloves of garlic provide similar effects.

Fresh and powdered garlic are popular food seasonings. The Food and Drug Administration considers the newer garlic oil, extract, and oleoresin products to be safe. You also can find garlic products promoted as "odorless" or "deodorized." These products may lack medicinal value because garlic's beneficial properties seem to be in allin, the chemical that gives garlic its distinctive odor.

Why people use this herb

- Asthma
- Athlete's foot
- Bacterial infections
- Constipation
- Diabetes
- Fungal infections
- Heavy-metal poisoning
- High blood pressure
- High cholesterol
- To ward off evil spirits
- Wounds

Common dose

Garlic comes as:

- tablets (garlic extract; 100, 320, 400, and 600 milligrams)
- tablets (allicin total potential; 2 and 5 milligrams)
- dried powder (400 to 1,200 milligrams)
- fresh bulb (2 to 5 grams)
- antiseptic oil
- fresh extract
- powdered, freeze-dried garlic powder
- garlic oil (essential oil).

Some experts recommend the following dose:

- To *lower cholesterol,* 600 to 900 milligrams taken orally daily; or an average of 4 grams (fresh garlic) or 8 milligrams (garlic oil) taken orally daily.

Side effects

Call your health care practitioner if you experience any of these possible side effects of garlic:

- dizziness
- irritation of the mouth, throat, and stomach
- nausea
- skin rash or other allergic reactions (such as asthma, rash, or chest tightness)

- sweating
- vomiting.

Chronic garlic use or excessive garlic doses may lead to decreased production of hemoglobin (a compound in red blood cells) and a resulting change in red blood cells.

This herb also can cause garlic odor and hypothyroidism (underactive thyroid).

Interactions

Combining herbs with certain drugs may alter their action or produce unwanted side effects. Tell your health care practitioner about any prescription or nonprescription drugs you're taking, especially:

- antiplatelet agents such as Persantine (garlic may increase their effects)
- blood thinners such as Coumadin (don't use garlic while taking these drugs).

Important points to remember

- Don't use garlic if you're sensitive to the herb or other members of the Liliaceae family.
- Avoid garlic if you have digestive tract problems, such as peptic ulcers or reflux disease.
- Don't take garlic if you're pregnant because it may stimulate the uterus.
- Remember that widely available cholesterol-lowering drugs have been proven safe and are more effective than garlic in reducing cholesterol.
- If you take garlic along with a drug to stop bleeding, report bleeding gums, easy bruising, tarry stools, and tiny red or purple spots on your skin.
- Report side effects to your health care practitioner promptly.

Other names for garlic

Other names for garlic include ail, allium, camphor of the poor, dasuan, knoblaunch, la-suan, nectar of the gods, poor-man's-treacle, rustic treacle, and stinking rose.

Products containing garlic are sold under such names as Garlic, Garlic-Power, Garlique, Kwai, Kyolic, Odorless Garlic Tablets, One a Day Garlic, and Sapec.

WHAT THE RESEARCH SHOWS

Although garlic is one of the oldest and most revered herbal remedies, research is still incomplete. Scientists don't know if garlic really helps to lower cholesterol or reduce deaths from coronary artery disease. Other potential garlic uses, such as to lower blood pressure, calm an upset stomach, or treat AIDS, haven't been fully evaluated.

Selected references

Berthold, H.K., et al. "Effect of a Garlic Oil Preparation on Serum Lipoproteins and Cholesterol Metabolism. A Randomized Controlled Trial," *JAMA* 279:1900-02, 1998.

Isaacsohn, J.L., et al. "Garlic Powder and Plasma Lipids and Lipoproteins. A Multicenter, Randomized, Placebo-Controlled Trial," *JAMA* 158:1189-94, 1998.

Jain, A.K., et al. "Can Garlic Reduce Levels of Serum Lipids? A Controlled Clinical Study," *American Journal of Medicine* 94:632, 1993.

McMahon, F.G., et al. "Can Garlic Lower Blood Pressure? A Pilot Study," *Pharmacotherapy* 13:406, 1993.

Gentian

Gentian has been used for centuries to treat mild to moderate digestive disorders. It has been approved for use in foods, cosmetics, and some antismoking products. During the summer, the herb is extracted from the roots and rhizome (underground stem) of 2- to 5-year-old *Gentiana lutea* L. plants. Another variety, called stemless gentian, is extracted from the entire plant of *Gentiana acaulis* L. Both types are approved food additives and used to flavor vermouth.

The herb's bitterness depends on how fast it's dried: the faster, the more bitter. Although no longer listed in the *United States Pharmacopoeia* (a legal compendium of drug standards), gentian can still be found in similar European compendiums, including the *British Pharmacopoeia*.

Common dose

Gentian comes as stemless gentian tea or extract, compound gentian infusion BP 1993, and concentrated compound gentian infusion BP 1993. Some experts recommend the following dose:

- As a *tea,* boil ½ teaspoon of coarsely powdered gentian root in ½ cup (120 milliliters) of water for 5 minutes. Strain the mixture and take 30 minutes before meals, up to four times daily. If the tea is strong and bitter, reduce the amount of herb.

Why people use this herb

- Heartburn
- Intestinal gas
- Irritable bowel syndrome
- Malaria
- Sharp intestinal pains
- To help curb smoking
- To stimulate the appetite

Side effects

Call your health care practitioner if you experience any of these possible side effects of gentian:

- headache
- nausea and vomiting (with overdose).

Interactions

Combining herbs with certain drugs may alter their action or produce unwanted side effects. Tell your health care practitioner about any prescription or nonprescription drugs you're taking.

Important points to remember

- Don't use gentian if you have high blood pressure.
- Avoid this herb if you're pregnant.

- Know that the best way to take gentian is by brewing a tea.
- Don't collect the herb in the wild because nonflowering *G. lutea* may be hard to distinguish from the poisonous white hellebore.

Other names for gentian

Other names for gentian include bitter root, feltwort, gall weed, pale gentian, stemless gentian, and yellow gentian.

A product containing gentian is sold as Angostura Bitters, a commercial cocktail flavoring containing an alcoholic extract of stemless gentian.

WHAT THE RESEARCH SHOWS

In one limited clinical trial, a small amount of gentian extract was effective in stimulating the appetite and aiding digestion. The herb's other uses haven't been tested or documented.

Selected references

Garnier, R., et al. "Acute Dietary Poisoning by White Hellebore (*Veratrum album*). Clinical and Analytical Data. A Propos of 5 Cases," *Annales de Medecine Interne* 136:125-28, 1985.

"Gentian," in *The Lawrence Review of Natural Products*. Edited by Dombek, C. St. Louis, Mo.: Facts and Comparisons, 1993.

Osol, A., ed. *The United States Dispensatory*, 27th ed. Philadelphia: Lippincott, Williams & Wilkins, 1973.

Ginger

Ginger, *Zingiber officinale*, is a perennial that grows in India, Jamaica, and China. The plant produces green-purple flowers resembling orchids. Most herbalists value the root more than the plant's other parts.

Common dose

Ginger comes as:

- root (530 milligrams)
- extract (250 milligrams)
- liquid, powder, and capsules (100 and 465 milligrams)
- chewable tablets (67.5 milligrams)
- tea.

The dose depends on the reason for taking ginger. For *nausea,* people in one study took 500 to 1,000 milligrams of powdered ginger orally or 1,000 milligrams of fresh ginger root orally.

Why people use this herb

- Arthritis
- As an antioxidant
- Bacterial infections
- Digestive problems
- Motion sickness
- Muscle pain and swelling
- Nausea
- Parasites
- To stimulate the heart and blood vessels
- Tumors

Side effects

Call your health care practitioner if you experience an irregular heartbeat from ginger overdose. Ginger also may cause slowing of the nervous system, leading to drowsiness and sedation.

Interactions

Combining herbs with certain drugs may alter their action or produce unwanted side effects. Tell your health care practitioner about any prescription or nonprescription drugs you're taking, especially blood thinners such as Coumadin.

Important points to remember

- Don't use ginger if you're pregnant.
- If you're taking blood thinners, check with your health care practitioner before using ginger because the herb may affect how fast your blood clots.

Other names for ginger

Another name for ginger is zingiber.

Products containing ginger are sold under such names as Cayenne Ginger, Gingerall, Ginger Peppermint Combo, Ginger Power, and Ginger Trips.

> **WHAT THE RESEARCH SHOWS**
>
> Although some studies support the therapeutic use of ginger, others don't. Scientists need to conduct more long-term studies of the herb's ability to stop vomiting, reduce swelling, and soothe the digestive tract.

Selected references

Bone, M., et al. "The Effect of Ginger Root on Post-operative Nausea and Vomiting After Major Gynecological Surgery," *Anesthesia* 45:669-71, 1990.

Fisher-Rasmussen, W., et al. "Ginger Treatment of Hyperemesis Gravidarum," *European Journal of Obstetrics, Gynecology, and Reproductive Biology* 38:19-24, 1990.

Mowrey, D.B., and Clayson, D.E. "Motion Sickness, Ginger and Psychophysics," *Lancet* 1:655-57, 1982.

Phillips, S., et al. "*Zingiber officinale* (Ginger)—An Antiemetic for Day Case Surgery," *Anesthesia* 48:715-7, 1993.

Srivastava, K.C., and Mustafa, T. "Ginger (*Zingiber officinale*) in Rheumatism and Musculoskeletal Disorders," *Medical Hypotheses* 39:342-48, 1992.

Ginkgo

A staple of Chinese herbal medicine for thousands of years, ginkgo biloba has aroused worldwide interest lately as a possible memory booster for people with Alzheimer's disease. In one study, some patients with Alzheimer's disease who took the herb showed modest memory improvements.

Ginkgo biloba extract comes from the fan-shaped leaves of the *Ginkgo biloba* tree (also called the maidenhair or kew tree). This ornamental deciduous tree dates back more than 200 million years. The extract is among the leading prescriptions in France and Germany, whose governments declared it an effective treatment for poor leg circulation in 1996 and recently approved it for treating dementia.

In the United States, ginkgo is available only as a dietary supplement. In 1997, it was the third-best-selling herbal product in U.S. health food stores. The seeds, reportedly edible, should be boiled first to remove toxic components.

Why people use this herb

- Asthma
- Blood vessel disease
- Dementia
- Hearing loss
- Impotence caused by use of Prozac and similar antidepressants
- Inner-ear disorders
- Irregular heartbeats
- Poor memory
- Premenstrual syndrome
- Senile macular degeneration (a type of vision loss related to aging)
- To enhance mental alertness and brain function

Common doses

Ginkgo biloba extract comes as:

- capsules (30, 40, 60, 120, 260, and 420 milligrams)
- tablets (30, 40, 60, 120, 260, and 420 milligrams)
- under-the-tongue spray (15 or 40 milligrams per spray)
- concentrated alcoholic extract of fresh leaf (80-milligram capsules).

Some experts recommend the following doses:

- For *dementia,* 120 to 240 milligrams daily taken orally in two or three equal doses.
- For *poor leg circulation, vertigo,* or *ringing in the ears (tinnitus),* 120 to 160 milligrams daily taken orally in two or three equal doses.

Side effects

Contact your health care practitioner if you experience any of these possible side effects of ginkgo:

- digestive upset, such as diarrhea, gas, nausea, or vomiting
- headache
- seizures
- skin irritation from contact with ginkgo biloba extract or the ginkgo fruit (the fruit pulp and seed coats contain substances related to those found in poison ivy)
- unusual bleeding or bruising.

Interactions

Combining herbs with certain drugs may alter their action or produce unwanted side effects. Tell your health care practitioner about any prescription or nonprescription drugs you're taking, especially blood thinners, such as Coumadin or aspirin.

Important points to remember

- Don't take ginkgo if you're allergic to ginkgo preparations.
- Avoid ginkgo if you're pregnant.
- Don't give this herb to children. Keep the seeds out of children's reach. A child who eats more than 50 gingko seeds may experience seizures.
- Call your health care practitioner at once if you experience excessive or unusual bleeding or bruising.
- Avoid contact with the fruit pulp or seed coats because of possible skin irritation.
- Know that using a crude dried leaf preparation or preparing the leaves yourself isn't recommended because of insufficient active ingredients.
- Be aware that applying potent ginkgo preparations to the skin or mucus membranes may cause irritation or blistering.

Other names for ginkgo

Other names for ginkgo include EGB 761, GBE, GBE 24, GBX, ginkgo biloba, ginkogink, LI 1370, rokan, sophium, tanakan, teboffortan, and tebonin.

Products containing ginkgo are sold under such names as Bioginkgo 24/6, Bioginkgo 27/7, Gincosan, Ginexin Remind, Ginkai, Ginkgoba, Ginkgo Go!, Ginkgold, Ginkgo Phytosome, Ginkgo Power, and Ginkoba.

WHAT THE RESEARCH SHOWS

Scientists believe ginkgo has a mild to moderate effect on blood vessels. Unfortunately, many of the clinical trials for this herb were flawed. Although preliminary studies suggest ginkgo may play a part in treating dementia and peripheral blood vessel disease, researchers haven't defined its specific role.

Selected references

Kanowski, S., et al. "Proof of Efficacy of the Ginkgo Biloba Special Extract EGB 761 in Outpatients Suffering from Mild to Moderate Primary Degenerative Dementia of the Alzheimer Type of Multi-Infarct Dementia," *Pharmacopsychiatry* 29:47-56, 1996.

Kobuchi, H., et al. "Ginkgo biloba Extract (EGB 761): Inhibitory Effect of Nitric Oxide Production in the Macrophage Cell Line RAW 264.7," *Biochemical Pharmacology* 53:897-903, 1997.

LeBars, P.L., et al. "A Placebo Controlled, Double-Blind Randomized Trial of an Extract of Ginkgo Biloba for Dementia," *JAMA* 278:1327-32, 1997.

Princemail, J., et al. "Superoxide Anion Scavenging Effect and Superoxide Dismutase Activity of Ginkgo biloba Extract," *Experientia* 45:708-12, 1989.

Ginseng

Used medicinally by Asians for 2,000 years, ginseng is now used regularly by about 6 million Americans. It comes from a plant called *Panax quinquefolius*. Ginseng has become so popular that the plant, once abundant in eastern North America, is threatened by aggressive harvesting for commercial sales.

***P. quinquefolius* is most commonly sought after for its root. However, other characteristics and root shapes make the plant more valuable. Ideal plants are at least 6 years old.**

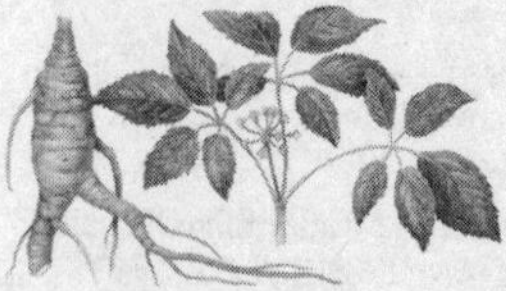

The Asian, Korean, or Japanese variety (*P. ginseng),* which grows in the wild, usually undergoes treatment such as drying or curing before it's sold. The American variety is less processed and therefore less valued.

Why people use this herb

- As an aphrodisiac
- As a sedative
- As a sleep aid
- Depression
- Diabetes
- Fluid retention
- High blood fat levels
- Impaired mental function
- Liver problems
- Overactive thymus gland
- To aid healing
- To boost the appetite
- To decrease mood swings
- To enhance physical and mental performance
- To heighten resistance to stress
- To improve mental concentration
- To increase stamina
- To soothe irritated or inflamed internal tissues or organs

Common doses

Ginseng comes as:

- capsules (100, 250, and 500 milligrams)
- tea bags containing 1,500 milligrams of ginseng root
- root extract (2 ounces in alcohol base)
- root powder (1 ounce, 4 ounces)
- oil
- unprocessed root (available in bulk by the pound).

Some experts recommend the following doses:

- 0.5 to 2 grams of dry ginseng root daily, or 200 to 600 milligrams of ginseng extract daily in one or two equal doses.
- For *improved well-being in frail elderly people,* 0.4 to 0.8 gram of root daily taken orally on a continual basis.

Side effects

Call your health care practitioner if you experience any of these possible side effects of ginseng:

- breast pain
- chest pain
- diarrhea
- headache
- high blood pressure symptoms, such as headache and blurred vision
- impotence
- insomnia
- itching
- nausea
- nervousness
- nosebleed
- rapid pulse
- skin eruptions (with ginseng abuse)
- vaginal bleeding
- vomiting.

Ginseng abuse syndrome may result from taking large ginseng doses at the same time with other stimulants, such as tea and coffee. Symptoms include diarrhea, high blood pressure, restlessness, insomnia, skin eruptions, depression, poor appetite, an unusual sense of well-being, and swelling. (However, experts disagree as to whether this syndrome really exists.)

Interactions

Combining herbs with certain drugs may alter their action or produce unwanted side effects. Tell your health care practitioner about any prescription or nonprescription drugs you're taking, especially:

- drugs that lower blood sugar, such as insulin, Amaryl, DiaBeta, Diabinese, Glucophage, Glucotrol, Precose, or Rezulin
- drugs to relieve depression called MAO inhibitors, such as Marplan and Nardil (don't use ginseng when taking these).

Important points to remember

- Consult your health care practitioner before using ginseng if you have heart or blood vessel disease, high or low blood pressure, or diabetes; if you're taking steroids; or if you have any other serious medical condition.

- Don't use the herb if you're pregnant or breast-feeding.
- Don't continue to take ginseng for a long time.

Other names for ginseng

Other names for ginseng include American ginseng, Asiatic ginseng, Chinese ginseng, five-fingers, g115, Japanese ginseng, jintsam, Korean ginseng, ninjin, Oriental ginseng, schinsent, seng and sang, tartar root, and Western ginseng.

Products containing ginseng are sold under such names as Bio Star, Cimexon, Gincosan, Ginsana, Ginsatonic, and Neo Ginsana.

WHAT THE RESEARCH SHOWS

Although ginseng seems to have therapeutic promise, researchers must test it more extensively to identify its advantages, side effects, and interactions with other drugs. In the meantime, medical experts caution that ingesting the plant carries certain risks, despite centuries of use.

Selected references

D'Angelo, L., et al. "A Double-Blind, Placebo-Controlled Clinical Study on the Effect of a Standardized Ginseng Extract on Psychomotor Performance in Healthy Volunteers," *Journal of Ethnopharmacology* 16:15-22, 1986.

Sotaniemi, E., et al. "Ginseng Therapy in Non-Insulin-Dependent Diabetic Patients," *Diabetes Care* 18:1373-75, 1995.

Wesnes, K.A., et al. "The Cognitive, Subjective, and Physical Effects of a Ginkgo Biloba/Panax Ginseng Combination in Healthy Volunteers with Neurasthenic Complaints," *Psychopharmacology Bulletin* 33:677-83, 1997.

Ginseng, Siberian

For medicinal use, Siberian ginseng is extracted from the root and root bark of *Eleutherococcus senticosus*. This plant belongs to the same family as panax or Chinese ginseng (Araliaceae). Some people describe Siberian ginseng as pungent, bittersweet, and warming.

Common dose

Siberian ginseng is available as powders, teas, tinctures, capsules, tablets, and oils. Some experts recommend the following dose:

- 500 to 2,000 milligrams taken orally daily.

Side effects

Call your health care practitioner if you experience any of these possible side effects of Siberian ginseng:

- diarrhea
- difficulty concentrating
- dizziness
- high blood pressure symptoms, such as headache and blurred vision
- increased agitation
- insomnia
- nervousness
- skin eruptions
- an unusual sense of well-being
- vaginal bleeding.

Why people use this herb

- Inflammation
- Insomnia caused by prolonged anxiety
- To improve exercise tolerance
- To increase stamina and stress tolerance
- To regulate blood pressure
- To stimulate the immune and circulatory systems

Interactions

Combining herbs with certain drugs may alter their action or produce unwanted side effects. Tell your health care practitioner about any prescription or nonprescription drugs you're taking, especially Lanoxin, a drug that slows the heart rate. Don't use Siberian ginseng when taking:

- hexobarbital
- vitamins B_1, B_2, and C.

Important points to remember

- Don't give this herb to children.
- Don't use Siberian ginseng if you're allergic to other ginsengs or to ingredients in the preparation.
- Know that most experts caution against using this herb for more than 3 weeks.

- Buy from a respected source. Siberian ginseng products aren't uniform in content and some contain less expensive plant products.
- Be aware that Siberian ginseng may be sold as a combination product with panax or Chinese ginseng, which may lead to side effects from that herb.
- Call your health care practitioner if you experience insomnia, nervousness, an unusual sense of well-being, skin eruptions, diarrhea, agitation, or abnormal menstrual bleeding.
- If you're diabetic, check your blood sugar carefully because Siberian ginseng may cause your blood sugar to drop too low.

Other names for Siberian ginseng

Other names for Siberian ginseng include *Acanthopanax senticosus*, devil's shrub, *Eleutherococcus senticosus, Hedera senticosa*, shigoka, and touch-me-not.

Products containing Siberian ginseng are sold under such names as Activex 40 Plus, Gincosan, Ginkovit, Ginseng Complex, Minadex Mix Ginseng, Panax Complex, Siberian Ginseng, and Vigoran.

Selected references

Bohn, B., et al. "Flow-Cytometric Studies with *Eleutherococcus senticosus* Extract as an Immunomodulatory Agent," *Arzneimittel-Forschung* 37:1193-96, 1987.

Dowling, E.A., et al. "Effect of *Eleutherococcus senticosus* on Submaximal and Maximal Exercise Performance," *Medicine and Science in Sports Exercise* 28:482-89, 1996.

Lewis, W.H., et al. "No Adaptogenic Response of Mice to Ginseng and Eleutherococcus Infusions," *Journal of Ethnopharmacology* 8:209-14, 1983.

Martinez, B., et al. "The Physiological Effects of Aralia, Panax and *Eleutherococcus senticosus* on Exercised Rats," *Japanese Journal of Pharmacology* 35:79-85, 1984.

WHAT THE RESEARCH SHOWS

Studies show that Siberian ginseng doesn't live up to claims that it improves stamina, boosts energy, and reduces stress. However, scientists believe the herb may help boost the immune system and protect against radioactivity. Larger studies are needed to explore these effects.

Research doesn't substantiate other claims for Siberian ginseng. What's more, no long-term studies have been done, so the herb's effects over time remain unknown. Thus, medical experts don't recommend using Siberian ginseng for more than 3 weeks.

Glucomannan

Tubers of the *Amorphophallus konjac* plant typically are harvested to yield glucomannan (also called konjac mannan). After reports of side effects, Australia stopped distribution of the tablet form of glucomannan in the mid-1980s.

Why people use this herb

- Constipation
- To aid weight loss
- To lower cholesterol
- To reduce blood sugar

Common doses

Glucomannan is available as:

- powder
- capsules
- tablets (600 milligrams).

Some experts recommend the following doses:

- To *lower cholesterol,* 3.9 grams taken orally daily for 4 weeks, stopped for 2 weeks, and then resumed for another 4 weeks. Or 100 milliliters of a 1% solution taken orally daily.
- To *reduce blood sugar levels,* 3.6 to 7.2 grams taken orally daily for 90 days.
- To *lose weight,* 1.5 grams taken orally twice daily for 8 weeks.

Side effects

Call your health care practitioner if you experience any of these possible side effects of glucomannan:

- diarrhea
- intestinal gas
- loose stools.

Glucomannan also may cause:

- blockage of the esophagus and lower digestive tract
- low blood sugar
- perforation of the esophagus. (Several people have had to undergo surgery to have the herb removed under general anesthesia.)

Interactions

Combining herbs with certain drugs may alter their action or produce unwanted side effects. Tell your health care practitioner about any prescription or nonprescription drugs you're taking, especially:

- drugs that lower blood sugar, such as insulin, Amaryl, DiaBeta, Diabinese, Glucophage, Glucotrol, Precose, or Rezulin

- drugs that reduce cholesterol, such as Baycol, Colestid, Lescol, Lipitor, Mevacor, Pravachol, Questran, or Zocor.

Important points to remember

- Don't use this herb if you're pregnant or breast-feeding.
- If you have diabetes and use glucomannan, be aware that you may need to reduce your insulin dosage. Check for changes in your blood sugar level.
- Take glucomannan a few hours apart from any other drug because it may alter drug absorption.
- Know that large doses can have a laxative effect.
- Report symptoms of esophageal or digestive tract blockage, such as constipation, a swollen or tense abdomen, appetite loss, abdominal pain, or nausea.
- Watch for the herb's effects on your bowel habits.
- Tell your health care practitioner if other drugs you're using seem less effective.
- Keep in mind that long-term effects of this herb aren't well known.

Other names for glucomannan

Other names for glucomannan include konjac and konjac mannan.

A product containing glucomannan is sold as Glucomannan.

WHAT THE RESEARCH SHOWS

Scientific studies show that glucomannan lowers cholesterol. However, modern drugs such as Mevacor, Pravachol, and Zocor do this more effectively. Nonetheless, scientists think the herb eventually may prove to be a valuable secondary treatment for high cholesterol. They must study it further to identify side effects.

Studies also show that glucomannan can lower blood sugar—but again, larger studies are needed. Information on the herb's effectiveness as a weight-loss aid are conflicting and hard to interpret.

Selected references

Doi, K., et al. "Treatment of Diabetes with Glucomannan (Konjac Mannan)," *Lancet* 1:987-88, 1979.

Fujiwara, S., et al. "Effect of Konjac Mannan on Intestinal Microbial Metabolism in Mice Bearing Human Flora and in Conventional F344 Rats," *Food and Chemical Toxicology* 29:601, 1991.

Huang, C.Y., et al. "Effect of Konjac Food on Blood Glucose Level in Patients With Diabetes," *Biomedical and Environmental Sciences* 3:123-31, 1990.

Kiriyama, S., et al. "Hypocholesterolemic Effect of Polysaccharides and Polysaccharide-Rich Foodstuffs in Cholesterol-Fed Rats," *Journal of Nutrition* 97:382, 1969.

Goat's rue

Goat's rue refers to the dried stalks, leaves, and flowers of *Galega officinalis* of the Leguminosae family. This perennial grows in damp meadows and river banks from Central Europe to Iran. Some sheep that grazed on it died, making researchers suspect that some chemicals it contains (galegine and paragalegine alkaloids) are poisonous.

Why people use this herb

- Diabetes
- Fever
- Plague
- Snakebites
- To increase breast milk flow

Common dose

Goat's rue comes as dried leaves. Some experts recommend the following dose:

- As *fluid extract,* mix 1 cup of boiling water with 1 teaspoon of dried leaves. Let it steep for 10 to 15 minutes and take orally twice daily.

Side effects

Call your health care practitioner if you experience headache, jitteriness, or weakness when using goat's rue.

Interactions

Combining herbs with certain drugs may alter their action or produce unwanted side effects. Tell your health care practitioner about any prescription or nonprescription drugs you're taking.

Important points to remember

- Avoid this herb if you're pregnant or breast-feeding unless a health care professional approves.
- Don't give goat's rue extract to infants or children.
- Discontinue goat's rue and contact your health care practitioner if you experience side effects.
- Be aware that this herb may turn your saliva yellowish green.

Other names for goat's rue

Other names for goat's rue include French honeysuckle and French lilac.

A product containing goat's rue is sold as Goat's Rue.

WHAT THE RESEARCH SHOWS

Medical experts don't recommend goat's rue for diabetics even though it was used to treat diabetes before oral diabetes drugs were developed. Also arguing against tradition, they caution breast-feeding women not to use the herb because effects on infants aren't known.

Selected references

Gresham, A.C.J., and Booth, K. "Poisoning of Sheep by Goat's Rue," *Veterinary Record* 129:197-98, 1991.

Remington, J.P., et al., eds. *The Dispensatory of the United States of America,* 20th ed. Philadelphia: Lippincott, Williams & Wilkins, 1918.

Goldenrod

In folklore, herbalists used goldenrod to mask the bitterness of medicines and to promote wound healing. As early as the mid-13th century, they used it to cure bladder stones. In the 1890s, the pharmaceutical company Parke-Davis marketed a fluid extract of goldenrod.

Active ingredients of goldenrod come from the flowers and leaves of *Solidago virgaurea*, a member of the Asteraceae family. The roots also are valued by herbalists.

More than 130 species of goldenrod grow wild all over the United States. Although the plant can cause allergic reactions, it's also mistakenly blamed for some reactions to ragweed, which blooms at the same time. Paradoxically, goldenrod has been used to treat allergy.

Why people use this herb

- Bladder stones
- Chronic diarrhea
- Exhaustion and fatigue
- Fluid retention
- General inflammation
- Kidney and intestinal inflammation
- Sore throat
- Spasms
- To induce abortion
- To prevent or treat kidney stones
- Urinary tract inflammation
- Wounds

Common doses

Goldenrod comes as an extract made with water or alcohol. Some experts recommend the following doses:

- As a *decoction*, mix 1 to 2 teaspoons (3 to 5 grams) of dried herb with 8 ounces of water. Boil the mixture, let stand for 2 minutes, and then strain and drink.
- As an *infusion*, mix 30 grams of the herb with 300 milliliters of water. Boil, cool, and strain as above. Take one tablespoon three or four times daily.

Side effects

Call your health care practitioner if you experience allergic reactions, such as asthma or hay fever (from extra pollens carried by goldenrod). This herb also can cause:

- poisoning, leading to weight loss, leg and abdominal swelling, digestive tract bleeding, and an enlarged spleen (related to parasites, fungus, and rust in the plant)

- vomiting, rapid breathing, and death (from ingesting the dried plant).

Interactions

Combining herbs with certain drugs may alter their action or produce unwanted side effects. Tell your health care practitioner about any prescription or nonprescription drugs you're taking.

Important points to remember

- Don't use goldenrod if you're pregnant or suspect you may be pregnant. The herb may cause miscarriage.
- Avoid this herb if you have allergies.
- Remember that goldenrod hasn't been proven effective in treating fluid retention, high blood pressure, or kidney stones.
- Don't delay seeking medical attention for high blood pressure or flank pain.

WHAT THE RESEARCH SHOWS

Scientists haven't documented the clinical effects of goldenrod in people. However, the German E Commission, which oversees herb use in Germany, has endorsed goldenrod when used to eliminate excess fluid, ease inflammation, and relieve muscle spasms.

Other names for goldenrod

Other names for goldenrod include Aaron's rod, blue mountain tea, sweet goldenrod, and woundwort.

No known products containing goldenrod are available commercially.

Selected references

Ghazaly, M., et al. "Study of the Anti-Inflammatory Activity of *Populus tremula, Solidago virgaurea* and *Fraxinus excelsior*," *Arzneimittel-Forschung* 42:333-36, 1992.

Tyler, V. *Herbs of Choice: The Therapeutic Use of Phytomedicinals*. New York: Pharmaceutical Products Press, Haworth Press Inc., 1994.

Wunderlin, R.P., and Lockey, R.F. "Questions and Answers," *JAMA* 260:3064-65, 1988.

Goldenseal

Goldenseal has been part of American folk medicine since Native Americans used the root to treat disease, paint their faces and skin, and dye their garments. The plant was so popular with pioneers and settlers that by the early 1900s, it had been harvested nearly into extinction. To save it, the U.S. Department of Agriculture published flyers promoting its cultivation. However, goldenseal is still scarce enough to bring farmers a high price for their crop.

More recently, the herb has been used—mistakenly—to hide illicit drug use in urine tests of people and racehorses. The bogus drug cover-up idea came from a fictional story of using the plant to conceal opiate ingestion.

Why people use this herb

- Appetite loss
- As an eye wash
- Cancer
- Conjunctivitis (inflammation of the eye's inner lining)
- Constipation
- Digestive disorders
- Ear discharge
- Fluid retention
- Gastritis (inflammation of the stomach lining)
- Inflammation
- Itching
- Menstrual pain
- Mouth sores
- Peptic ulcer
- Ringing, buzzing, roaring, or clicking in the ear (tinnitus)
- To clean wounds
- To control bleeding after childbirth
- Tuberculosis

The main ingredient in goldenseal products is the root of a bright yellow plant called *Hydrastis canadensis*. The herb gets its name from the golden-yellow scars, shaped like old-fashioned wax letter seals, that develop when a stem breaks off.

Common doses

Goldenseal comes as:

- capsules (250, 350, 400, 404, 470, 500, 535, and 540 milligrams)
- tablets (250, 350, 400, 404, 470, 500, 535, and 540 milligrams)
- ethanol and water extract
- dried ground root powder
- tincture
- tea.

Some experts recommend the following doses:

- As *ethanol and water extract,* 250 milligrams taken orally three times daily.
- As *dried root,* 0.5 to 1 gram of dried root ingested three times daily.

Side effects

Call your health care practitioner if you experience any of these possible side effects of goldenseal:

- diarrhea
- mouth sores
- nausea
- nervous system depression, causing excessive sleepiness or sedation, slow breathing, and reduced mental alertness
- numbness, prickling, or tingling in the arms and legs
- paralysis (with high doses)
- seizures
- skin inflammation
- slow pulse
- stomach cramping and pain
- vomiting.

Goldenseal also can cause:

- dangerous heart rhythms called asystole and heart block
- decreased white blood cells
- respiratory depression.

Taking large doses can cause death or overdose symptoms such as stomach upset, nervousness, depression, exaggerated reflexes, seizures, respiratory paralysis, and heart and blood vessel collapse.

Interactions

Combining herbs with certain drugs may alter their action or produce unwanted side effects. Don't use goldenseal when taking:

- blood thinners such as Coumadin
- drugs that depress the nervous system, such as alcohol and benzodiazepines
- drugs that lower blood pressure
- heart drugs called beta blockers, such as Inderal
- heart drugs called calcium channel blockers, such as Calan and Procardia
- Lanoxin.

Important points to remember

- Don't use goldenseal if you have heart or blood vessel disease, especially high blood pressure, heart failure, or irregular heartbeats.
- Don't use this herb if you're pregnant.

- Avoid driving and other hazardous activities until you know how goldenseal affects you.
- Be aware that most medical experts believe this herb could be toxic.

Other names for goldenseal

Other names for goldenseal include eye balm, eye root, goldsiegel, ground raspberry, Indian dye, Indian turmeric, jaundice root, yellow paint, yellow puccoon, and yellow root.

Products containing goldenseal are sold under such names as Golden Seal Extract, Golden Seal Extract 4:1, Golden Seal Power, Golden Seal Root, Nu Veg Golden Seal Root, and Nu Veg Golden Seal Herb.

WHAT THE RESEARCH SHOWS

Goldenseal's therapeutic effects haven't been adequately studied. Scientists believe the herb carries a significant toxicity risk, and even some herbalists don't endorse it for any disorder. Nonetheless, goldenseal and its components have promising properties, which need to be put through comprehensive, controlled studies.

Selected references

Preininger, V. "The Pharmacology and Toxicology of the Papaveraceae Alkaloids," in *The Alkaloids*, vol 15. Edited by Maske, R.H.F., and Holmes, H.L. New York: Academic Press, 1975.

Swanston-Flatt, S.K., et al. "Evaluation of Traditional Plant Treatments for Diabetes: Studies in Streptozotocin Diabetic Mice," *Acta Diabetologica Latina* 26:51-55, 1989.

Gossypol

Gossypol comes from seeds, roots, and stems of the cotton plant, *Gossypium hirsutum*, which grows throughout the southern United States. Seeds of the *Gossypium* species vary widely in their gossypol content.

In other uses, gossypol is processed out of commercial cottonseed oil. Some people consider gossypol-free cottonseed flour a low-cost, abundant protein source. The flour is used in baked goods, snacks, and livestock feed. Chinese studies conducted in the 1950s first identified gossypol as an antifertility drug.

Common dose

Gossypol is available as an extract. Some experts recommend the following dose:

- As a *male contraceptive,* 20 milligrams taken daily for 60 to 90 days until the sperm count drops to a threshold of 4 million sperm per milliliter; then maintenance doses of approximately 50 milligrams weekly.

Why people use this herb

- To aid labor and delivery
- To prevent pregnancy
- To promote normal menstruation

Side effects

Call your health care practitioner if you experience any of these possible side effects of gossypol:

- diarrhea
- hair discoloration
- rapid muscle fatigue, muscle weakness, and paralysis.

This herb also can cause:

- circulation problems
- heart failure
- kidney damage (with high doses)
- malnutrition
- too little potassium in the blood.

Cotton seeds are potentially toxic and may cause death. Domesticated animals have been poisoned by feed containing cotton seeds.

Interactions

Combining herbs with certain drugs may alter their action or produce unwanted side effects. Don't use gossypol while taking diuretics such as Lasix or drugs that can cause kidney damage.

Important points to remember

- Don't use gossypol if you're pregnant or breast-feeding.
- If you have kidney disease, check with your health care practitioner before using this herb.
- If you're thinking of using gossypol for birth control, know that proven contraceptive alternatives are available.
- Be aware that long-term gossypol use may cause permanent infertility.

WHAT THE RESEARCH SHOWS

Gossypol shows promise as an oral contraceptive for men and as a vaginal spermicide in women. However, the oral preparation may cause permanent sterility. Scientists must conduct more studies to determine an appropriate dose and administration route and to track side effects. Women who are considering using gossypol as a vaginal spermicide should keep in mind that researchers haven't thoroughly studied the herb's safety and effectiveness.

Other names for gossypol

Other names for gossypol include American upland cotton, common cotton, cotton, upland cotton, and wild cotton.

No known products containing gossypol are available commercially.

Selected references

Liang, X.S., et al. "Developing Gossypol Derivatives with Enhanced Antitumor Activity," *Investigational New Drugs* 13:3:181-86, 1995.

Ratsula, K., et al. "Vaginal Contraception with Gossypol: A Clinical Study," *Contraception* 27:571, 1983.

Royer, R.E., et al. "Comparison of the Antiviral Activities of 3-azido-3-deoxythymidine and Gossylic Iminolactone Against Clinical Isolates of HIV-1," *Pharmacology Research* 31:49-52, 1995.

Shidaifat, F., et al. "Gossypol Arrests Human Benign Prostatic Hyperplastic Cell Growth at G_0/G_1 Phase of the Cell Cycle," *Anticancer Research* 17:1003-09, 1997.

Gotu kola

Sri Lankans believed gotu kola promoted longevity because they saw elephants chewing leaves of the plant it comes from, *Centella asiatica*. This plant that originated in Madagascar now grows in India, Sri Lanka, and South Africa. Some people mistakenly consider gotu kola a stimulant because they confuse its name with kola nuts, koa, or cola—all of which contain caffeine.

Why people use this herb

- Birth control
- Cancer
- Chronic liver disorders
- High blood pressure
- Leg swelling
- Mental fatigue
- Psoriasis (scaly, raised skin patches)
- Rheumatism
- Skin ulcers
- To reduce scars
- Varicose veins
- Wounds

Common dose

Gotu kola comes as:

- capsules (221, 250, 435, 439, 441, and 450 milligrams)
- tinctures
- creams.

Some experts recommend the following dose:

- 0.6 gram of the dried leaf taken three times daily, or a 450-milligram capsule taken once daily.

Side effects

Call your health care practitioner if you experience any of these possible side effects of gotu kola:

- burning sensation (with topical use)
- drowsiness
- itching
- sedation (with large doses)
- skin inflammation.

Gotu kola also can cause high cholesterol and high blood sugar.

Interactions

Combining herbs with certain drugs may alter their action or produce unwanted side effects. Don't use gotu kola while taking:

- drugs that lower blood sugar, such as insulin, Amaryl, DiaBeta, Diabinese, Glucophage, Glucotrol, Precose, or Rezulin
- drugs that reduce cholesterol, such as Baycol, Colestid, Lescol, Lipitor, Mevacor, Pravachol, Questran, or Zocor.

Important points to remember

- Don't take gotu kola if you're pregnant or breast-feeding.
- Avoid this herb if you have a history of skin inflammation.
- Know that some gotu kola ingredients have depressed animals' nervous systems, causing slow breathing and reduced alertness.
- Be aware that the herb may cause a burning sensation when applied to the skin.
- Keep in mind that most health care practitioners recommend using tested contraceptives for birth control instead of gotu kola.
- If you use gotu kola, tell your health care practitioner about any planned or suspected pregnancy.
- Don't use this herb for more than 6 weeks at a time.

WHAT THE RESEARCH SHOWS

Gotu kola seems to have promise in aiding wound healing and treating certain skin disorders. But more research in people must be done to determine if it's safe and to define its long-term effects.

Other names for gotu kola

Other names for gotu kola include centella, hydrocotyle, Indian pennywort, Indian water navelwort, talepetrako, and TECA (titrated extract of *Centella asiatica*).

Products containing gotu kola are sold under such names as Gingko/Gotu Kola Supreme, Gotu Kola Gold Extract, and Gotu Kola Herb.

Selected references

Bosse, J-P., et al. "Clinical Study of a New Antikeloid Agent," *Annals of Plastic Surgery* 3:13-21, 1979.

Natarajan, S., et al. "Effect of Topical Hydrocotyle *Asiatica* in Psoriasis," *Indian Journal of Dermatology* 18:82-85, 1973.

Pointel, J.P., et al. "Titrated Extract of *Centella asiatica* (TECA) in the Treatment of Venous Insufficiency of the Lower Limbs," *Angiology* 38:46-50, 1987.

Grapeseed; Pinebark

Grapeseed is extracted from the seeds of *Vitis vinifera*. Pinebark comes from the bark of the European coastal pine tree, *Pinus maritima* or *P. nigra*. Both herbs contain proanthocyanidins, a chemical marketed as Pycnogenol.

Why people use this herb

- Cancer
- Inflammation
- Poor circulation
- Varicose veins

Common dose

Grapeseed and pinebark come as:

- tablets (25 to 300 milligrams)
- capsules (25 to 300 milligrams).

Some experts recommend the following dose:

- As *tablets* or *capsules,* 25 to 300 milligrams taken orally daily for up to 3 weeks, followed by a maintenance dose of 40 to 80 milligrams taken orally daily.

Side effects

Call your health care practitioner if you experience unusual symptoms when taking grapeseed or pinebark.

Interactions

Combining herbs with certain drugs may alter their action or produce unwanted side effects. Tell your health care practitioner about any prescription or nonprescription drugs you're taking.

Important point to remember

- If you have a circulation problem, call your health care practitioner immediately if your hands or feet become cold or pale while you're using grapeseed or pinebark.

Other names for grapeseed and pinebark

Other names for grapeseed include *Vitis coignetiae* and *Vitis vinifera.* Other names for pinebark include muskat, *Pinus maritima*, and *Pinus nigra.*

Products containing grapeseed and pinebark are sold under such names as Mega Juice, NutraPack, and Pycnogenol.

WHAT THE RESEARCH SHOWS

Although grapeseed extract is popular in Europe, it hasn't been studied adequately in people for medical experts to recommend its medicinal use. The same holds true for pinebark.

Selected reference

Covington, T.R., ed. *The Handbook of Nonprescription Drugs*. Washington, D.C.: American Pharmaceutical Association, 1996.

Green tea

The Chinese have used green tea leaf and its extracts for thousands of years. Green tea is prepared from the steamed and dried leaves of *Camellia sinensis*, a large shrub with evergreen leaves native to eastern Asia. Unlike black tea, green tea comes from leaves that have been withered, rolled, fermented, and dried. Because of the curing process, green tea's properties closely resemble those of the fresh leaf.

About 30 countries grow tea. Next to water, tea is the most frequently consumed beverage worldwide. It's considered one of the safest beverages because the water is boiled.

Common doses

Green tea comes as teas and capsules. Studies suggest possible effects from drinking 6 to 10 cups daily or taking 3 capsules of green tea extract.

Side effects

Call your health care practitioner if you experience asthma or other allergic reactions when using green tea.

Why people use this herb

- As a stimulant
- Fluid retention
- To fight infection
- To prevent atherosclerosis (plaque buildup in the arteries)
- To prevent cancer
- To prevent dental cavities
- To prevent high cholesterol

Interactions

Combining herbs with certain drugs may alter their action or produce unwanted side effects. Tell your health care practitioner about any prescription or nonprescription drugs you're taking, especially Adriamycin, a cancer chemotherapy drug.

Also, don't use green tea if you drink milk. Milk may reduce the tea's antioxidant effects.

Important points to remember

- Don't drink green tea if you've experienced "green tea asthma" or other tea allergies.
- Remember that green tea contains caffeine.

Other names for green tea

Other names for green tea include matsu-cha and tea.

Green tea is sold by various manufacturers.

WHAT THE RESEARCH SHOWS

Asian research suggests green tea has potential in preventing cancer and atherosclerosis (hardening of the arteries). These reports and the herb's widespread use over thousands of years suggest green tea is relatively safe. Still, researchers must conduct more studies on people to investigate claims that the herb can prevent cancer.

Selected references

Ahmad, N., et al. "Green Tea Constituent Epigallocatechin-3-gallate and Induction of Apoptosis and Cell Cycle Arrest in Human Carcinoma Cells," *Journal of the National Cancer Institute* 89:1881-86, 1997.

Hibasami, H., et al. "Induction of Apoptosis in Human Stomach Cancer Cells by Green Tea Catechins," *Oncology Research* 5:527-29, 1998.

Imai, K., et al. "Cancer-Preventative Effects of Drinking Green Tea Among a Japanese Population," *Preventive Medicine* 26:769-75, 1997.

Yang, T.T., and Koo, M.W. "Hypocholesterolemic Effect of Chinese Tea," *Pharmacology Research* 35:505-12, 1997.

Ground ivy

In parts of England, people refer to ground ivy as alehoof because it was used in medieval times to flavor and clarify ale. Ground ivy comes from *Glechoma hederacea*. This plant with kidney-shaped leaves and purple-blue flowers is one of Great Britain's most common wild plants.

Common dose

Ground ivy is available as an infusion or a tincture made from leaves and flowers. Some experts recommend the following dose:

- 14 to 28 grains prepared as a fluid extract taken orally three times daily.

Why people use this herb

- Diarrhea
- Digestive disorders
- Ear, nose, and throat disorders
- Nasal allergies
- To reduce phlegm in allergies, bronchitis, hay fever, and sinus inflammation

Side effects

Call your health care practitioner if you experience unusual symptoms when using ground ivy.

Interactions

Combining herbs with certain drugs may alter their action or produce unwanted side effects. Tell your health care practitioner about any prescription or nonprescription drugs you're taking.

Important points to remember

- Be aware that little information supports therapeutic use of ground ivy.
- Remember that tested drugs are available to treat the complaints for which some people use this herb.

WHAT THE RESEARCH SHOWS

Ground ivy seems to be well tolerated, and research suggests it's safe in low doses. But more studies must be done on people before medical experts can recommend this herb.

Other names for ground ivy

Other names for ground ivy include alehoof, cat's-foot, creeping Charlie, *Glechoma hederacea*, haymaids, and hedgemaids.

No known products containing ground ivy are available commercially.

Selected reference

Grieve, M. *A Modern Herbal*. New York: Barnes & Noble, Inc., 1996.

Guarana

Various cultures have used guarana, partly for its high caffeine content (which exceeds that of coffee or tea). In the 19th century, the French popularized a guarana drink. Others have mixed it with alcohol for a unique beverage.

Guarana is a dried paste made from the crushed seeds of *Paullinia cupana* (also called *P. sorbilis*), a woody vine or shrub native to Brazil and the Amazon basin. During guarana processing, small particles of the seed husk remain in the final product, giving the herb a bitter, chocolate-like taste. The plant is cultivated widely because of its market value as a caffeine source and an ingredient in soft drinks, nutritional supplements, and medicinal products.

In Central and South America, parts of the guarana plant are used to poison fish. The Amazon Indians crush the seeds and combine them with cassava flour to make a paste. They roll the paste into sticks, dry them, and grind them on a bone inside the tongue of a large fish or on a stone, making a powder that they mix with water and drink.

Many South Americans still consume guarana daily. The herb is a main ingredient in several herbal weight-loss products and soft drinks. The Food and Drug Administration considers guarana a safe food additive.

Common doses

Guarana provides the caffeine in many soft drinks, including Josta, Dark Dog Lemon, and Guts, and is an ingredient in nutritional supplements, candies, and chewing gum. Guarana also comes as teas, alcoholic extracts, elixirs, capsules, and tablets of various strengths.

The dose depends on the product and batch. Single doses commonly contain 200 to 800 milligrams of guarana. Daily intake of guarana shouldn't exceed 3 grams of guarana powder or its equivalent taken orally.

Why people use this herb

- As an aphrodisiac
- Diarrhea
- Itchy skin
- To aid weight loss and body-building
- To curb the appetite
- To prevent dysentery
- To prevent malaria
- To stimulate the nervous system

A maximum daily caffeine intake of approximately 250 milligrams (3 to 5 grams of guarana) has been suggested for nonpregnant adults. Daily doses of up to 1 gram of caffeine have been used without side effects, although some people have withdrawal symptoms when they stop using the herb.

Side effects

Call your health care practitioner if you experience any of these possible side effects of guarana:

- increased urine formation and excretion
- insomnia.

Excessively large guarana doses can cause:

- agitation
- anxiety
- diarrhea
- headache
- irregular heartbeats
- irritability
- nausea
- rapid pulse
- seizures
- tremors
- vomiting.

Taking more than 1 gram of caffeine may cause toxic symptoms, such as agitation, irritability, tremors, irregular heartbeats, and seizures. An oral dose of 5 to 10 grams of caffeine may cause death.

Abrupt withdrawal after regular daily consumption of guarana may lead to anxiety, headache, and irritability.

Interactions

Combining herbs with certain drugs may alter their action or produce unwanted side effects. Tell your health care practitioner about any prescription or nonprescription drugs you're taking, especially:

- Adenocard
- Antabuse
- antibiotics called fluoroquinolones, such as Cipro, Floxin, Neg-Gram, or Noroxin
- birth-control pills

- heart drugs called beta blockers, such as Inderal
- iron (wait 1 hour after meals before taking guarana)
- Lithobid
- Neo-Synephrine
- Tagamet
- Theo-Dur (don't use guarana when taking this drug)
- tobacco.

Important points to remember

- Don't use this herb if you're pregnant or breast-feeding.
- Avoid guarana or consult your health care practitioner about using it if you have heart or blood vessel disease, stomach ulcers, chronic headache, or diabetes.
- If you're taking Theo-Dur, seek medical advice before using guarana.
- If you have irregular heartbeats, know that guarana and other caffeine-containing products can worsen your symptoms.
- Reduce your guarana intake if you have symptoms of excessive caffeine use—tremors, irritability, headache, and palpitations.
- Be aware that guarana may worsen high blood pressure, hiatal hernia, acid reflux disease, and peptic ulcer disease.

Other names for guarana

Other names for guarana include Brazilian cocoa, guarana gum, guarana paste, and zoom.

Products containing guarana are sold under such names as Guarana Plus, Guarana Rush, Happy Motion, Superguarana, and Zoom.

WHAT THE RESEARCH SHOWS

Although guarana is probably as safe as coffee, tea, and colas, it may provide unwanted extra caffeine. Many products, including weight-loss and body-building supplements, contain guarana as an unlisted ingredient. Guarana elixirs may contain more caffeine than powdered guarana products.

Selected references

Bempong, D.K., and Houghton, P.J. "Dissolution and Absorption of Caffeine from Guarana," *Journal of Pharmacy and Pharmacology* 44:769-71,1992.

DeSimone, E.M., and Scott, D.M. "Nicotine and Caffeine Abuse," in *Applied Therapeutics: The Clinical Use of Drugs*, 6th ed. Edited by Young, L.Y., and Koda-Kimble, M.A. Vancouver, Wash.: Applied Therapeutics, 1995.

Henman, A.R. "Guarana (*Paullinia cupana* var. *sorbilis*): Ecological and Social Perspectives on an Economic Plant of the Central Amazon Basin," *Journal of Ethnopharmacology* 6:311-38, 1982.

Gum arabic

Gum arabic comes from the *Acacia senegal* tree. Its quality varies with growing conditions and gum extraction method (beetle attack, extreme drought, or tapping). In 1977, the United States imported more than 11,000 tons of gum arabic—most of it used to add body and texture to processed food products. The herb also is added to nonprescription and prescription drugs as a preservative.

Common doses

Gum arabic comes as:

- powder (20 grams per package)
- gum
- syrup (10% gum arabic).

Some experts recommend the following doses:

- To *reduce cholesterol,* 9.7 to 50 grams of powdered gum arabic taken daily.
- To *reduce dental plaque,* chew gum arabic.

Why people use this herb

- Burns
- Common cold
- Cough
- Dental plaque
- Diarrhea
- Dysentery
- Gonorrhea
- High cholesterol
- Infections
- Inflammation
- Kidney failure
- Leprosy
- Sore nipples
- Sore throat

Side effects

Call your health care practitioner if you experience any of these possible side effects of gum arabic:

- bloating
- intestinal gas
- more frequent bowel movements
- skin inflammation from exposure to gum arabic preservative.

Intravenous injection of gum arabic may cause kidney and liver damage.

Interactions

Combining herbs with certain drugs may alter their action or produce unwanted side effects. Tell your health care practitioner about any prescription or nonprescription drugs you're taking.

Important points to remember

- Don't use this herb if you're pregnant or breast-feeding.
- Don't neglect regular dental care in favor of this herb.
- Keep in mind that direct contact with gum arabic can cause skin inflammation.

Other names for gum arabic

Other names for gum arabic include *acacia*, acacia arabica gum, acacia gum, *Acacia senegal*, acacia ver, Egyptian thorn, *Gummae mimosae*, and senega.

No known products containing gum arabic are available commercially.

WHAT THE RESEARCH SHOWS

Research suggests gum arabic may be useful as a chewing gum to fight dental plaque, but more studies are needed to determine its appropriate dose and role in treatment. People prone to allergic reactions should use this herb cautiously. Studies have found that gum arabic isn't effective in reducing high cholesterol.

Selected references

Bliss, D.Z., et al. "Supplementation with Gum Arabic Fiber Increases Fecal Nitrogen Excretion and Lowers Serum Urea Nitrogen Concentration in Chronic Renal Failure Patients Consuming a Low-Protein Diet," *American Journal of Clinical Nutrition* 63:392-98, 1996.

Clark, D.T., et al. "The Effects of *Acacia arabica* Gum on the In Vitro Growth and Protease Activities of Periodontopathic Bacteria," *Journal of Clinical Periodontology* 20:238-43, 1993.

Haskell, W.L., et al. "Role of Water-Soluble Dietary Fiber in the Management of Elevated Plasma Cholesterol in Healthy Subjects," *American Journal of Cardiology* 69:433-39, 1992.

Jensen, C.D., et al. "The Effect of Acacia Gum and a Water-Soluble Dietary Fiber Mixture on Blood Lipids in Humans," *Journal of the American College of Nutrition* 12:147-54, 1993.

Hawthorn

Used in Europe to treat heart failure, hawthorn comes from the berries, flowers, or leaves of *Crataegus* species (commonly *C. laevigata, C. monogyna,* or *C. folium).* More than 300 *Crataegus* species exist worldwide in the temperate parts of North America, Asia, and Europe.

Germany's Federal Institute for Drugs and Medical Devices has approved hawthorn leaf and flower extracts for treating mild heart failure. It hasn't approved hawthorn berry extracts because their effectiveness hasn't been proven. Still, some companies advertise berry preparations as a nutritional supplement to strengthen and invigorate the heart and circulatory system.

Why people use this herb

- Arteriosclerosis (hardening of the arteries)
- Buerger's disease (a condition of blocked, inflamed blood vessels)
- Heart failure
- High blood pressure
- Rapid pulse

Common dose

Hawthorn comes as:
- biologic extracts (4 milligrams per milliliter of vitexin-2-0-rhamnoside)
- berry capsules (510 milligrams)
- extended-release capsules (300 milligrams)
- berry leaves (80 milligrams).

Some experts recommend the following dose:
- 160 to 900 milligrams of a standardized extract containing 2.2% flavonoids or 18.75% oligomeric procyanidines, taken orally in two or three doses.

Side effects

Call your health care practitioner if you experience any of these possible side effects of hawthorn:
- fatigue
- nausea
- sweating.

High doses of hawthorn can cause low blood pressure, irregular heartbeats, and sedation.

Interactions

Combining herbs with certain drugs may alter their action or produce unwanted side effects. Tell your health care practitioner about any prescription or nonprescription drugs you're taking, especially:

- alcohol and other drugs that slow the nervous system, such as cold and allergy drugs, sedatives, tranquilizers, and narcotic pain relievers
- drugs that lower blood pressure
- heart drugs called cardiac glycosides, such as Lanoxin
- nitrates.

Important points to remember

- Don't take hawthorn if you're allergic to other members of the Rosaceae plant family.
- Avoid this herb if you're pregnant or breast-feeding.
- Use hawthorn only under medical supervision.
- Avoid driving and other hazardous activities until you know how the herb affects you.
- If hawthorn doesn't stop your symptoms after 6 weeks, consult your health care practitioner.
- Seek emergency medical treatment if you experience shortness of breath or chest pain that spreads to your arm, lower jaw, or upper abdomen.

Other names for hawthorn

Other names for hawthorn include crataegus extract, li 132, may, maybush, and whitethorn.

Products containing hawthorn are sold under such names as Cardiplant, Hawthorne Berry, Hawthorne Formula, Hawthorne Heart, Hawthorne Phytosome, and Hawthorne Power.

WHAT THE RESEARCH SHOWS

Several recent foreign studies suggest hawthorn may be effective in treating mild to moderate heart failure. However, long-term studies showing prolonged survival for heart patients haven't been done. Experts recommend focusing future studies on determining whether hawthorn improves patients' heart failure symptoms, quality of life, and survival.

Selected references

Hanak, T.H., and Bruckel, M.H. "Behandlung Von Leichten Stabilen Formen der Angina Pectoris mit Crataegutt Novo," *Therapiewoche* 33:4331-33, 1983.

Lianda, L., et al. "Studies on Hawthorn and its Active Principle. I. Effect on Myocardial Ischemia and Hemodynamics in Dogs," *Journal of Traditional Chinese Medicine* 4:283-88, 1984.

Schmidt, U., et al. "Efficacy of the Hawthorn (*Crataegus*) Preparation LI 132 in 78 Patients with Chronic Congestive Heart Failure Defined as NYHA Functional Class II," *Phytomedicine* 1:17-24, 1994.

Hellebore, American

American (green) hellebore comes from the dried roots of the perennial called *Veratrum viride*. Related species include *V. album* (white hellebore), *V. californicum, V. officinale* (Cevadilla), and *V. japonicum*.

Veratrine, a chemically similar Mexican herb, was listed in some national drug directories 100 years ago. Still used as a soothing lotion and to kill parasites, it has been linked to birth defects in grazing animals who eat it in the wild. However, in preliminary test tube research, veracintine, a hellebore derivative, killed leukemia cells.

Why people use this herb

- Epilepsy
- High blood pressure, including acute high blood pressure episodes and toxemia of pregnancy (eclampsia)
- Kidney disease
- Peritonitis (inflammation of the abdominal cavity's lining)
- Pneumonia
- Pulmonary edema
- Seizures
- Sharp stabbing pains
- To induce vomiting

Common dose

Hellebore comes as fluid extract, tincture, and powder. Some experts recommend the following dose:

- For *heart "sedation,"* 1 to 3 minims of fluid extract taken orally every 2 to 3 hours until the pulse rate slows. Or 1 to 2 grains of powder or 10 to 30 minims of tincture taken orally. Intravenous doses are unknown.

Side effects

Call your health care practitioner if you experience any of these possible side effects of hellebore:

- abdominal pain and bloating
- bad taste in the mouth
- fainting
- irregular heartbeats
- labored breathing
- muscle weakness
- nausea
- numbness, prickling, or tingling in the arms and legs
- pale skin
- salivation

- seizures
- shortness of breath
- slow pulse
- sneezing (if inhaled)
- sweating
- vomiting.

American hellebore also can cause:
- high or low blood pressure
- increased muscle tone
- paralyzed eye muscles.

All parts of the plant are poisonous if eaten. However, most cases haven't been fatal because of the rapid vomiting that occurs and poor intestinal absorption of the plant's chemicals. Overdose symptoms include:
- abdominal pain
- burning throat
- diarrhea
- fainting
- loss of consciousness
- nausea
- paralysis
- reduced vision
- shortness of breath
- spasms.

Interactions
Combining herbs with certain drugs may alter their action or produce unwanted side effects. Tell your health care practitioner about any prescription or nonprescription drugs you're taking.

WHAT THE RESEARCH SHOWS

Although once used extensively to treat high blood pressure, American hellebore and its derivatives are no longer preferred for this purpose because of their dangerous effects. What's more, we now have safer and more tolerable high blood pressure drugs.

Important points to remember

- Don't use American hellebore if you have high blood pressure or another type of heart or blood vessel disease.
- Avoid this herb if you're pregnant.
- Know that American hellebore is considered highly toxic.

Other names for American hellebore

Other names for American hellebore include false hellebore, green hellebore, Indian poke, itch-weed, and swamp hellebore.

A product containing hellebore is sold as Cryptenamine.

Selected references

Anon. "Veratrum Alkaloids in the Therapy of Myasthenia Gravis," *Canadian Medical Association Journal* 96:1534-35, 1967.

Arena, J.M., and Drew, R.H., eds. *Poisoning: Toxicology, Symptoms, Treatments,* 5th ed. Springfield, Ill: Charles C. Thomas Publisher, 1986.

Fogh, A., et al. "Veratrum Alkaloids in Sneezing-Powder: A Potential Danger," *Journal of Toxicology. Clinical Toxicology* 20:175-79, 1983.

Hellebore, black

An ornamental garden plant, black hellebore also is used as a homeopathic herb. "Hellebore" comes from the Greek *elein* (to injure) and *bora* (food)—which describes the herb's toxic nature. Active components of black hellebore come from the dried root of the perennial called *Helleborus niger*. The herb sometimes is called Christmas rose because it produces white flowers in the winter.

Common dose

Black hellebore comes as a fluid or solid extract and a powdered root. Some experts recommend the following dose:

- As a *laxative,* 1 to 10 drops of fluid extract taken orally, 1 to 2 grains of solid extract taken orally, or 10 to 20 grains of powder taken orally.

Side effects

Call your health care practitioner if you experience any of these possible side effects of black hellebore:

- abdominal pain
- burning sensation in the mouth
- diarrhea
- eye irritation
- irregular heartbeats
- low blood pressure symptoms, such as dizziness and weakness
- nasal irritation
- salivation
- shortness of breath
- skin inflammation
- slow heartbeat
- sneezing
- vomiting.

Using contaminated black hellebore can cause respiratory failure.

Why people use this herb

- Anxiety
- As an anesthetic
- Cancer
- Constipation
- Epilepsy
- Fluid retention
- Heart failure
- Intestinal worms
- Lack of menstruation
- Meningitis (inflammation of the lining of the brain and spinal cord)
- Psychoses and other mental disorders
- Skin sores
- Sleeping sickness
- To induce abortion
- Toxemia of pregnancy (eclampsia)

Interactions

Combining herbs with certain drugs may alter their action or produce unwanted

side effects. Tell your health care practitioner about any prescription or nonprescription drugs you're taking.

Important points to remember

- Avoid black hellebore if you're pregnant or breast-feeding.
- Know that this herb is considered toxic. Eating the plant may burn your mouth and throat and cause salivation, vomiting, diarrhea, and abdominal pain.

WHAT THE RESEARCH SHOWS

Although some cancer patients apparently use black hellebore to help stimulate their immune systems, researchers haven't tested this effect on people. In fact, medical experts warn against using this herb because it's a poison with no proven benefits.

Other names for black hellebore

Other names for black hellebore include christe herbe, Christmas rose, Easter rose, and melampode.

No known products containing black hellebore are available commercially.

Selected references

Bussing, A., and Schweizer, K. "Effects of Phytopreparation from *Helleborus niger* on Immunocompetent Cells In Vitro," *Journal of Ethnopharmacology* 59:139-46, 1998.

Erickson, R.O. "Protoanemonin as a Mitotic Inhibitor," *Science* 108:533, 1948.

Holden, M., et al. "Range of Antibiotic Activity of Protoanemonin," *Proceedings of the Society for Experimental Biology and Medicine* 66:54, 1947.

Hops

Used by some people as a sedative-hypnotic, hops are most familiar as a beer ingredient, where they add a bitter taste and act as a preservative. The hops plant, *Humulus lupulus*, belongs to the Cannabaceae family (the same genus as *Cannabis sativa/indica*, or marijuana). A perennial vine, it grows up to 20 feet (6 meters) long. Fruits or flowers appear in conelike leafy bracts at the base of the flower stalk, and typically measure 2 to 4 inches (5 to 10 cm) long.

Common dose

Hops come in herbal tea preparations. Both solid and liquid forms are gaining in popularity, and some people apparently smoke dried hops. No specific dose is recommended because hops commonly are used in combination with other herbs or as a tea. However, based on combination products, the approximate dosage may be 2 to 4 milligrams of the extract.

Side effects

Call your health care practitioner if you experience any of these possible side effects of hops:

- airway irritation and bronchitis (with inhalation)
- blisters
- mental slowness
- sedation
- severe allergic reaction (chest tightness, wheezing, hives, itching, and rash) and allergic skin rash.

Why people use this herb

- As a hypnotic or sedative
- Depression
- Menopause symptoms
- Pain
- Tapeworms, pinworms, and other worm infections
- To ease muscle spasms
- To stimulate the digestive system

Interactions

Combining herbs with certain drugs may alter their action or produce unwanted side effects. Tell your health care practitioner about any prescription or nonprescription drugs you're taking, especially drugs that slow the nervous system, including:

- alcohol
- anticholinergics such as atropine
- antidepressants such as Prozac
- antihistamines

- antipsychotic drugs such as Haldol
- anxiety medications, such as Ativan and Valium.

Don't use hops when taking:

- drugs metabolized by the liver's cytochrome P-450 system, such as certain antibiotics (including Ery-Tab and Nizoral), Coumadin, Inderal, nonsteroidal anti-inflammatory drugs (including Advil and Naprosyn), Theo-Dur, and Tylenol
- phenothiazine-type drugs such as Thorazine.

Important points to remember

- If you have an estrogen-related cancer, such as breast, uterine, or cervical cancer, check with your health care practitioner before using hops.
- Use hops with caution if you regularly consume alcohol or are taking a drug that slows the nervous system, such as a cold or allergy drug, a sedative, a tranquilizer, a narcotic pain reliever, a barbiturate, a drug for seizures, or a muscle relaxant.
- Note that the herb loses potency when stored. Only 15% remains after 9 months.
- Avoid driving and other hazardous activities until you know how hops affect you.

WHAT THE RESEARCH SHOWS

Medical experts believe hops probably are safe when used infrequently for insomnia by people who don't take other drugs and who don't have preexisting medical conditions. Although the herb has estrogen-like effects, its use in treating menopause is less established than its use in treating insomnia. Medical experts don't recommend hops because they don't have enough information to determine what dose to use or to evaluate the herb's safety and benefits.

Other names for hops

Products containing hops are sold under such names as Avena Sativa Compound in Species Sedative Tea, HR 129 Serene, HR 133 Stress, Melatonin with Vitamin B_6, Snuz Plus, and Stress Aid. Hops also is available as single-ingredient compounds.

Selected references

Gerhard, U., et al. "Vigilance-Decreasing Effects of Two Plant-Derived Sedatives," *Schweizerische Rundschau für Medizin Praxis* 85:473-81, 1996.

Mannering, G.J., and Shoeman, J.A. "Murine Cytochrome P4503A is Induced by 2-methyl-3-buten-2-ol, 3 methyl-1-pentyn-3-ol (meparfynol), and Tert-amyl Alcohol," *Xenobiotica* 26:487-93, 1996.

Yasukawa, K., et al. "Humulon, a Bitter in the Hop, Inhibits Tumor Promotion by 12-O-tetradecanoylphorbol-13-acetate in Two-Stage Carcinogenesis in Mouse Skin," *Oncology* 52:156-58, 1995.

Zava, D.T., et al. "Estrogen and Progestin Bioactivity of Foods, Herbs, and Spices," *Proceedings of the Society for Experimental Biology and Medicine* 217:369-78, 1998.

Horehound

Herbalists typically make horehound extracts from the fresh or dried leaves and flowering tops of *Marrubium vulgare.* Native to Europe and Asia, this plant has been naturalized to the United States and other parts of North America. In Europe, a variety called white horehound serves as a natural food flavoring source and is added to liqueurs, candy, and cough drops.

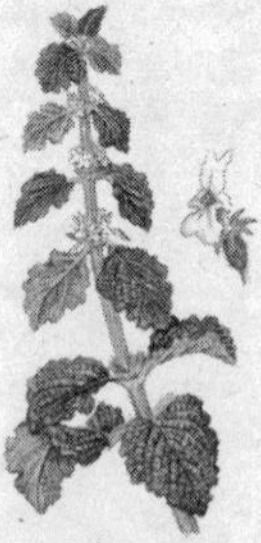

Why people use this herb

- As a digestive aid
- As an expectorant
- Cough
- Fluid retention
- Intestinal parasites
- Sore throat
- To induce sweating

Common doses

Horehound comes as capsules of fluid extract (300 milligrams), lozenges, syrup, tea, powder, and candies. Some experts recommend the following doses:

- For *cough and throat ailments,* 10 to 40 drops of extract taken orally in warm water up to three times daily; or 1 to 2 grams of the powder or an infusion taken orally three times daily; or lozenges taken orally as needed.

Side effects

Call your health care practitioner if you experience any of these possible side effects of horehound:

- diarrhea
- irregular heartbeats
- low blood sugar symptoms, such as shakiness, weakness, difficulty concentrating, anxiety, and cool, pale skin.

Horehound also may cause miscarriage.

Interactions

Combining herbs with certain drugs may alter their action or produce unwanted side effects. Don't use horehound while taking:

- certain antidepressants (consult your health care practitioner)
- drugs for irregular heartbeats
- drugs for migraine, such as D.H.E. 45, Ergostat, and Imitrex

- drugs that lower blood sugar, such as insulin, Amaryl, DiaBeta, Diabinese, Glucophage, Glucotrol, Precose, and Rezulin
- drugs used to halt vomiting, such as Kytril or Zofran.

Important points to remember

- Don't use horehound if you're pregnant or breast-feeding.
- Avoid this herb if you have diabetes or irregular heartbeats.
- Be aware that black horehound *(Ballota nigra)* sometimes is mixed into compounds that claim to contain only white horehound.

WHAT THE RESEARCH SHOWS

Horehound has a long history as a cough remedy and flavoring agent, but research doesn't support other uses. Medical experts recommend avoiding large doses because the herb may have harmful effects on the heart rhythm and blood sugar.

Other names for horehound

Other names for horehound include common horehound, hoarhound, marrubium, marvel, and white horehound.

Products containing horehound are sold under such names as Horehound Herb and Hore Hound Tea.

Selected reference

Roman, R.R., et al. "Hypoglycemic Effect of Plants Used in Mexico as Antidiabetics," *Archives of Medical Research* 23:59, 1992.

Horse chestnut

In Europe, horse chestnut has been used to treat varicose veins and water retention. Horse chestnut extract (sometimes called *Hippocastani semen)* is made from the seeds of *Aesculus hippocastanum*, a member of the Hippocastanaceae family. Herbalists use bark from young branches because older bark is poisonous.

Common dose

Horse chestnut comes as extract using aescin (a mixture of certain compounds) to standardize the concentration. Some experts recommend the following dose:

- 100 to 150 milligrams of the aescin component taken orally in either one or two equal daily doses.

Why people use this herb

- Diarrhea
- Enlarged prostate
- Fever
- Hemorrhoids
- Phlebitis (vein inflammation)
- Varicose veins

Side effects

Call your health care practitioner if you experience any of these possible side effects of horse chestnut:

- allergic reaction
- hives
- itching
- muscle spasms
- nausea
- vomiting.

Horse chestnut also can cause:

- kidney damage
- severe bleeding and bruising, shock, and liver damage.

Interactions

Combining herbs with certain drugs may alter their action or produce unwanted side effects. Tell your health care practitioner about any prescription or nonprescription drugs you're taking, especially blood thinners such as Coumadin and aspirin.

Important points to remember

- Don't use horse chestnut if you're pregnant or breast-feeding.
- If you're allergic to other members of the horse chestnut family or have a bleeding disorder, check with your health care practitioner before using this herb.

- Know that this herb may turn your urine red.
- Report unusual bleeding or bruising, yellow-tinged skin or eyes, fatigue, or fever.
- Be aware that the fruit, leaves, and older bark of the horse chestnut plant are poisonous. Use only products that come from the seeds or bark of young branches.
- Tell your health care practitioner if other drugs you're taking seem less effective after you start using horse chestnut.
- Check for aspirin in nonprescription or prescription drugs, because it interacts with horse chestnut.
- Don't confuse this herb with the buckeye tree, also called horse chestnut.

WHAT THE RESEARCH SHOWS

Researchers may test horse chestnut for treating varicose veins because most people with the condition don't like to wear the therapeutic compression stockings often prescribed. Horse chestnut may be a more acceptable alternative.

Other names for horse chestnut

Other names for horse chestnut include aescin, chestnut, and escine.

Products containing horse chestnut are sold under such names as Horse Chestnut Extract, Venostasin Retard, and Venostat.

Selected references

Diehm, C., et al. "Comparison of Leg Compression Stocking and Oral Horse Chestnut Seed Extract in Patients with Chronic Venous Insufficiency," *Lancet* 347:292-94, 1996.

Diehm, C., et al. "Medical Edema Protection—Clinical Benefits in Patients With Deep Vein Incompetence. A Placebo-Controlled, Double-Blind Study," *Vasa* 21:188-92, 1992.

Kreysel, H.W., et al. "A Possible Role of Lysosomal Enzymes in the Pathogenesis of Varicosis and the Reduction in Their Serum Activity by Venostatin," *Vasa* 12:377-82, 1983.

Rehn, D., et al. "Comparative Clinical Efficacy and Tolerability of Oxerutins and Horse Chestnut Extract in Patients With Chronic Venous Insufficiency," *Arzneimittel-Forschung* 5:483-87, 1996.

Horseradish

A common food seasoning, horseradish comes from the root of a large, leafy perennial called *Armoracia rusticana*. Some people mix horseradish with toxic substances to prevent accidental poisoning of domesticated animals. Certain chemicals in the herb are used in diagnostic tests for blood sugar and joint disorders.

Why people use this herb

- Certain infections
- Fluid retention
- Inflamed joints

Common dose

Horseradish comes as fresh root, powder, and semisolid paste for use as a condiment or spice. Some experts recommend the following dose:

- For *all uses,* 2 to 4 grams of fresh root taken orally before meals.

Side effects

Call your health care practitioner if you experience any of these possible side effects of horseradish:

- allergic reaction
- bloody diarrhea, vomiting (with large amounts)
- severe irritation of the nose and throat lining.

Interactions

Combining herbs with certain drugs may alter their action or produce unwanted side effects. Tell your health care practitioner about any prescription or nonprescription drugs you're taking, especially:

- anticholinergic drugs such as atropine
- cholinergic drugs, such as Mestinon, Prostigmin, or Urecholine.

Important points to remember

- Don't use horseradish medicinally if you're pregnant or breast-feeding.
- If you have thyroid disease, consult your health care practitioner before using horseradish.
- Be aware that the horseradish plant is poisonous. In animals, poisoning has led to collapse.
- Don't grow wild horseradish—you may confuse it with pokeweed root, which is toxic.

Other name for horseradish

Another name for horseradish is pepperrot.

No known medicinal products containing horseradish are available commercially.

> **WHAT THE RESEARCH SHOWS**
>
> Scientific studies don't support the medicinal use of horseradish. Until medical experts learn more about the effects of consuming large amounts, they recommend eating no more than the amount normally used to season foods.

Selected references

Leiner, I.E. *Toxic Constituents of Plant Foodstuffs*. New York: Academic Press, 1980.

Shiozawa, S., et al. "Presence of HLA-DR Antigen on Synovial Type A and B Cells: An Immunoelectron Microscopic Study in Rheumatoid Arthritis, Osteoarthritis and Normal Traumatic Joints," *Immunology* 50:587, 1983.

Sjaastad, O.V., et al. "Hypotensive Effects in Cats Caused by Horseradish Peroxidase Mediated by Metabolites of Arachidonic Acid," *Journal of Histochemistry and Cytochemistry* 32:1328-30, 1984.

Horsetail

Horsetail comes from the tall, hollow stems of *Equisetum arvense*. Resembling wetland rushes, this plant has scale-like leaves and no flowers.

The Food and Drug Administration says horsetail's safety is "undefined." Some horsetail products contain thiaminase, a poison that cancels out the action of the nutrient thiamine to cause thiamine deficiency (which can lead to permanent nervous system damage). Children reportedly have been poisoned by using the hollow stems as whistles or blowguns. In Canada, manufacturers must prove that their horsetail products are thiaminase-free.

Why people use this herb

- As a styptic (to stop bleeding)
- Cancer
- Fever
- Fluid retention
- Gonorrhea
- Gout
- Indigestion
- Rheumatism
- To strengthen tissues in tuberculosis patients

Common doses

Horsetail comes as a liquid extract. Goldenrod-Horsetail Compound, a blend of liquid extracts, contains 22.5% goldenrod flowering tips, 22.5% corn silk, 22.5% horsetail, 22.5% pipsissewa leaf, and 10% juniper berry. Some experts recommend the following doses:

- For *short-term use,* 20 to 40 drops in water taken orally three to five times daily.
- For *extended use,* 20 to 40 drops in water taken orally two or three times daily.

Side effects

Call your health care practitioner if you experience any of these possible side effects of horsetail:

- allergic reaction
- fever
- irregular heartbeats
- muscle weakness
- poor coordination
- seborrheic dermatitis (greasy skin scales)
- weight loss.

Interactions

Combining herbs with certain drugs may alter their action or produce unwanted side effects. Tell your health care practitioner about any prescription or nonprescription drugs you're taking, especially:

- diuretics (don't use horsetail when taking these)
- nervous system stimulants, such as nicotine replacement products used as an aid to smoking cessation.

Important points to remember

- Avoid horsetail if you're pregnant or breast-feeding.
- Don't use large amounts of horsetail because it can cause nicotine poisoning.
- Keep this herb out of reach of children and pets.
- Remember that horsetail contains nicotine.

WHAT THE RESEARCH SHOWS

Research shows that horsetail has a weak diuretic effect. But medical experts don't recommend it for this use because it can be toxic and because safer, more effective diuretics are available. Claims that horsetail products can aid urination and strengthen hair, bone, nails, and connective tissue haven't been explored.

Other names for horsetail

Other names for horsetail include bottle brush, dutch rush, paddock pipes, pewterwort, scouring rush, and shave grass.

A product containing horsetail is sold as Goldenrod-Horsetail Compound.

Selected reference

Hamon, N.W., and Awang, D.V.C. "Horsetail," *Canadian Pharmaceutical Journal* 125:399-401, 1992.

Hyssop

Hyssop comes from *Hyssopus officinalis,* a plant of the Labiatae family that has aromatic leaves and clusters of blue flowers. Many French liqueurs, including Chartreuse and Benedictine, contain the volatile oil of hyssop. Some fragrances contain the essential oil.

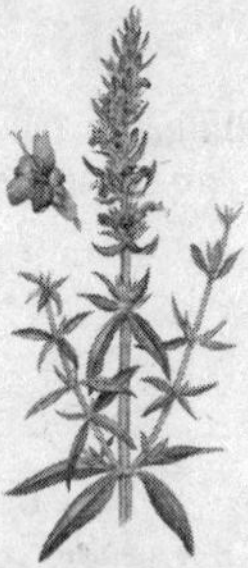

Why people use this herb

- Anxiety
- Asthma
- Bronchitis
- Burns
- Cold sores
- Common cold
- Cough
- Genital herpes sores
- Hysteria
- Indigestion
- Intestinal gas
- Petit mal seizures (a form of epilepsy)
- Sore throat
- Wounds

Common doses

Hyssop comes as a commercial or fluid extract, tincture, and oil. Fresh or dried flowering tops are used to prepare teas or compresses. Some experts recommend the following doses:

- As a *tea,* infuse 1 to 2 teaspoons of dried hyssop in 1 cup of boiling water for 10 to 15 minutes. Drink three times daily for cough, or gargle three times daily for sore throat.
- As a *tincture,* 1 to 4 milliliters taken orally three times daily.

Side effects

Call your health care practitioner if you experience any of these possible side effects of hyssop:

- diarrhea
- upset stomach.

Overdose of hyssop oil may cause seizure-like muscle spasms.

Interactions

Combining herbs with certain drugs may alter their action or produce unwanted side effects. Tell your health care practitioner about any prescription or nonprescription drugs you're taking.

Important points to remember

- Don't use hyssop if you're pregnant.

- Know that children ages 2 to 12 and elderly adults should use low-strength preparations.
- Don't give hyssop to children under age 2.
- Keep hyssop out of reach of children and pets.
- Check with your health care practitioner if you plan to use the herb more than 3 days in a row.
- Don't confuse this herb with giant hyssop, hedge hyssop, prairie hyssop, or wild hyssop.

WHAT THE RESEARCH SHOWS

Medical experts generally recognize hyssop as safe but advise people to seek medical supervision when using it more than 3 days in a row. They suspect—but aren't certain—that the herb acts as an expectorant in treating cough and bronchitis and reduces intestinal gas in such disorders as bloating and irritable bowel.

No evidence supports external use of hyssop in treating burns, wounds, and other infections. Although hyssop extracts have inhibited HIV in test tubes, no studies show that the herb is useful in treating AIDS.

Other names for hyssop

Hyssop has no other names.

No known products containing hyssop are available commercially.

Selected reference

Kaplan, K.W., et al. "Inhibition of HIV Replication by *Hyssop officinalis* Extracts," *Antiviral Research* 14:323-37, 1990.

Iceland moss

Iceland moss, which goes by the botanical name *Cetraria islandica*, is a lichen with green algae and a web of root filaments. It grows mainly on Iceland's mountains and heathlands. The lichen may be gathered throughout the year but is most abundant between May and September. After the moss is cleaned and dried, the whole plant is used for extraction.

Iceland moss has been exported to manufacturers of herbal medicines (particularly in Germany) and has been used in European medicines to treat minor ailments. Iceland is one of the least polluted countries in the world, and the purity of its plants is desirable. Iceland moss is grown organically and fertilizers aren't used where many of these plants are found. However, lichens lack roots, making Iceland moss susceptible to contamination by radioactivity and heavy metals. Fallout from the Chernobyl accident contaminated lichen in most of Europe. Fortunately, Iceland's radioactivity level was almost negligible.

Why people use this herb

- Asthma
- Cough
- Digestive disorders, such as gastritis (stomach inflammation)
- Stomach ulcers
- Throat irritation
- Tuberculosis

Common doses

Iceland moss comes as throat lozenges, capsules, and creams. Some experts recommend the following doses:

- As a *decoction,* mix 1 teaspoonful of shredded moss in 1 cup of cold water, boil for 3 minutes, and take orally twice daily. Or take 1 to 2 milliliters of the tincture orally three times daily.

Side effects

Call your health care practitioner if you experience any unusual symptoms when taking Iceland moss. Large doses or prolonged use may lead to:

- digestive tract irritation
- liver damage
- nausea.

Interactions

Combining herbs with certain drugs may alter their action or produce unwanted side effects. Tell your health care practitioner about any prescription or nonprescription drugs you're taking.

Important points to remember

- Don't use Iceland moss if you're pregnant or breast-feeding.
- Know that medical experts don't recommend this herb for any use because it hasn't been adequately tested on people.
- If you use Iceland moss, watch for poisoning symptoms— abdominal pain, diarrhea, nausea, vomiting, bleeding, and changes in urine, stool, or skin color.

WHAT THE RESEARCH SHOWS

Iceland moss derivatives show promise as immune system and anti-tumor drugs. Someday, they may play a role in treating *Helicobacter pylori*, an infection linked to stomach ulcers and inflammation. Although more human studies must be done, the extracts seem to be relatively safe when used in small amounts.

Other names for Iceland moss

Other names for Iceland moss include *Cetraria*, consumption moss, Iceland lichen, and *Lichen islandicus*.

A product containing Iceland moss is sold as Iceland Moss.

Selected references

Ingolfsdottir K., et al. "Immunologically Active Polysaccharide From *Cetraria islandica*," *Planta Medica* 60:527-31, 1994.

Ingolfsdottir, K., et al. "In Vitro Evaluation of the Antimicrobial Activity of Lichen Metabolites as Potential Preservatives," *Antimicrobial Agents and Chemotherapy* 28:289-92, 1985.

Ingolfsdottir, K., et al. "In Vitro Susceptibility of *Helicobacter pylori* to Protolichesterinic Acid From the Lichen *Cetraria islandica*," *Antimicrobial Agents and Chemotherapy* 41:215-17, 1997.

Indigo

Indigo comes from the leaves and branches of a group of plants called *Indigofera*. Many *Indigofera* species grow worldwide, but only a few (such as *I. tinctoria* and *I. suffruticosa*) grow in the United States.

***I. tinctoria* is the source of natural blue indigo dye, which has been used for hundreds of years. (All commercially available indigo is now prepared synthetically.) *I. tinctoria* also is thought to be the active ingredient in a traditional Chinese medicine used to treat chronic myelocytic leukemia.**

Why people use this herb

- Bleeding disorders
- Boils
- Carbuncles (pockets of infected, pus-containing abscesses or boils under the skin)
- Diabetes
- Fever
- Hemorrhoids
- Inflammation
- Infant seizures
- Mumps
- Ovarian cancer
- Pain
- Scorpion bites
- Stomach cancer
- To induce vomiting
- To purify the liver

Common dose

Indigo comes as tablets and a blue powder. Experts disagree on what dose to take.

Side effects

Call your health care practitioner if you experience any of these possible side effects of indigo:

- eye irritation
- skin inflammation from direct contact with indigo dyes.

Indospicine, a component of *I. spicata*, may cause liver damage and can harm an embryo or a fetus. In animals, it has caused cleft palate and embryo death.

Interactions

Combining herbs with certain drugs may alter their action or produce unwanted side effects. Tell your health care practitioner about any prescription or nonprescription drugs you're taking.

Important points to remember

- Keep indigo away from your eyes. Flush your eyes with water if contact occurs.
- If you suspect you're pregnant or if you're planning a pregnancy, check with your health care practitioner before using this herb.

WHAT THE RESEARCH SHOWS

Researchers haven't substantiated therapeutic claims for indigo—used alone or combined with other ingredients. Until indigo is tested on people, medical experts can't recommend this herb.

Other names for indigo

Other names for indigo include common indigo, Indian indigo, and qingdai.

No known products containing indigo are available commercially.

Selected reference

Han, R. "Highlight on the Studies of Anticancer Drugs Derived From Plants in China," *Stem Cells* 12:53-63, 1994.

Irish moss

The term Irish moss usually refers to a seaweed called *Chondrus crispus* or to a mixture of *C. crispus* and *Mastocarpus stellatus*. The herb can be collected at low tide on the rocky Atlantic coastlines of northwestern Europe and Canada.

Carrageenan, a seaweed gum processed from Irish moss, is found in a wide range of products. The French use degraded carrageenan (changed by acid or heat) in peptic ulcer medicines. In the United States, carrageenan is used in milk products (chocolate milk, ice cream, sherbets, cottage cheese, evaporated milk, puddings, yogurts, and infant formulas) and to thicken sauces, gravies, jams, and jellies. It's also an ingredient in various herbal drinks, weight-loss products, fruit juices, and aloe vera lotions. Irish moss is used extensively as a binder, emulsifier, or stabilizer in toothpastes, hand lotions, creams, and tablets. Because food-grade carrageenan isn't absorbed, experts believe it's nontoxic.

Why people use this herb

- Bronchitis
- Common cold
- Gastritis (inflammation of the stomach lining)
- Tuberculosis
- Ulcers

Common dose

Although available as tablets in some countries, Irish moss usually is taken as a decoction. Some experts recommend the following dose:

- As a *decoction,* add 1 ounce of dried plant to 1 to 1½ pints of boiling water. Simmer gently and strain the liquid. If desired, sweeten with lemon, cinnamon, or honey. Take two or three times daily in 1-cup doses.

Side effects

Call your health care practitioner if you experience any of these possible side effects of Irish moss:

- bleeding
- cramping
- diarrhea
- low blood pressure symptoms, such as dizziness or weakness.

Irish moss also can cause infection. In animals, it has caused stomach ulcers and kidney disease.

Interactions

Combining herbs with certain drugs may alter their action or produce unwanted side effects. Tell your health care practitioner about any prescription or nonprescription drugs you're taking, especially drugs that lower blood pressure.

Don't use Irish moss when taking:

- blood thinners such as Coumadin
- other drugs you take by mouth.

Important points to remember

- Don't use Irish moss if you're pregnant or breast-feeding.
- Avoid this herb if you have active peptic ulcer disease or a history of peptic ulcer disease.
- If you use Irish moss, rise slowly from a sitting or lying position to reduce dizziness.
- Watch for symptoms of abnormal bleeding, such as easy bruising, bleeding gums, tarry stools, and nosebleed.
- Know that carrageenan is considered safe only in the small amounts normally found in foodstuffs and commercial creams and lotions. Researchers haven't tested its effects on people who use larger amounts.

Other names for Irish moss

Other names for Irish moss include carrageen, carrageenan, chondrus, chondrus extract, and Irish moss extract.

Products containing Irish moss are sold by various manufacturers.

WHAT THE RESEARCH SHOWS

Although carrageenan, the main derivative of Irish moss, is widely used in the pharmaceutical and food industries, researchers haven't confirmed its value in treating disease. Until more studies are done, medical experts can't recommend this herb.

Selected references

Anderson, W., and Soman, P.D. "Degraded Carrageenan and Duodenal Ulceration in the Guinea Pig," *Nature* 3:101-2, 1965.

Evans, P.R.C., et al. "Blind Trial of a Degraded Carrageenan and Aluminum Hydroxide Gel in the Treatment of Peptic Ulceration," *Postgraduate Medical Journal* 41:48-52, 1965.

Grahnen, A., et al. "Doxycycline Carrageenate—An Improved Formulation Providing More Reliable Absorption and Plasma Concentrations at High Gastric pH than Doxycycline Monohydrate," *European Journal of Clinical Pharmacology* 46:143-46, 1994.

Jaborandi tree

Jaborandi or pilocarpus refers to leaves of *Pilocarpus jaborandi* (*Pernambuco jaborandi*), *P. microphyllus* (Maranham jaborandi), or *P. pinnatifolius* (Paraguay jaborandi). The plant is native to northern and northeastern Brazil.

Common doses

Leaves from the jaborandi tree come as a powder, an essential oil, a fluid extract, and a tincture. Pilocarpine, the herb's main active ingredient, is available in many prescription products, including:

- tablets (5 milligrams)
- eye medications ranging from 0.25% to 10% solutions, a 4%-solution gel, and eye inserts of 20 micrograms and 40 micrograms.

Some experts recommend the following doses:

- For *glaucoma,* 1 to 2 drops applied three or four times daily. (See the pilocarpine package insert for specific dosage information.)
- For *dry mouth,* 15 to 30 milligrams taken orally daily (100 milligrams orally is considered a fatal dose.).
- For *general daily use,* powdered leaves, 5 to 60 grains (0.324 to 3.9 grams); fluid extract, 10 to 30 drops; or tincture, ½ to 1 dram (1.75 to 3 milliliters).

Why people use this herb

- Baldness
- Deafness
- Diabetes
- Dry mouth
- Fluid retention
- Glaucoma
- Increased pressure within the eye
- Intestinal weakness
- Jaundice
- Kidney disease
- Nausea
- Pleurisy (inflammation of the lung sac)
- Psoriasis (scaly, raised skin patches)
- Rheumatism
- Syphilis
- To induce sweating
- To make the pupils contract (as for treating glaucoma)
- Tonsillitis
- To stimulate saliva secretion

Side effects

Call your health care practitioner if you experience any of these possible side effects of jaborandi tree:

- headache
- nausea
- salivation
- slow pulse

- sweating
- vision changes
- vomiting
- watery eyes.

Jaborandi tree may cause pilocarpine poisoning, which leads to symptoms such as headache, vision problems, increased eye tearing, sweating, labored breathing, stomach spasms, nausea, vomiting, diarrhea, and an unusually fast or slow pulse. In extreme cases, pulmonary edema and shock may occur.

Interactions

Combining herbs with certain drugs may alter their action or produce unwanted side effects. Tell your health care practitioner about other drugs you're taking, especially:

- Antilirium
- Aricept
- heart drugs called beta blockers, such as Inderal
- other prescription drugs that contain pilocarpine
- other substances that act like this herb (such as arecoline, methacholine, and muscarine)
- Tensilon.

Don't use jaborandi tree when taking:

- atropine
- Atrovent
- heart drugs called cardiac glycosides, such as Lanoxin
- iron-containing preparations
- Transderm-Scōp.

Important points to remember

- Don't take jaborandi tree if you're allergic to pilocarpine or if you have uncontrolled asthma, acute inflammation of the iris, or angle-closure glaucoma.
- Avoid this herb if you're pregnant or breast-feeding.
- Don't take large doses because this herb can damage your liver, especially if you already have liver disease.
- Check with your health care practitioner before using jaborandi tree, especially if you have serious heart or blood vessel disease, a mental or psychiatric disorder, abnormality of the urinary or genital tract, gallstones, or kidney stones.

- Be aware that excessive sweating may lead to dehydration if you don't drink plenty of fluids while using jaborandi tree.
- Immediately report pain in your upper right torso, jaundice, and fever. These are symptoms of liver injury.
- Know that this herb may cause vision changes, especially at night, that reduce your ability to drive safely.

WHAT THE RESEARCH SHOWS

Pilocarpine, which comes from jaborandi tree, is a well-documented treatment for glaucoma and dry mouth. However, researchers haven't tested unprocessed jaborandi leaves for any therapeutic use.

Other names for jaborandi tree

Other names for jaborandi tree include arruda brava, arruda do mato, indian hemp, jaborandi, jamguarandi, juarandi, pernambuco jaborandi, and *Pilocarpus jaborandi.*

Products containing jaborandi tree are sold under such names as Jaborandi, Wonder Gel, and X-Tablets.

Selected references

Brown, J.H., and Taylor, P. "Muscarinic Receptor Agonists and Antagonists," in *Goodman and Gilman's The Pharmacological Basis of Therapeutics,* 9th ed. Edited by Hardman, J.G., and Limbird, L.E. New York: McGraw-Hill Book Co., 1996.

Claus, E.P. *Pharmacognosy*, 3rd ed. Philadelphia: Lea & Febiger, 1956.

Jamaican dogwood

Central and South American fishermen use ingredients found in Jamaican dogwood to stun fish. Although the herb doesn't seem to have this effect on people and other mammals, the European Council has rejected it as a natural food flavoring.

Why people use this herb

- Asthma
- Insomnia
- Kidney pain
- Labor pain
- Lack of menstrual flow
- Migraine
- Nerve pain
- Sharp intestinal pain
- Toothache
- Whooping cough

Jamaican dogwood, or *Piscidia erythrina*, grows in the West Indies and northern parts of South America. It has been transplanted to Mexico, Texas, and Florida. The plant isn't related to the common dogwood found in the eastern United States.

Common doses

Jamaican dogwood comes as:

- dried preparations of root or bark
- tinctures (45% alcohol)
- fluid extracts (30% to 60% alcohol)
- unprocessed bark strips.

Some experts recommend the following doses:

- As a *dried product,* 2 to 4 grams taken orally in equal doses daily, or simmer 1 teaspoonful for 10 minutes in 1 cup of water and drink.
- As a *tincture,* 5 to 15 milliliters taken daily, usually as 2 to 3 milliliters at a time.
- As an *extract,* 1 to 2 drams taken daily, starting with 5 to 20 drops. Increase the dose cautiously.
- To *relieve pain* or *muscle spasms,* take three to five times daily.
- As a *sleep aid,* take at bedtime.

Side effects

Call your health care practitioner if you experience any of these possible side effects of Jamaican dogwood:

- drowsiness or sedation
- nausea
- stomach upset
- sweating, salivation, and tremors (with overdose).

Interactions

Combining herbs with certain drugs may alter their action or produce unwanted side effects. Don't use Jamaican dogwood while drinking alcohol or taking other drugs that slow the nervous system, such as:

- barbiturates
- cold and allergy drugs
- muscle relaxants
- narcotic pain relievers
- sedatives
- seizure medications
- tranquilizers.

Important points to remember

- Don't use this herb if you're pregnant or breast-feeding.
- Avoid Jamaican dogwood if you have heart or blood vessel disease.
- Know that this herb hasn't been studied extensively on people, and no evidence suggests it does any good.
- If you use Jamaican dogwood, avoid driving and other hazardous activities until you know how the herb affects you.
- Remember that some chemicals in the plant may cause cancer.

WHAT THE RESEARCH SHOWS

Information on Jamaican dogwood is scarce. Medical experts caution against using the herb until studies prove it's safe.

Other names for Jamaican dogwood

Other names for Jamaican dogwood include fishfuddle, fish poison tree, and West Indian dogwood.

A product containing Jamaican dogwood is sold as Willow-Meadowsweet Compound.

Selected reference

Della-Loggia, R., et al. "Isoflavones as Spasmolytic Principles of *Piscidia erythrina*," *Progress in Clinical Biological Research* 280:365-68, 1988.

Jambul

Jambul is extracted from the fruits, seeds, and leaves of *Syzygium cuminii*. Native to India and Sri Lanka, this tree grows 50 to 80 feet high and has edible berries. A related species, *S. jambos*, has been used for treating diabetes.

Why people use this herb

- Diabetes
- Diarrhea
- Dysentery
- Fever
- Inflammation

Common dose

Jambul comes as tea or decoctions made from seeds or dried leaves. Experts disagree on what dose to take.

Side effects

Call your health care practitioner if you experience unusual symptoms when using jambul.

Interactions

Combining herbs with certain drugs may alter their action or produce unwanted side effects. Don't use jambul while drinking alcohol or taking other drugs that slow the nervous system, such as:

- barbiturates
- cold and allergy drugs
- muscle relaxants
- narcotic pain relievers
- sedatives
- seizure medications
- tranquilizers.

Important points to remember

- Don't use jambul if you're pregnant or breast-feeding.
- If you use this herb, report changes in your behavior or coordination to your health care practitioner.

Other names for jambul

Other names for jambul include black plum, *Eugenia cyanocarpa, Eugenia jambolana,* jamba, jambolão, jambool, jambu, jambula, jambulon plum, java plum, and syzygium jambolanum.

No known products containing jambul are available commercially.

WHAT THE RESEARCH SHOWS

Although herbalists say jambul is effective in treating diabetes, diarrhea, and dysentery, little clinical evidence supports these claims. Some animal studies suggest jambul may be valuable for certain traditional uses, but human studies haven't been done.

Selected references

Chakraborty, D., et al. "A Neuropsychopharmacologic Study of *Syzygium cuminii*," *Planta Medica* 2:139-43, 1986.

Chaudhuri, A.K., et al. "Anti-inflammatory and Related Actions of *Syzygium cuminii* Seed Extract," *Phytotherapy Research* 4:5-10, 1990.

Teixeria, C.C., et al. "Effect of Tea Prepared From the Leaves of *Syzygium jambos* on Glucose Tolerance in Nondiabetic Patients," *Diabetes Care* 13:907-8. 1990.

Teixeria, C.C., et al. "The Effect of *Syzygium cumini* (L.) Seeds on Post-Prandial Blood Glucose Levels in Nondiabetic Rats and Rats with Streptozotocin-Induced Diabetes Mellitus," *Journal of Ethnopharmacology* 56:209-13, 1997.

Jimsonweed

Jimsonweed *(Datura stramonium)* grows in fields, roadside ditches, and refuse sites. Herbalists use the leaves, flowering tops, roots, and sometimes the seeds. However, all plant parts are toxic, especially the seeds. Most countries restrict the herb. In the United States, it's considered illegal except when prescribed.

Why people use this herb

- As a hallucinogen
- Asthma
- Muscle spasms
- Parkinson's disease
- To cause the pupils to enlarge
- To relax muscles of the digestive, bronchial, and urinary tracts
- Whooping cough

Common dose

Jimsonweed comes in an oral form and as a suppository. Some people smoke it in cigarettes, burn it in powders, or inhale its fumes.

Some experts previously recommended a dose of 75 milligrams. For adults, estimated lethal doses for the chemicals in jimsonweed are 10 milligrams of atropine and 2 to 4 milligrams of scopolamine.

Side effects

Call your health care practitioner if you experience any of these possible side effects of jimsonweed:

- blurred vision
- difficulty swallowing and speaking
- dilated pupils
- dry, hot, flushed skin
- dry mucous membranes
- fever
- high blood pressure symptoms, such as headache and blurred vision
- low blood pressure symptoms, such as dizziness and weakness
- mental changes, such as confusion, disorientation, loss of short-term memory, visual and auditory hallucinations, and psychosis
- poor muscle coordination
- rapid pulse
- thirst
- unusual eye sensitivity to light
- urine retention.

Eating this herb can cause coma, seizures, respiratory failure, heart and blood vessel collapse, and death. Eating 50 to 100 seeds can cause severe intoxication or death.

Interactions

Combining herbs with certain drugs may alter their action or produce unwanted side effects. Don't use jimsonweed while taking:

- antihistamines (used for treating colds, allergies, and hay fever)
- L-dopa
- Norpace
- other anticholinergic drugs such as atropine
- other drugs that interact with atropine and Levsin, such as antihistamines and Nizoral
- phenothiazines (used for anxiety, nausea, vomiting, or psychosis) such as Thorazine
- Procan SR
- Quinaglute Dura-tabs
- Symmetrel
- thiazide diuretics, such as Naturetin, Diuril, HydroDIURIL, Renese, and Metahydrin
- tricyclic antidepressants.

Important points to remember

- Avoid jimsonweed if you're pregnant or breast-feeding.
- Don't use this herb if you have glaucoma, a rapid pulse, overactive thyroid, a digestive or urinary tract blockage, or myasthenia gravis.
- Know that health care practitioners advise against eating jimsonweed.

WHAT THE RESEARCH SHOWS

Studies show jimsonweed is less effective than conventional treatments for asthma, whooping cough, and muscle spasms. Until this herb is studied on people and researchers explore the many poisoning reports, medical experts discourage its use. Also, keep in mind that nonprescription use of jimsonweed is illegal.

Other names for jimsonweed

Other names for jimsonweed include angel's trumpet, angel tulip, apple-of-Peru, devil weed, devil's-apple, devil's trumpet, Estramonio, green dragon, gypsyweed, inferno, Jamestown weed, loco seeds, locoweed, mad apple, moon weed, stramoine, stechapfel, stinkweed, thorn apple, tolguacha, trumpet lily, and zombie's cucumber.

No known products containing jimsonweed are available commercially.

Selected references

Clause, E.P. *Pharmacognosy*, 4th ed. Philadelphia: Lea & Febiger, 1961.
Ellenhorn, M.J. *Ellenhorn's Medical Toxicology—Diagnosis and Treatment of Human Poisoning,* 2nd ed. Baltimore: Williams & Wilkins Co., 1997.

Jojoba

Jojoba oil comes from *Simmondsia chinesis* and *S. californica* seeds. Apaches, other American Southwest Indians, and Israeli immigrants have been using this herb for many years to treat external conditions, such as to promote hair growth and relieve skin problems. Jojoba is an ingredient in some creams, facial scrubs, ointments, lotions, and lipsticks.

Common dose

Jojoba comes as an unprocessed wax (jojoba oil), hydrogenated jojoba wax, jojoba butter, and wax beads. No recommended dose exists.

Side effects

Call your health care practitioner if you experience skin irritation from direct contact.

Eating jojoba seeds has caused poisoning.

Interactions

Combining herbs with certain drugs may alter their action or produce unwanted side effects. Tell your health care practitioner about any prescription or nonprescription drugs you're taking.

Why people use this herb

- Acne
- Athlete's foot
- Chapped skin
- Cuts
- Dandruff
- Dry scalp
- Dry skin
- Eczema (a type of skin inflammation)
- Mouth sores
- Pimples
- Psoriasis (scaly, raised skin patches)
- Seborrhea (greasy, yellowish skin scales)
- Skin abrasions
- To promote hair growth
- Warts
- Wrinkles

Important point to remember

- Know that jojoba oil is for external use only.

WHAT THE RESEARCH SHOWS

Despite numerous claims regarding jojoba's effectiveness in treating skin and scalp disorders, no studies have been done to back up these claims. However, a long history of external use suggests jojoba oil is relatively safe.

Other names for jojoba

Other names include deernut, goatnut, and pignut.

Various manufacturers sell products containing jojoba as cosmetics and hair treatments.

Selected reference

Mallet, J.F., et al. "Antioxidant Activity of Plant Leaves in Relation to Their Alpha-Tocopherol Content," *Food and Chemical Toxicology* 49:1:61, 1994.

Juniper

Herbalists use the dried ripe fruit of the plant *Juniperus communis* (family Cupressaccae), also called female cones or berries. Some people also use the heartwood and tops. Juniper should be used fresh because it's so abundant.

Common doses

Juniper comes as capsules, tablets, an oral liquid, and an essential oil. Some experts recommend the following doses:

- For *intestinal gas* and *sharp intestinal pains,* 0.05 to 0.2 milliliter of juniper oil.

Studies have used the following doses:

- For *low blood sugar,* 250 to 500 milligrams per kilogram of body weight taken daily.
- To *reduce inflammation,* 0.2 milligram per milliliter.
- To *combat bacteria,* 20 milligrams per milliliter.

Why people use this herb

- Fluid retention in children
- Intestinal gas
- Intestinal pain
- Kidney infection
- Swelling caused by kidney obstruction
- Wound infections

Side effects

Call your health care practitioner if you experience any of these possible side effects of juniper:

- blisters
- diarrhea (with large amounts)
- skin burning or redness.

Juniper also may irritate the urinary tract, especially the kidneys. *Juniper sabina,* a closely related species, has been used to induce abortion, although studies don't support this use.

Interactions

Combining herbs with certain drugs may alter their action or produce unwanted side effects. Tell your health care practitioner about any prescription or nonprescription drugs you're taking.

Important points to remember

- Don't use juniper if you're pregnant.
- Avoid this herb if you have kidney disease.

- Check with your health care practitioner before using juniper if you are elderly, have diabetes, or have a history of skin irritation or allergic reactions.
- Don't apply juniper to open wounds or skin abrasions.
- Be aware that this plant and others in the Juniper class are considered poisonous and can cause diarrhea and urinary tract irritation. Tell your health care practitioner about significant diarrhea or burning on urination.
- Know that more potent juniper preparations may cause skin and mucous membrane irritation or blistering.
- Don't use juniper instead of prescribed diuretics.

Other names for juniper

Other names for juniper include a'ra'r a'di, ardic, baccal juniper, common juniper, dwarf, gemener, genievre, ground juniper, hackmatack, harvest, horse savin, juniper mistletoe, *Juniperi fructus*, yoshu-nezu, and zimbro.

Products containing juniper are sold under such names as Cold-Plus, Cornsilk Buchu Formula, Formula 600 Plus for Men, Naturalvite, PMS Aid, Regeneration Softgels, and SKB.

Selected references

Clark, A.M., et al. "Antimicrobial Properties of Heartwood, Bark/Sapwood and Leaves of *Juniperus* Species," *Phytotherapy Research* 4:15-19, 1990.

Ritch-Krc, E.M., et al. "Carrier Herbal Medicine; Traditional and Contemporary Plant Use," *Journal of Ethnopharmacology* 52:85-94, 1996.

Swanston-Flatt, S., et al. "Traditional Plant Treatments for Diabetes. Studies in Normal and Streptozotocin Diabetic Mice," *Diabetologia* 33:462-64, 1990.

Tunon, N. H., et al. "Evaluation of Anti-inflammatory Activity of Some Swedish Medicinal Plants. Inhibition of Prostaglandin Biosynthesis and PAF-Induced Exocytosis," *Journal of Ethnopharmacology* 48:61-76, 1995.

WHAT THE RESEARCH SHOWS

Most information about juniper comes from animal studies. The traditional use of this plant as a diuretic and for kidney infections hasn't been studied in people, although evidence suggests it may work like the drug streptomycin to combat infections. Most promising is the plant's effect on lowering blood sugar, but scientists must conduct studies on people before juniper can be used as an oral antidiabetic drug.

Karaya gum

Karaya gum is the dried sap of *Sterculia urens* and other *Sterculia* species. Native to India and Pakistan, this softwood tree grows to a height of about 30 feet. All parts of the tree ooze a soft gum when injured. To gather the gum, people cut the trunk, let the gum seep out, then wash and dry the gum.

Use of karaya gum became widespread in the early 1900s, when it began to replace a substance called tragacanth gum in many products. Currently, the food and pharmaceutical industries use karaya gum as a bulk ingredient and emulsifying agent.

Common dose

Karaya gum powder is used to form gels or pastes for bases in food, cosmetics, and pharmaceuticals. The dose is expressed as a percentage of karaya gum used in the final product.

Side effects

Call your health care practitioner if you experience any of these possible side effects of karaya gum:

- abdominal pain
- choking (seek immediate treatment)
- diarrhea.

Why people use this herb

- As a denture adhesive
- Constipation
- Sore throat
- To clean dentures
- Warts

Interactions

Combining herbs with certain drugs may alter their action or produce unwanted side effects. Tell your health care practitioner about any prescription or nonprescription drugs you're taking.

Important points to remember

- Don't use karaya gum if you're pregnant or breast-feeding.
- Use only small amounts of karaya gum if you're prone to a condition called gastric outlet obstruction (ask your health care practitioner).
- Know that using large amounts of karaya gum may lower blood sugar levels. If you have diabetes, consult your health care practitioner and watch for low blood sugar symptoms.
- If you're using other drugs, take them at least 2 hours before or after ingesting karaya gum.

WHAT THE RESEARCH SHOWS

Research suggests karaya gum has little effect—good or bad. Its use as a bulk laxative appears safe and may be effective, but large, controlled clinical studies haven't been done.

Other names for karaya gum

Other names for karaya gum include *Bassora tragacanth*, Indian tragacanth, kadaya, kadira, katila, kullo, mucara, *Sterculia*, and sterculia gum.

No known herbal products containing karaya gum are available commercially.

Selected references

Anderson, D.M. "Evidence for the Safety of Gum Karaya (*Sterculia* spp.) as a Food Additive," *Food Additives and Contaminants* 6:189, 1989.

Bart, B.J. "Salicylic Acid in Karaya Gum Patch as a Treatment for Verruca Vulgaris," *Journal of the American Academy of Dermatology* 20:74-76, 1989.

Kava

A kava drink is a popular beverage in the South Pacific islands, reportedly because it makes people feel tranquil, sociable, and euphoric. Historically, island women chewed the leaves and root stalks of the kava plant into a pulpy mass, spat the contents into a bowl, and mixed them with water, coconut milk, or other fruit juices. After straining the mixture, they served it at weddings, births, funerals, and other ceremonial rites of passage.

Now, the plant is ground and pulverized instead of chewed. This modern version of the kava cocktail probably isn't as potent as the earlier one, because chewing is thought to enhance the effects of the plant's active ingredients.

Kava comes from the dried root of *Piper methysticum,* a member of the black pepper family (Piperaceae). This large shrub with broad, heart-shaped leaves is native to many South Pacific islands. Although kava is a depressant, it isn't fermented, doesn't contain alcohol, and is neither an opiate nor a hallucinogen. It doesn't seem to be addictive either, although some people may become psychologically dependent on it.

Common doses

Kava comes as a drink prepared from pulverized roots, tablets, capsules, or extract. The dose usually depends on how much of a component called kavapyrone the preparation contains. Most studies used 70 to 240 milligrams of kavapyrone daily. One study used 90 to 110 milligrams of dried kava extract given three times daily to treat anxiety. Doses of freshly prepared kava beverages average 400 to 900 grams weekly.

Why people use this herb

- Anxiety
- Asthma
- Depression
- Insomnia
- Muscle spasms
- Pain
- Psychosis
- Rheumatism
- Seizures
- Venereal disease
- Wounds

Side effects

Call your health care practitioner if you experience any of these possible side effects of kava:

- changes in muscle control
- poor judgment
- vision problems.

Continuous heavy use of this herb can cause:

- changes in blood chemistry
- dry, flaking, discolored skin
- exaggerated kneecap reflex
- pulmonary hypertension
- reddened eyes
- shortness of breath
- weight loss.

Interactions

Combining herbs with certain drugs may alter their action or produce unwanted side effects. Don't use kava while drinking alcohol or when taking:

- benzodiazepines or other nervous system depressants
- L-dopa
- Nembutal
- Xanax.

Important points to remember

- Don't use kava if you're pregnant or breast-feeding.
- Don't give kava to children under age 12.
- Before using kava, check with your health care practitioner if you have kidney disease, a low platelet count, or an abnormal white blood cell count.
- Avoid using kava with drugs that cause mood changes.
- Be aware that long-term kava use may cause significant side effects.
- Know that taking kava with food aids its absorption.

Other names for kava

Other names for kava include ava, awa, kava-kava, kawa, kew, sakau, tonga, and yagona.

Products containing kava are sold under such names as Aigin, Antares, Ardeydystin, Cefkava, Kavasedon, Kavasporal, Kavatino, Laitan, Mosaro, Nervonocton N, Potter's Antigian Tablets, and Viocava.

Selected references

Almeida, J.C., et al. "Coma from the Health Food Store: Interaction Between Kava and Alprazolam," *Annals of Internal Medicine* 125:940, 1996.

Dobelis, I.N. *Magic and Medicine of Plants*. Pleasantville, N.Y: Reader's Digest Association, Inc., 1986.

Norton, S.A., et al. "Kava Dermopathy," *Journal of the American Academy of Dermatology* 31:89-97, 1994.

Volz, H.P., et al. "Kava-kava Extract WS-1490 versus Placebo in Anxiety Disorders—A Randomized Placebo Controlled 25-week Outpatient Trial," *Pharmacopsychiatry* 30:1-5,1997.

WHAT THE RESEARCH SHOWS

Limited evidence from a few small studies supports kava's use in treating anxiety, stress, and restlessness. Long-term heavy use of the herb can cause significant side effects. More testing must be done to establish appropriate kava doses and evaluate the herb's benefits.

Kelp

Kelp comes from fronds of the tall, brown algae called *Laminaria digitata, L. japonica, L. saccharina,* and *Macrocystis pyrifera,* which grow in the sea along the northern Atlantic and Pacific coasts. Although some people have used natural stents or kelp "tents" to keep the cervix open in women during childbirth, contamination of these tents has caused infection and led to a halt in their use.

Why people use this herb

- As an iodine source
- High blood pressure
- Obesity
- Rheumatism
- To induce abortion
- To prevent breast cancer
- To thin the blood
- Tumors

Common dose

Kelp comes as:

- capsules (380 micrograms, 640 milligrams, and 660 milligrams)
- tablets (150 and 225 micrograms)
- a water extract or powder.

Some experts recommend the following dose:

- One tablet or capsule daily, providing 500 to 650 milligrams of ground kelp. This quantity provides approximately 250 micrograms of elemental iodine (about 150% of the recommended daily allowance).

Side effects

Call your health care practitioner if you experience any of these possible side effects of kelp:

- acne
- bleeding.

This herb also can cause:

- arsenic poisoning (if contaminated)
- bone marrow changes that affect red blood cells
- high blood pressure
- low platelet count.

Interactions

Combining herbs with certain drugs may alter their action or produce unwanted side effects. Don't use kelp while taking drugs that lower blood pressure. If you have abnormal blood clotting or a platelet defect or if you take aspirin, don't use kelp when taking blood thinners, such as Coumadin.

Important points to remember

- If you're pregnant, check with your health care practitioner before using kelp. Applying the herb to your skin may affect the cervix and placenta. Also know that kelp "tents" used to dilate the cervix during delivery have been linked to fetal death.
- Don't use this herb if you're breastfeeding.
- Don't use kelp if you're prone to heart failure or high blood pressure.
- If you feel ill when using large amounts of kelp daily, have your health care practitioner check for arsenic poisoning.
- If you use kelp and take a blood thinner, notify your health care practitioner if you experience bleeding symptoms, such as unexplained bruises, bleeding gums, or blood in the stool.

Other names for kelp

Other names for kelp include brown algae, horsetail, *Laminaria,* sea girdles, seaweed, sugar wrack, and tangleweed.

Products containing kelp are sold under such names as Kelp and Kelp Norwegian.

Selected references

Agress, R.L., and Benedetti, T.J. "Intrauterine Fetal Death During Cervical Ripening with *Laminaria*," *American Journal of Obstetrics and Gynecology* 141:587, 1981.

Okai, Y., et al. "Identification of Heterogenous Antimutagenic Activities in the Extract of Edible Brown Seaweeds, *Laminaria japonica* (Makonbu) and *Undaria pinnatifida* (Wakame) by the Umu Gene Expression System in *Salmonella typhimurium*," *Mutation Research* 303: 63-70, 1993.

Teas, J. "The Dietary Intake of *Laminaria*, a Brown Seaweed, and Breast Cancer Prevention," *Nutrition and Cancer* 4: 217-22, 1983.

Walkin, O., and Douglas, D.E. "Health Food Supplements Prepared From Kelp—A Source of Elevated Urinary Arsenic," *Clinical Toxicology* 8:325-31, 1975.

WHAT THE RESEARCH SHOWS

Scientific studies don't support the use of kelp for cancer prevention. No research has been done to evaluate kelp and blood thinners.

Kelpware

Kelpware comes from *Fucus vesiculosus* (of the Fucaceae family), a brownish green seaweed that grows on rocky areas along the northern coasts of the Atlantic and Pacific oceans. Several species found along the French coastline are used to make kelpware tablets.

Product quality can vary widely. Some products contain eight times as much iodine as others, depending on the plant's origin. *F. vesiculosus* accumulates cadmium and lead in various plant parts, probably because of the heavy metal content of sea water.

Why people use this herb

- Fatty degeneration of the heart
- Goiter (an abnormally large thyroid)
- Inflammatory bladder disease
- Kidney disease
- Menstrual irregularities
- Obesity

Common doses

Kelpware comes as dried plant, soft extract prepared with 45% alcohol, liquid extract, tablets, and softgel formulation with lecithin and B_6. Some experts recommend the following doses:

- For *obesity,* mix 16 grams of bruised plant with 1 pint of water and take 2 fluid ounces orally three times daily.
- As *soft extract,* 200 to 600 milligrams taken orally.
- As *liquid extract,* 4 to 8 milliliters taken orally before meals.
- As *tablets,* three tablets (3.75 grains) taken orally daily, then increase gradually up to 24 tablets daily.

Side effects

Call your health care practitioner if you experience any of these possible side effects of kelpware:

- chronic excessive thirst
- excessive urination.

This herb also can cause:

- high blood sugar
- increased blood creatinine, which may damage the liver.

Interactions

Combining herbs with certain drugs may alter their action or produce unwanted side effects. Tell your health care practitioner about any prescription or nonprescription drugs you're taking, especially:

- aspirin
- blood thinners such as Coumadin.

Important points to remember

- Don't use kelpware if you're pregnant or breast-feeding.
- Avoid this herb if you have cancer, diabetes, a kidney disorder, severe liver disease, heart failure, recent heart attack; if you're elderly; or if you're taking drugs known to cause liver damage.
- If you take thyroid hormone replacement therapy, Lithobid, Cordarone, or a blood thinner, check with your health care practitioner before using kelpware.
- Don't give kelpware to children.
- Know that kelpware may cause symptoms of cadmium, lead, arsenic, or bromide poisoning.
- Be aware that kelpware products may contain iodine.

Other names for kelpware

Other names for kelpware include black-tang, bladder fucus, bladderwrack, blasen-tang, quercus marina, sea wrack, sea-oak, and seetang.

Products containing kelpware are sold under such names as Kelp, Kelp Combination Tabs, Kelp/Lecithin/B6, Kelp Natural Iodine, and Pacific Kelp.

WHAT THE RESEARCH SHOWS

Although kelpware seems to work as a blood thinner, medical experts don't recommend it because it hasn't been tested on people. Most experience with the herb comes from Europe.

As an obesity treatment, kelpware has been criticized. Generally, it's not used to treat life-threatening obesity.

Selected references

Conz, P.A., et al. "*Fucus vesiculosus*: A Nephrotoxic Alga?" *Nephrology Dialysis Transplantation* 13:526-27, 1998.

Criado, M.T., and Ferreiros, C.M. "Selective Interaction of *Fucus vesiculosus* Lectin-like Mucopolysaccaride with Several *Candida* Species," *Annales de Microbiologie* 134:149-54, 1983. Abstract.

Criado, M.T., and Ferreiros, C.M. "Toxicity of an Algal Mucopolysaccharide for *Escherichia coli* and *Neisseria meningitidis* Strains," *Revista Espanola de Fisiologia* 40:227-30, 1984. Abstract.

Dhrig, J., et al. "Anticoagulant Fucoidan Fractions from *Fucus vesiculosus* Induce Platelet Activation in Vitro," *Thrombosis Research* 85:479-91, 1997.

Khat

Chewing khat is a popular form of drug abuse in East Africa, where it's consumed in daily social gatherings and is deeply rooted in cultural tradition (especially among men in Yemen). East Africans consider the red form of the herb superior to the white, which contains less of a component called cathinone.

Khat's effects reportedly are more intense than caffeine's but less intense than those of "speed" and other amphetamines. The sweet-tasting leaves cause dryness of the mouth and throat, usually creating a thirst for large amounts of fluids.

Khat comes from the raw leaves and tender twigs of *Catha edulis*. A member of the staff-tree family (Celastraceae) native to East Africa and the highlands of the Arabian peninsula, the tree grows to a height of 80 feet.

Common dose

Khat comes as raw leaves. Some experts recommend the following dose:

- 100 to 200 grams of raw leaf chewed at a time.

Side effects

Call your health care practitioner if you experience any of these possible side effects of khat:

- decreased sex drive (in men)
- fast pulse
- irregular heartbeats
- large pupils
- migraine
- mouth sores
- overheating and sweating
- reduced appetite
- unusual sense of well-being.

This herb also can cause:

- bleeding in the brain
- decreased pressure within the eye
- gum disease
- heart stoppage

Why people use this herb

- Depression
- Fatigue
- Obesity
- To improve the appetite
- Ulcers

- high blood pressure
- liver damage
- low sperm count and reduced sperm motility
- oral cancers
- pulmonary edema
- stomach and esophagus inflammation.

Chronic khat use may impair performance on perceptual-visual memory and decision speed tests. Khat overdose may lead to hyperactivity, aggressiveness, mania, psychoses, and hallucinations.

Interactions

Combining herbs with certain drugs may alter their action or produce unwanted side effects. Don't use khat if you're taking:

- decongestants
- drugs for irregular heartbeats
- drugs that lower blood pressure
- drugs used to relieve depression called MAO inhibitors (such as Marplan and Nardil)
- heart drugs called beta blockers (such as Inderal).

WHAT THE RESEARCH SHOWS

Medical experts believe khat has little, if any, medicinal value. What's more, researchers have gathered many reports of side effects stemming from khat abuse and overuse. On the positive side, though, khat seems less likely than amphetamines to cause addiction, tolerance, and psychological dependence.

Important points to remember

- Don't use khat if you have heart or blood vessel disease, kidney disease, or high blood pressure.
- Avoid this herb if you're pregnant or breast-feeding because it may cause birth defects.
- Know that if you use khat for a long time and then quit, you may experience withdrawal symptoms, such as depression and sedation. However, researchers doubt that people can become physically dependent on or addicted to khat.
- Be aware that medical experts warn against chewing khat leaves or khat products because the herb may impair nutrition, disrupt the digestive system, and lead to oral cancer.

- Know that elderly people are more likely to have side effects from khat.

Other names for khat

Other names for khat include cat, chat, gad, kaht, kat, miraa, and tschut.

No known products containing khat are available commercially.

Selected references

Elmi, A.S. "The Chewing of Khat in Somalia," *Journal of Ethnopharmacology* 8:163-76, 1983.

Islam, M.W., et al. "An Evaluation of the Male Reproductive Toxicity of Cathinone," *Toxicology* 603:223-34, 1990.

Khella

Active components of khella, including khellin, come from the fruits and seeds of *Ammi visnaga*. A member of the carrot family (Umbelliferae), this plant is native to Egypt and other Middle Eastern countries.

Why people use this herb

- Abdominal cramps
- Angina
- Gallbladder pain
- High cholesterol
- Painful menstruation
- Psoriasis (scaly, raised skin patches)
- To treat severe allergic reactions
- To prevent allergic reactions
- To prevent bronchial asthma
- Vitiligo (smooth, white skin patches)

Common doses

Khella comes as capsules, tablets, teas, and injectable preparations. Some experts recommend the following doses:

- Take an average daily dose of 20 milligrams of khellin.
- For *angina,* 30 to 300 milligrams. (Sources typically are standardized to 12% khellin content.)

Side effects

Call your health care practitioner if you experience any of these possible side effects of khella:

- allergic reactions (such as itching)
- mild sensitivity to sunlight
- sleeplessness.

This herb also can cause:

- elevated liver enzymes
- skin cancer in people predisposed to such cancer.

With prolonged use or overdose, khella may cause:

- constipation
- headache
- nausea
- poor appetite
- vertigo
- vomiting.

Interactions

Combining herbs with certain drugs may alter their action or produce unwanted side effects. Don't use khella while taking:

- blood thinners such as Coumadin
- heart drugs called calcium channel blockers (such as Calan and Procardia)
- other drugs that lower blood pressure.

Important points to remember

- Avoid khella if you're pregnant or breast-feeding.
- If you have liver disease, check with your health care practitioner before using khella.
- Before you take khella for angina symptoms, have your health care practitioner conduct a complete heart examination.
- Know that khella can dramatically enhance the effects of drugs that lower blood pressure.
- If you use khella while taking a blood thinner, watch for symptoms of bleeding (such as unexplained bruises, bleeding gums, or blood in the stool). Report these to your health care practitioner.
- Be aware that khellin applied to the skin increases the cancer-causing effects of ultraviolet light and sunlight.

Other names for khella

Other names for khella include ammi, bishop's weed, khellin, visnaga, and visnagin.

A product containing khella is sold as Khella.

WHAT THE RESEARCH SHOWS

Khella seems to expand blood vessels, working like such drugs as Calan and Procardia. The herb also may be valuable in preventing bronchial and allergic reactions and is being studied for other disorders. However, until these effects are tested on people, medical experts discourage khella use except under a health care professional's supervision.

Selected references

Borges, M.L., et al. "Photophysical Properties and Photobiological Activity of the Furanochromes Visnagin and Khellin," *Photochemistry and Photobiology* 67:184-91, 1998.

Harvengt, C., and Desanger, J.P. "HDL Cholesterol Increase in Normolipaemic Subjects on Khellin: A Pilot Study," *International Journal of Clinical Pharmacology Reseach* 3:363, 1983.

Jansen, T., et al. "Provocation of Porphyria Cutanea Tarda by KUVA-therapy of Vitiligo," *Acta Dermato-Venereologica* 75:232-33, 1995.

Lowe, W., et al. "A Khellin-like 7,7'glycerol-bridged Bischromone with Anti-Anaphylactic Activity," *Archive der Pharmazie* (Weinheim) 327:255-59, 1994.

Osher, H.L., et al. "Khellin in the Treatment of Angina Pectoris," *New England Journal of Medicine* 244:315-21, 1951.

Lady's mantle

Lady's mantle is extracted from the roots, leaves, and flowers of *Alchemilla mollis, A. vulgaris,* and other members of this species. Native to Europe, the plant also grows in the northeastern United States and Canada.

Now used in some herbal cleansing creams and other cosmetics, lady's mantle is rich in folklore. The plant's name, *Alchemilla,* comes from the word "alchemy" because people believed the herb could produce miraculous cures. It has also been linked with the Virgin Mary because the lobes of its leaves resemble the scalloped edges of a cloak.

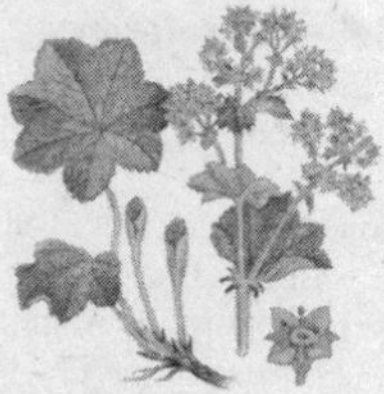

Common dose

Lady's mantle comes in compounded extracts and teas. Some experts recommend the following dose:

- As an *infusion* or *tea,* steep 2 teaspoons of dried herb in 1 cup of boiling water. Take the tea (2 to 4 milliliters) orally three times daily.

Why people use this herb

- Diarrhea
- Menstrual bleeding, cramps, and irregularity
- To aid blood clotting
- Wounds

Side effects

Call your health care practitioner if you experience unusual symptoms when using lady's mantle. Tannins in this herb may lead to liver damage.

Interactions

Combining herbs with certain drugs may alter their action or produce unwanted side effects. Tell your health care practitioner about any prescription or nonprescription drugs you're taking.

Important points to remember

- Don't use lady's mantle if you're breast-feeding or pregnant.
- Know that little information about this herb is available.
- If you use lady's mantle, report weakness, fatigue, or jaundice to your health care practitioner.

Other names for lady's mantle

Other names for lady's mantle include *Alchemilla,* bear's foot, dew-cup, leontopodium, lion's-foot, nine hooks, and stellaria.

Various manufacturers sell products containing this herb under the name Lady's Mantle.

> **WHAT THE RESEARCH SHOWS**
>
> Clinical studies don't support the use of lady's mantle for any condition. Human studies must be done to determine if the herb is safe or effective.

Selected references

Filipek, J. "Effect of *Alchemilla xantochlora* Water Extract on Lipid Peroxidation and Superoxide Anion Scavenging Activity," *Pharmazie* 47:717-18, 1992.

Jonadet, M., et al. "Flavonoids Extracted from *Ribes nigrum* L. and *Alchemilla vulgaris* L.: 1. In vitro Inhibitory Activities on Elastase, Trypsin and Chymotrypsin. 2. Angioprotective Activities Compared In Vivo," *Journal of Pharmacology* 17:21-27, 1986.

Swanson-Flatt, S.K., et al. "Traditional Plant Treatments for Diabetes. Studies in Normal and Streptozotocin Diabetic Mice," *Diabetologia* 33:462-64, 1990.

Lady's slipper, yellow

Native American healers used yellow lady's slipper to treat flu, hysteria, and certain other illnesses. Today, lady's slipper is combined with another herb, valerian root (*Valerian officinalis*), in products that claim to have calming effects.

Lady's slipper comes from the root of the orchid, *Cypripedium pubescens, C. calceolus,* or other species. These plants are sparsely located throughout North American and European forests.

Common doses

Yellow lady's slipper comes as liquid extract, powdered root, dried rhizome (underground stem), teas, and tinctures. Some experts recommend the following doses:

- As *dried rhizome* or *root,* 2 to 4 grams taken orally three times daily.
- As *liquid extract,* 2 to 4 milliliters (1:1 water and 45% alcohol) taken orally three times daily.

Why people use this herb

- As a mild hypnotic or sedative
- Epilepsy
- Headache
- Hysteria
- Low-grade fever
- Muscle spasms
- "Nervous depression" caused by stomach disorders
- Nervousness
- Sharp, stabbing pains

Side effects

Call your health care practitioner if you experience any of these possible side effects of yellow lady's slipper:

- giddiness
- headache
- mental excitement leading to hallucinations
- restlessness
- skin inflammation.

Interactions

Combining herbs with certain drugs may alter their action or produce unwanted side effects. Don't use lady's slipper while taking:

- Larodopa
- Permax
- Requip.

Important points to remember

- Don't use lady's slipper if you have plant allergies.
- Avoid lady's slipper if you're pregnant or breast-feeding.
- If you're bothered by headaches or have a history of mental illness, don't take this herb without consulting your health care practitioner.
- Don't drive or perform other activities that require alertness until you know how lady's slipper affects you.

WHAT THE RESEARCH SHOWS

Researchers haven't adequately studied lady's slipper in people. Consequently, medical experts don't recommend this herb for any therapeutic use.

Other names for lady's slipper

Other names for lady's slipper include American valerian, moccasin flower, nerveroot, Noah's ark, whippoorwill's shoe, and yellow Indian shoe.

No known products containing lady's slipper are available commercially.

Selected reference

Sanchez, T.R., et al. "The Delivery of Culturally Sensitive Health Care to Native Americans," *Journal of Holistic Nursing* 14:295-307, 1996.

Lavender

Although used in small concentrations to flavor food, lavender is cultivated mainly as an ingredient in perfumes or potpourris and for decorations. Some people believe its scent has a calming effect. France is a major producer of lavender products.

Lavender comes from the flowering tops and stalks of *Lavandula officinalis* and other *Lavandula* species. Native to the Mediterranean area, lavender is cultivated widely in American gardens for its color and fragrance. Lavandin, a popular variety, is a hybrid of spike lavender and true lavender.

Common doses

Lavender comes as oils, flowers, and leaves. Some experts recommend the following doses:

- As a *tea,* steep 1 to 2 teaspoons of the herb in 150 milliliters of hot water for approximately 10 minutes.
- As an *oil,* place 1 to 4 drops of oil on a sugar cube and take orally.
- As an *astringent for external use,* add 20 to 100 grams of lavender to 7.7 gallons (20 liters) of water (to avoid too strong a scent).

Why people use this herb

- Insomnia
- Migraine
- Muscle strain
- Restlessness
- Sharp stabbing pains
- To stimulate the appetite
- Upper abdominal discomfort caused by nervousness

Side effects

Call your health care practitioner if you experience unusual symptoms when taking lavender. Consuming large doses may cause:

- constipation
- euphoria, mental dullness, confusion, and drowsiness
- headache
- nausea
- nervous system depression, causing excessive sleepiness or drowsiness, slow breathing, and reduced mental alertness
- skin inflammation
- small pupils
- vomiting.

Interactions

Combining herbs with certain drugs may alter their action or produce unwanted side effects. Don't use lavender when drinking alcohol or taking drugs that cause sedation, such as:

- benzodiazepines (for instance, Ativan, Dalmane, Halcion, Restoril, or Valium)
- narcotic pain relievers.

Important points to remember

- Don't take lavender if you're pregnant or breast-feeding.
- Know that lavender oil is potentially poisonous. Large doses can cause narcotic-like effects. Don't consume more than 2 drops of the volatile oil.
- Before using lavender as a sleep aid, consider such alternatives as behavior modification, light therapy, and a regular bedtime to combat insomnia. Also be aware that prescription sedative and hypnotic drugs have known risks and benefits, whereas lavender doesn't.

Other names for lavender

Other names for lavender include aspic, echter lavendel, English lavender (*Lavandula angustifolia),* esplieg, French lavender, garden lavender, lavanda, lavande commun, lavandin, nardo, Spanish lavender *(L. stoechas*), spigo, spike lavender, and true lavender.

Products containing lavender are sold under such names as Lavender and Lavender Flowers.

Selected references

Nelson, R.R.S. "In-Vitro Activities of Five Plant Essential Oils Against Methicillin-Resistant *Staphylococcus aureus* and Vancomycin-Resistant *Enterococcus faecium*," *Journal of Antimicrobial Chemotherapy* 40:305-06, 1997.

Ziegler, J. "Raloxifene, Retinoids, and Lavender: 'Me Too' Tamoxifen Alternatives," *Journal of the National Cancer Institute* 88:1100-02, 1996.

WHAT THE RESEARCH SHOWS

Although lavender has been used medicinally for centuries, scientific studies haven't shown its value in treating any disease or condition. Until controlled studies with people are done, medical experts won't recommend this herb.

Licorice

Used medicinally since Roman times, licorice is still popular in Chinese herbal medicine. The "licorice candy" sold in the United States usually is flavored with anise oil and doesn't actually contain licorice. Besides serving as a flavoring and sweetener for bitter drugs, licorice is an ingredient in some tobacco products, chewing gums, candies, beverages, toothpastes, and shampoos.

Most licorice remedies come from the roots of *Glycyrrhiza glabra,* a perennial low-growing shrub native to the Mediterranean region. Spanish licorice is the most common variety, but *G. glabra* plants are widely cultivated in the United States, Russia, Spain, Turkey, Greece, India, Italy, Iran, and Iraq.

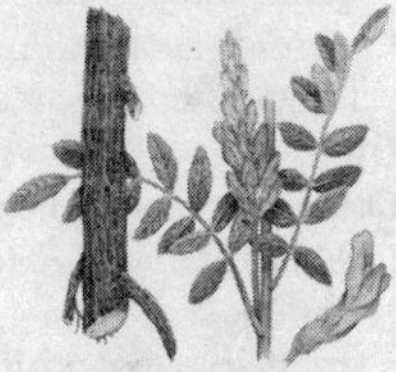

Common dose

Licorice comes as:
- capsules (100 to 520 milligrams)
- tablets (7 milligrams of licorice root plus 333 milligrams of garlic concentrate)
- liquid extracts
- teas
- tobacco products
- chewing gums
- throat lozenges
- candy.

Some experts recommend the following dose:
- For *peptic ulcer,* take 200 to 600 milligrams orally daily for no more than 4 to 6 weeks. Or make a tea by placing 2 to 4 grams of licorice in ½ cup of boiling water and simmering for 5 minutes. Cool and strain the tea, then drink three times daily after consuming food.

Why people use this herb
- Addison's disease (a life-threatening endocrine disorder)
- Cold sores
- Common cold
- Cough
- Eczema (a type of skin inflammation)
- Mouth sores
- Stomach pain

Side effects

Call your health care practitioner if you experience any of these possible side effects of licorice:

- headache
- muscle weakness
- swelling (from salt and fluid retention).

Licorice also may cause:
- heart failure (with overdose)
- high blood pressure
- a muscle disorder called rhabdomyolysis.

Interactions

Combining herbs with certain drugs may alter their action or produce unwanted side effects. Tell your health care practitioner about prescription or nonprescription drugs you're taking, especially:
- Claritin
- Procan SR
- quinidine
- steroids such as Prednisone
- topical steroid salves and lotions.

Don't use licorice when taking:
- Aldactone
- diuretics
- drugs that lower blood pressure
- Lanoxin.

Important points to remember

- Don't use licorice if you have high blood pressure; irregular heartbeats; or cerebrovascular, kidney, or liver disease.
- Don't use this herb if you're pregnant or breast-feeding.
- Be aware that licorice can be poisonous when used in high doses for long periods.
- Know that a single large dose of licorice is less likely to make you sick than long-term use of smaller amounts.
- Keep in mind that symptoms of licorice poisoning may be subtle. Report headache, lethargy, swelling, and irregular heartbeats to your health care practitioner.

Other names for licorice

Other names for licorice include Chinese licorice, licorice root, Persian licorice, Russian licorice, Spanish licorice, and sweet root.

> **WHAT THE RESEARCH SHOWS**
>
> Researchers have studied licorice extensively as a treatment for peptic ulcers. They've found that it performs no better than established drugs, may cause more side effects, and can be poisonous if taken in large doses for a long time.
>
> However, glycyrrhetic acid, a chemical made from the licorice plant, shows promise in enhancing the effects of steroid preparations applied to the skin.

Products containing licorice are sold under such names as Full Potency Licorice Root Vegicaps, Licorice ATC Concentrate, Licorice and Garlic, Licorice Root Extract, Licorice Root Tea, Natural Arthro-Rx, Solaray Licorice Root, Tea with Mint, and Tummy Soother.

Selected references

Bardhan, K.D., et al. "Clinical Trial of Deglycyrrhizinised Licorice in Gastric Ulcer," *Gut* 19:779-82, 1978.

LaBrooy, S.J., et al. "Controlled Comparison of Cimetidine and Carbenoxolone Sodium in Gastric Ulcer," *BMJ* 1:1308-09, 1979.

Marks, I.N. "Current Therapy in Peptic Ulcer," *Drugs* 20:283-99, 1980.

Maxton, D.G., et al. "Controlled Trial of Pyrogastrone and Cimetidine in the Treatment of Reflux Oesophagitis," *Gut* 31:351-54, 1990.

Lily of the valley

Lily of the valley has been used traditionally for heart conditions—a use that medical experts consider dangerous. In Germany, the flowers are mixed with raisins to make a wine.

Why people use this herb

- As a heart "tonic"
- As an antidote to poisonous gas
- Heart valve disease
- Seizures
- To help burns heal and prevent scar formation

The herb comes from the leaves, roots, and flowers of *Convallaria majalis*. This low-growing perennial is native to Europe and cultivated throughout North America. The essential oils of the highly aromatic flowers have been used in perfumes and cosmetics. However, the Food and Drug Administration considers lily of the valley an unsafe and poisonous plant.

Common dose

Lily of the valley is available as extracts. Experts disagree on what dose to take.

Side effects

Call your health care practitioner if you experience any of these possible side effects of lily of the valley:

- abdominal pain and cramping
- burning pain in the mouth and throat
- cold, clammy skin
- diarrhea
- dizziness
- enlarged pupils
- excessive salivation
- hallucinations
- headache
- irregular heartbeats
- nausea
- paralysis
- skin inflammation from contact with the leaves
- urinary urgency
- vomiting.

This herb also can cause:

- coma
- death
- heart failure
- too much potassium in the blood, leading to weakness, nausea, diarrhea, intestinal pain, and a slow pulse.

Interactions

Combining herbs with certain drugs may alter their action or produce unwanted side effects. Don't use lily of the valley while taking:

- heart drugs called beta blockers (such as Inderal)
- heart drugs called calcium channel blockers (such as Calan and Procardia)
- Lanoxin.

Important points to remember

- Know that taking any part of this plant is inadvisable.
- Never use lily of the valley for a heart condition because it may be toxic and experts don't agree on a safe dose.

Other names for lily of the valley

Other names for lily of the valley include *Convallaria*, Jacob's ladder, ladder-to-heaven, lily constancy, lily convalle, male lily, May lily, muguet, and Our-Lady's-tears.

No known products containing lily of the valley are available commercially.

WHAT THE RESEARCH SHOWS

Medical experts don't recommend lily of the valley. When used to treat heart failure and other heart conditions, this highly toxic, poorly studied herb might have effects similar to those of Lanoxin and other prescription drugs. But there's little reason to take it because those tested, proven drugs are widely available.

Selected reference

Swanston-Flatt, S.K., et al. "Traditional Plant Treatments for Diabetes: Studies in Normal and Streptozotocin Diabetic Mice," *Diabetologia* 33:462-64, 1990.

Lobelia

Because lobelia has nicotine-like effects, some people have used it to help them stop smoking. Lobelia comes primarily from the dried leaves and tops of *Lobelia inflata*. This plant, with long clusters of showy flowers, is native to moist woodlands in eastern North America. Other species include *L. berlandieri*, *L. cardinalis*, and *L. siphilitica*.

Common dose

Lobelia comes as:

- capsules (395 milligrams)
- tablets (2 milligrams)
- lozenges (1 milligram)
- extract.

Why people use this herb

- As a smoking cessation aid
- Asthma
- Bronchitis
- Muscle spasms
- To induce vomiting

Some experts recommend the following dose:

- As a *smoking deterrent,* 0.5 to 2 milligrams in tablets or lozenges. The usual dose is 2 milligrams taken orally after each meal with ½ glass of water for no more than 6 weeks. Oral doses up to 8 milligrams have been used but caused significant stomach upset. Daily oral doses of lobeline (an alkaloid in the herb) exceeding 20 milligrams are considered poisonous.

Side effects

Call your health care practitioner if you experience any of these possible side effects of lobelia:

- coughing
- dizziness
- fluid retention
- nausea and vomiting (with higher doses)
- palpitations
- seizures
- severe heartburn
- stomach pain
- sweating
- tremors.

Lobelia also may cause:

- death (from respiratory depression and respiratory muscle paralysis)
- increased blood pressure
- respiratory slowing (with high doses) or stimulation (with low doses)
- slow pulse.

Interactions

Combining herbs with certain drugs may alter their action or produce unwanted side effects. Don't use lobelia while taking drugs used for nicotine therapy.

Important points to remember

- Don't use lobelia if you're pregnant or breast-feeding.
- Don't give this herb to children.
- Be aware that an overdose of lobeline (an alkaloid in lobelia) causes such symptoms as an irregular heartbeat, extreme sweating, dizziness (from low blood pressure), muscle twitching, seizures, chills, and coma.
- If you have liver or kidney problems, check with your health care practitioner before using this herb.
- To help stop smoking, medical experts recommend smoking cessation programs, counseling, behavior modification, nicotine replacement, and other drugs instead of lobelia.
- Don't use any product containing lobeline for more than 6 weeks because researchers have no information about long-term use.

Other names for lobelia

Other names for lobelia include asthma weed, bladderpod, cardinal flower, eyebright, gagroot, great lobelia, Indian pink, Indian tobacco, pukeweed, rapuntium inflatum, and vomitwort.

Products containing lobelia are sold under such names as Bantron Tablets, Lobelia Capsules, Lobelia Extract, Lobeline Lozenges, and Lobidram Computabs.

WHAT THE RESEARCH SHOWS

Because it's similar to nicotine, lobeline, an alkaloid in lobelia, has been used to help people stop smoking. However, no long-term data are available and no clinical trials have been done. Lobeline can cause more serious side effects than other smoking cessation treatments. Therefore, medical experts don't recommend it.

Selected references

Damaj, M.I., et al. "Pharmacology of Lobeline, a Nicotine Receptor Ligand," *Journal of Pharmacology and Experimental Therapeutics* 282:410-19, 1997.

Rapp, G.W., and Olen, A.A. "A Critical Evaluation of a Lobeline-Based Smoking Deterrent," *American Journal of Medical Sciences* 230:9-14, 1955.

Westfall, T.C., and Meldrum, M.J. "Ganglionic Blocking Agents," in Craig, C.R., and Stizel, R.E. *Modern Pharmacology,* 2nd ed. Boston: Little, Brown and Company, 1986.

Lovage

Lovage comes from the roots and seeds of lovage varieties called *Levisticum officinale* and *L. radix*. Found in southern Europe, these plants have been naturalized to the United States. Lovage oil is used as a fragrance in some cosmetics, lotions, and soaps.

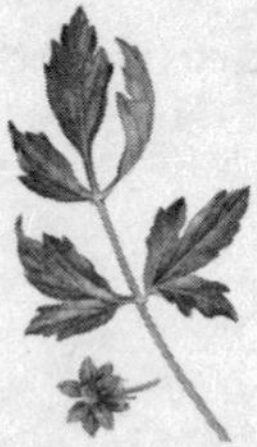

Common dose

Lovage comes as an herbal tea and an essential oil. Some experts recommend the following dose:

- As a *tea,* pour 1 cup (150 milliliters) of boiling water into 1.5 to 3 grams of finely cut lovage root. Drain after 15 minutes. Drink 4 to 8 grams daily.

Side effects

Call your health care practitioner if you experience skin changes from light exposure when using lovage.

Interactions

Combining herbs with certain drugs may alter their action or produce unwanted side effects. Don't use lovage while taking blood thinners such as Coumadin.

Why people use this herb

- As a sedative
- Fluid retention
- Intestinal gas
- Menstrual irregularity
- Muscle spasms
- Stomach pain
- To dissolve phlegm
- To prevent kidney stones
- Urinary tract inflammation

Important points to remember

- Don't use lovage if you're pregnant or breast-feeding.
- Know that lovage may aggravate plant allergies.
- If you're using lovage as a diuretic, remember that swollen ankles and legs may indicate heart failure or another potentially dangerous condition that calls for a complete medical examination.
- Remember that proven diuretics are available to use instead of lovage.

Other names for lovage

Other names for lovage include *Aetheroleum levistici*, *Angelica levisticum, Hipposelinum levisticum,* maggi plant, sea parsley, and smellage.

WHAT THE RESEARCH SHOWS

Although some evidence suggests lovage can ease muscle spasms and cause sedation in animals, scientists haven't done enough studies on people. Therefore, medical experts don't recommend this herb.

No known products containing lovage are available commercially.

Selected reference

Gijbels, M.J.M., et al. "Phthalides in the Essential Oil From Roots of *Levisticum officinale*," *Planta Medica* 44:207-11, 1982.

Lungwort

Historically, lungwort has been used to treat lung ailments. In fact, the herb gets its name from the spotted leaves of *Pulmonaria officinalis,* which resemble the surface of a lung. *P. officinalis* is a member of the Borage family.

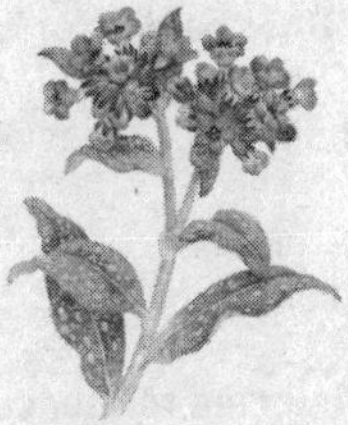

Common doses

Lungwort comes as tablets and extracts. Some experts recommend the following doses:

- As a *tincture,* 1 to 4 milliliters taken orally three times daily.
- As an *infusion,* steep 1 to 2 teaspoons of dried herb in boiling water, and drink three times daily.

Why people use this herb

- Bronchitis
- Cough
- Diarrhea
- Digestive tract bleeding
- Excessive menstruation
- Flu
- Hemorrhoids
- Hoarseness
- Tuberculosis
- Wounds.

Side effects

Call your health care practitioner if you experience any of these possible side effects of lungwort:

- prolonged bleeding
- skin inflammation
- upset stomach.

Interactions

Combining herbs with certain drugs may alter their action or produce unwanted side effects. Don't use lungwort while taking blood thinners such as Coumadin.

Important points to remember

- Don't use lungwort if you're pregnant or breast-feeding.
- If you have a history of digestive tract bleeding, low platelet count, or allergies, check with your health care practitioner before using lungwort.
- Know that medical experts recommend using conventional drug therapy for asthma, bronchitis, and emphysema instead of lungwort.

WHAT THE RESEARCH SHOWS

Scientists don't understand the chemical basis for lungwort's effects on the respiratory system. Because they haven't tested the herb on people, medical experts don't consider it safe or effective.

Other names for lungwort

Other names for lungwort include Jerusalem cowslip, Jerusalem sage, lung moss, lungs of oak, and spotted comfrey.

A product containing lungwort is sold as Lungwort Compound (formerly Bleeders Blend).

Selected reference

Byshevskii, A., et al. "Nature, Properties and the Mechanism of the Effect of Blood Coagulation of the Preparation Obtained from *Pulmonaria officinalis*," *Gematologiia Transfuziologiia* 35:6-9, 1990.

Madder

Madder-dyed cloth has been found on Egyptian mummies. The herb also colored the red trousers of French soldiers and Turkish fezzes. Because alizarin, a red dye obtained from the roots of the madder plant, stains living bone red, medical researchers in the 1800s used the herb to trace bone development and bone cell function. (Eventually, synthetic alizarin replaced the natural product.)

Madder consists of the dried roots of *Rubia tinctorum*. The plant is native to parts of the Mediterranean, Europe, and Asia and cultivated in some areas of North America.

Common doses

Madder comes as dried root and fluid extract. Some experts recommend the following doses:

- As an *infusion* or a *decoction from dried root,* 1 to 2 grams taken orally four times daily for up to 2 months.
- 20 drops of the fluid extract or 1 capsule (from dried root tincture) taken orally three times daily for up to 2 months.

Why people use this herb

- Bladder stones
- Jaundice
- Kidney stones
- Lack of menstruation
- Paralysis
- Sciatica (severe hip and leg pain)

Side effects

Call your health care practitioner if you notice red-tinged breast milk, perspiration, saliva, tears, or urine.

Madder has caused intestinal and liver tumors in rats.

Interactions

Combining herbs with certain drugs may alter their action or produce unwanted side effects. Tell your health care practitioner about any prescription or nonprescription drugs you're taking.

Important points to remember

- Don't use madder if you're pregnant or breast-feeding because lucidin, found in madder, may cause mutations and cancer.
- Be aware that madder may stain your contact lenses.

Other names for madder

Other names for madder include dyer's-madder, garance, krapp, madder root, and robbia.

Products containing madder are sold under such names as Nephrubin, Rubia Teep, Rubicin, and Uralyt.

WHAT THE RESEARCH SHOWS

Researchers haven't tested madder on people so they don't know if it has medicinal value. However, they suspect the herb may harm DNA. For this reason, medical experts strongly discourage its use.

Selected references

Berg, W., et al. "Influence of Anthraquinones on the Formation of Urinary Calculi in Experimental Animals," *Urologe* [A] 15:188-91, 1976. Abstract, author's translation.

Blomeke, B., et al. "Formation of Genotoxic Metabolites from Anthraquinone Glycosides Present in *Rubia tinctorum* L.," *Mutation Research* 265:263-72, 1992. Abstract.

Ino, N., et al. "Acute and Subacute Toxicity Tests of Madder Root, Natural Colorant Extracted from Madder (*Rubia tinctorum*), in (C57BL/6 X C3H) F1 Mice," *Toxicology and Industrial Health* 11:449-58, 1995. Abstract.

Poginsky, B, et al. "Evaluation of DNA-Binding Activity of Hydroxyanthraquinones Occurring in *Rubia tinctorum* L.," *Carcinogenesis* 12:1265-71, 1991. Abstract.

Male fern

Greek physicians recommended male fern as a delousing potion as far back as 103 A.D. Today, London's Foods Standards Committee cautions against using the herb as a flavoring agent in foods.

Male fern comes from the dried rhizomes (underground stems) and roots of *Dryopteris filix-mas*, a perennial fern found in Europe, Asia, North America, South America, and northern Africa. Herbalists treat fresh rhizomes with ether to produce the herb's active components. When stored, rhizomes lose their herbal value in about 6 months.

Why people use this herb

- Intestinal tapeworms

Common doses

Male fern comes as extract, an extract draught (4 grams of male fern extract), and capsules (single- or combination-product). Some experts recommend the following doses:

- For *adults* (after fasting), 3 to 6 milliliters taken orally.
- For *children over age* 2, 0.25 to 0.5 milliliter per year of age taken orally. The maximum dose is 4 milliliters taken in equal doses.
- For *children up to age* 2, no more than 2 milliliters taken orally in equal doses.

Some people have received 50 milliliters of male fern draught through a stomach tube to reduce digestive tract intolerance to the herb. This treatment may need to be repeated every 7 to 10 days. Male fern may be given as capsules but is considered more effective as a draught.

Side effects

Call your health care practitioner if you experience any of these possible side effects of male fern:

- abdominal cramps
- diarrhea
- headache
- nausea
- shortness of breath
- vomiting.

Male fern also may increase bilirubin and albumin levels in the blood.

Severe poisoning from the herb may cause respiratory failure, seizures, optic nerve pain, heart failure, coma, and death.

Interactions

Combining herbs with certain drugs may alter their action or produce unwanted side effects. Don't use male fern within 1 to 2 hours of taking an antacid. Don't use male fern when taking:

- fats and oils, such as castor oil
- Prevacid
- Prilosec.

Important points to remember

- Don't use male fern if you're elderly or debilitated.
- Avoid male fern if you're pregnant or breast-feeding.
- Don't give this herb to infants.
- Avoid male fern if you have anemia, ulcers, or a disease of the heart, liver, or kidney.
- If you're taking prescribed drugs to treat a liver condition, check with your health care practitioner before using male fern.
- Take the herb on an empty stomach.

Other names for male fern

Other names for male fern include bear's paw, erkek egrelti, helecho macho, knotty brake, shield fern, sweet brake, and wurmfarn.

Products containing male fern are sold under such names as Aspidium Oleoresin, Bontanifuge, Extractum Filicis, Extractum Filicis Aethereum, Extractum Filicis Maris Tenue, Male Fern Oleoresin, and Paraway Plus.

Selected reference

Alterio, D.L. "Treatment of Taeniasis with Ether Extract of Male Fern Administered by Duodenal Intubation," *Tropical Diseases Bulletin* 66:831, 1969.

WHAT THE RESEARCH SHOWS

Male fern shows promise in treating tapeworms. But researchers don't know if the herb is effective by itself or only when used with other treatments, such as a low-residue diet and laxatives. Medical experts point out that prescription tapeworm treatments are much safer than male fern. Nonetheless, if such drugs fail, a person may want to consider using male fern after weighing its possible benefits against its side effects.

Mallow

People have been eating young mallow leaves and shoots since the 8th century B.C. The Spanish captured the herb's importance in the adage, "A kitchen garden and mallow, sufficient medicines for a home." Mallow comes from the dried leaves and flowers of *Malva sylvestris*, a member of the mallow family (Malvaceae) that's related to the hibiscus. Recently, researchers have begun to examine mallow's structural and molecular properties.

Why people use this herb

- As a skin astringent
- Bronchitis
- Constipation
- Cough
- Digestive tract irritation
- Hoarseness
- Laryngitis
- Mouth and throat irritation
- Pain from skin abrasions and insect stings
- Swelling and allergic skin irritation
- Teething pain
- To eliminate toxins
- Tonsillitis
- Vaginal irritation

Common dose

Mallow comes as dried herb and fluid extract. Some experts recommend the following dose:

- Eat 5 grams of the chopped, dried herb daily, or take an infusion orally.

Side effects

Call your health care practitioner if you experience unusual symptoms when using mallow.

Interactions

Combining herbs with certain drugs may alter their action or produce unwanted side effects. Tell your health care practitioner about any prescription or nonprescription drugs you're taking.

Important points to remember

- Avoid mallow if you're pregnant or breast-feeding.
- Don't confuse this herb with the similar-sounding marshmallow (*Althaea officinalis*), described on pages 350 and 351.

Other names for mallow

Other names for mallow include blue mallow, cheeseflower, cheeseweed, field mallow, fleurs de mauve, high mallow, *Malva parviflora*, malve, and zigbli.

Products containing mallow are sold under such names as Malvedrin and Malveol.

WHAT THE RESEARCH SHOWS

No studies support the use of mallow for any medical condition. Because the herb contains tannin, medical experts think it may work as a skin astringent. However, they don't recommend long-term or heavy use.

Selected references

Farina, A., et al. "HPTLC and Reflectance Mode Densitometry of Anthocyanins in *Malva silvestris* L.: A Comparison with Gradient-Elution Reversed-Phase HPLC," *Journal of Pharmceutical and Biomedical Analysis* 14:203-11, 1995. Abstract.

Gonda, R., et al. "Structure and Anticomplementary Activity of an Acidic Polysaccharide from the Leaves of *Malva sylvestris* var. *mauritiana*," *Carbohydrate Research* 198:323-29, 1990. Abstract.

Tomoda, M., et al. "Plant Mucilages. XLII. An Anticomplementary Mucilage from the Leaves of *Malva sylvestris* var. *mauritiana*." *Chemical and Pharmaceutical Bulletin* (Tokyo) 37:3029-32, 1989. Abstract.

Marigold

Marigold's botanical name, *Calendula officinalis*, reflects the fact that the plant seems to be in bloom the first day of each calendar month. Herbal components come from the small, bright yellow-orange flower heads of *C. officinalis*. Researchers have also examined the shoots and leaves for active compounds.

An annual, this plant is native to southern Europe and the eastern Mediterranean and now grows in many parts of the United States and Canada. It probably originated in Egypt, where it was valued as a rejuvenating herb. During the American Civil War, field doctors reportedly used marigold leaves on open wounds.

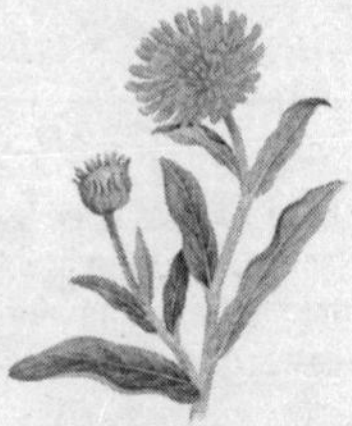

Why people use this herb

- As an antiseptic
- As a skin treatment during aromatherapy
- Bedsores
- Chapped lips
- Cracked nipples from breast-feeding
- Leg ulcers
- Skin inflammation
- To aid digestion
- To enhance bile production
- To promote skin healing
- Varicose veins

Common doses

Marigold comes as an ointment of 5% flower extract, an infusion, and a mouthwash. Some experts recommend the following doses:

- As an *ointment,* apply to the skin.
- As a *tincture* or *tea,* take 1 to 4 milliliters orally daily.

Side effects

Call your health care practitioner if you experience an allergic reaction when using marigold.

Interactions

Combining herbs with certain drugs may alter their action or produce unwanted side effects. Tell your health care practitioner about any prescription or nonprescription drugs you're taking.

Important points to remember

- Don't use marigold if you're pregnant or breast-feeding.
- Don't confuse *C. officinalis* with other ornamental marigolds, such

as *Tagetes patula* (French marigold), *T. erecta* (African marigold), or *T. minuta* (Inca marigold). Known for their ability to repel insects and earthworms, these plants are found in many vegetable gardens.

- Know that marigold carries a risk of allergic reactions.

Other names for marigold

Other names for marigold include calendula, garden marigold, and pot marigold.

> **WHAT THE RESEARCH SHOWS**
>
> Marigold has been used for centuries to aid skin healing—apparently without causing problems. Although some animal tests support its healing and anti-inflammatory effects, the herb hasn't been tested on people. More research must be done to confirm other claims for marigold's medicinal uses.

No known products containing marigold are available commercially.

Selected references

Akihisa, T., et al. "Triterpene Alcohols from the Flowers of Compositae and their Anti-Inflammatory Effects," *Phytochemistry* 43:1255-60, 1996.

Chew, B.P., et al. "Effects of Lutein from Marigold Extract on Immunity and Growth of Mammary Tumors in Mice," *Anticancer Research* 16:3689-94, 1996.

Kalvatchev, Z., et al. "Different Effects of Phorbol Ester Derivatives on Human Immunodeficiency Virus 1 Replication in Lymphocytic and Monocytic Human Cells," *Acta Virologica* 41:289-92, 1997.

Zitterl-Eglseer, K., et al. "Anti-Oedematous Activities of the Main Triterpendiol Esters of Marigold (*Calendula officinalis* L.)," *Journal of Ethnopharmacology* 57:139-44, 1997.

Marjoram

Early Greeks believed marjoram was cultivated by Aphrodite, the Greek goddess of love. The herb is still added to love potions and placed in hope chests or under a woman's pillow to ensure a happy marriage. The Food and Drug Administration regards marjoram as generally safe.

Typically, products identified as marjoram are the dried leaves and flowering tops of *Origanum majorana* L., a member of the mint family (Labiatae). However, similar species exist. The name "wild marjoram" usually refers to *O. vulgare*, more commonly known as oregano.

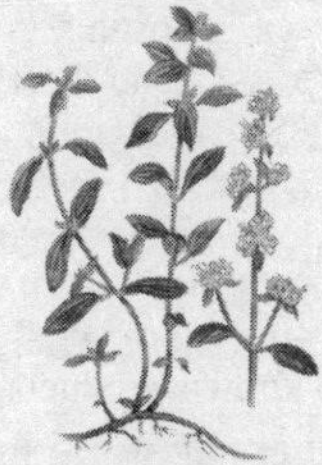

Common doses

Marjoram comes as dried or powdered leaves and a tea. Some experts recommend the following doses:

- As a *tea,* steep 1 to 2 teaspoons of dried leaves and flower tops for 10 minutes in 1 cup of boiling water. Drink no more than 3 cups daily.
- As a *tincture,* ½ to 1 teaspoon taken orally three times daily.

Side effects

Call your health care practitioner if you experience unusual symptoms when using marjoram.

Although apparently no one has been harmed by consuming marjoram, product labels on certain preparations of the essential oil warn against internal use. The marjoram ingredients thymol and hydroquinone may be poisonous.

Interactions

Combining herbs with certain drugs may alter their action or produce unwanted side effects. Tell your health care practitioner about any prescription or nonprescription drugs you're taking.

Why people use this herb

- As a snakebite antidote
- Bruises
- Certain cancers
- Conjunctivitis (infection of the eye's inner lining)
- Cough
- Headache
- Insomnia
- Lack of menstruation
- Menstrual cramps
- Motion sickness
- Muscle and joint pain
- Nausea
- Sharp intestinal pains in infants
- To prevent intestinal gas
- To stimulate digestion

Important points to remember

- If you're pregnant, don't use marjoram in amounts larger than those commonly used in cooking. An overdose carries a slight risk of uterine contractions.
- Be aware that researchers don't know if the herb is safe for infants and children.
- Avoid using the volatile oil.
- Know that the content of some active marjoram components varies among plants and products and that the volatile oil content may decrease with age.
- Reduce your dose or discontinue the herb if you experience nausea, vomiting, or diarrhea. Consult your health care practitioner if nausea and diarrhea last more than a few days.
- Keep marjoram away from the eyes.
- Know that medical experts caution against consuming more marjoram than you'd normally find in foods.
- Be aware that thyme, not marjoram, is the source of the essential oils called "Oil of Marjoram" and "Wild Marjoram Oil."

Other names for marjoram

Other names for marjoram include common marjoram, knotted marjoram, oleum majoranae (oil), oregano, sweet marjoram, and wild marjoram.

WHAT THE RESEARCH SHOWS

Marjoram extracts help ease spasms, which may account for their use in treating nausea, sharp intestinal pains, and menstrual cramps. The herb is considered a safe food additive, so consuming moderate amounts in food or tea probably won't cause harm—and may even relieve nausea, sharp intestinal pains, and cramps.

In the test tube, certain marjoram components (thymol and carvacrol) help fight bacteria, viruses, and fungi. However, their concentrations vary widely, making them unreliable for treating infections. As a toothache remedy, marjoram's effects may come from thymol's ability to combat oral bacteria. Still, medical experts recommend conventional drugs instead to treat suspected oral infections.

Little evidence supports marjoram's other therapeutic claims. Experts caution people to restrict marjoram to oral intake or topical use on the skin. They warn against applying it to open wounds, rashes, or the eye.

Products containing marjoram are sold under such names as Marjoram and Sweet Marjoram Essential Oil.

Selected references

Assaf, M.H., et al. "Preliminary Study of Phenolic Glycosides from *Origanum majorana*; Quantitative Estimation of Arbutin; Cytotoxic Activity Of Hydroquinone," *Planta Medica* 53:343-45, 1987.

Van Den Broucke, C.O., and Lemli, J.A. "Antispasmodic Activity of *Origanum compactum*," *Planta Medica* 38:317-31, 1980.

Marshmallow

Unprocessed marshmallow comes from the dried roots of *Althaea officinalis,* a perennial herb native to Europe that also grows in the United States. Some herbalists use the flowers and leaves as well as the roots.

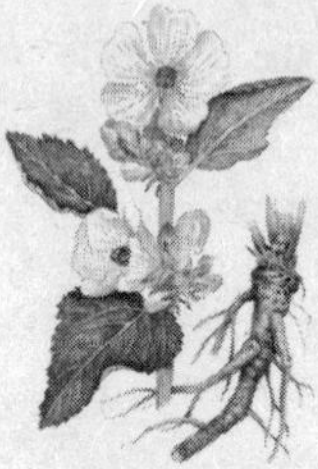

Why people use this herb

- As a cough suppressant
- Constipation
- Gastritis (inflammation of the stomach lining)
- Irritable bowel syndrome
- Minor abrasions
- Peptic ulcer
- Skin inflammation
- Throat irritation

Common doses

Marshmallow comes as whole dried root, dried leaves or flowers, capsules containing powdered root, and extracts. Some experts recommend the following doses:

- As the *crude root* or a *formulation,* 6 grams taken orally daily.
- As the *leaf,* 5 grams taken orally daily.

Side effects

Call your health care practitioner if you experience unusual symptoms when using marshmallow.

Interactions

Combining herbs with certain drugs may alter their action or produce unwanted side effects. If you take other drugs, stagger their administration times with marshmallow's because the herb may slow drug absorption. Also, don't use marshmallow if you take insulin because it may make your blood sugar drop too low.

Important point to remember

- Avoid this herb if you're pregnant or breast-feeding.

Other names for marshmallow

Other names for marshmallow include althaea root, althea, mortification root, and sweetweed.

No known medicinal products containing marshmallow are available commercially.

WHAT THE RESEARCH SHOWS

Without adequate research showing that marshmallow is effective, medical experts don't recommend it for any condition or disease. They advise people to eat only the amounts normally found in food.

Selected references

Recio, M.C., et al. "Antimicrobial Activity of Selected Plants Employed in the Spanish Mediterranean Area, Part II," *Phytotherapy Research* 3:77-80, 1989.

Tomoda, M., et al. "Hypoglycemic Activity of Twenty Plant Mucilages and Three Modified Products," *Planta Medica* 53:8-12, 1987.

Mayapple

Mayapple fruit is an ingredient in some drinks, marmalades, and jellies. Herbal mayapple preparations come from extracts of the rhizomes (underground stems) of *Podophyllum peltatum*. This perennial herb grows wild in North American forests. Don't confuse it with *Mandragora officinarum*, also called "mandrake," which is native to the Mediterranean area and causes different effects.

Why people use this herb

- As a stimulant
- Cancer
- Genital and anal warts
- Liver congestion
- Plantar warts
- To cause bowel evacuation
- To induce vomiting
- Tumors

Common doses

Mayapple comes as:

- dried root
- prescription-only resinous extract (0.5% podophyllotoxin in alcohol)
- concentrated tincture (5% to 25% solution in alcohol or compound benzoin tincture).

A mayapple component is available commercially in various synthetic anticancer drugs.

Some experts recommend the following doses:

- As a *powdered root,* 10 to 30 grains taken orally daily.
- As a *tincture,* 1 to 10 drops taken orally once or twice daily.
- As *5% to 25% solution in alcohol* or *compound benzoin tincture,* apply to warts once a week. Leave on for 1 to 6 hours, then wash off. If symptoms don't improve after 4 weeks, consider other treatment.
- As a *resin,* apply to warts twice daily for 3 days in a row. Don't wash the resin off. Repeat application at weekly intervals for up to 5 weeks. Treat a small number of warts at one time.

Side effects

Call your health care practitioner if you experience any of these possible side effects of mayapple:

- abdominal pain
- diarrhea
- dizziness when rising from a sitting or lying position (from low blood pressure)

- irritation of the skin, eyes, or mucous membranes (when using the resin)
- nausea
- nervous system effects, such as acute psychotic reactions, poor muscle coordination, confusion, dizziness, hallucinations, muscle weakness, seizures, and stupor
- numbness, prickling, or tingling in the arms and legs
- rapid pulse
- vomiting.

This herb also can cause:

- breathing stoppage
- coma
- decreased reflexes
- kidney failure
- liver damage
- low blood cell counts
- urine retention.

Except for the ripe fruits, the entire mayapple plant is toxic. Eating the herb or putting it on your skin may lead to severe systemic poisoning. Applying the resin to widespread skin lesions can cause serious nervous system problems and even death.

Interactions

Combining herbs with certain drugs may alter their action or produce unwanted side effects. Tell your health care practitioner about any prescription or nonprescription drugs you're taking.

Important points to remember

- Don't use mayapple if you're pregnant or breast-feeding.
- Avoid this herb if you have diabetes or poor circulation or if you use steroids.
- Don't put the resin on a crumbly or bleeding wart, an unusual wart with hair growing from it, or on a recently biopsied wart, mole, or birthmark.
- Know that mayapple can cause extremely violent laxative and nervous system effects.
- Be aware that mayapple resin and tincture are for external use only. Consult your health care practitioner before using them.
- Keep the resin away from your eyes.

- Immediately report unusual bruising, bleeding, or infection.
- Keep mayapple products out of reach of children and pets.

WHAT THE RESEARCH SHOWS

Researchers have documented mayapple's ability to stop cell division. Consequently, this herb has many established uses, such as in treating tumors and venereal warts. However, the ability to stop cell division also contributes to the herb's toxicity. Other therapeutic claims for mayapple, including its use as a liver remedy, remain unproven.

Other names for mayapple

Other names for mayapple include devil's-apple, hog apple, Indian apple, mandrake, umbrella plant, and wild lemon.

Products containing mayapple are sold under such names as Condylox, Podocon-25, Podofilm, Warix, and Wartec.

Selected references

Dobb, G.J., et al. "Coma and Neuropathy After Ingestion of Herbal Laxative Containing Podophyllin," *Medical Journal of Australia* 140:495, 1984.

Rate, R.G., et al. "Podophyllin Toxicity," *Annals of Internal Medicine* 90:723, 1979.

Meadowsweet

Meadowsweet was among the ancient Druids' most sacred herbs, although no one knows if they used it medicinally. In the Middle Ages, cooks used it to flavor a beverage called mead. In Europe, meadowsweet is still used as a food flavoring.

In the late 1800s, some aspirin products contained meadowsweet. In fact, some people believe the word *aspirin* comes from meadowsweet's alternative botanical name, *Spiraea ulmaria*.

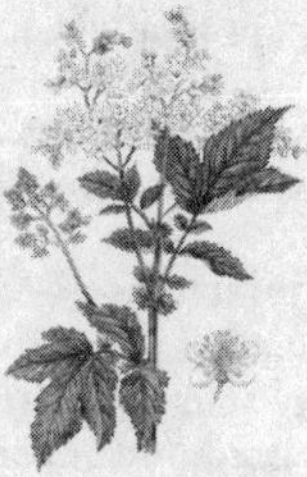

Meadowsweet comes from the dried flowers, stems, and leaves of *Filipendula ulmaria* (also called *S. ulmaria*, as mentioned above*)*. A member of the rose family (Rosaceae), this hardy perennial is native to Europe and Asia. It's grown in the United States as an ornamental plant. The Food and Drug Administration lists it as an herb of undefined safety.

Why people use this herb

- Arthritis
- Bladder inflammation
- Cancer
- Chills
- Common cold
- Diarrhea
- Fluid retention
- Gastritis (inflammation of the stomach lining)
- Headache
- Heartburn
- Indigestion
- Irritable bowel syndrome
- Joint pain
- Peptic ulcer
- Rheumatism
- Sprains
- Tendinitis
- To induce sweating
- Toothache

Common doses

Meadowsweet comes as:

- tablets of dried herb (300 milligrams)
- infusion
- powder
- fluid extract
- tincture.

Some experts recommend the following doses:

- For *diarrhea,* 1 cup of decoction taken orally two or three times daily.
- As *dried flowers,* 2.5 to 3.5 grams taken orally up to three times daily.
- As *dried herb,* 2 to 6 grams taken orally up to three times daily.
- As *liquid extract,* 1.5 to 6 milliliters taken orally up to three times daily.

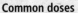

- As an *oral infusion,* 100 milliliters taken orally every 2 hours.
- As *powder,* ½ teaspoon with a small amount of water taken orally three times daily.
- As a *tincture* (1:5 in 25% alcohol), 2 to 4 milliliters taken orally up to three times daily.

Side effects

Call your health care practitioner if you experience unusual symptoms when taking meadowsweet. This herb may cause sudden contraction of lower airway muscles.

Avoid meadowsweet if you're allergic to aspirin. Salicin, an aspirin ingredient, may be linked to birth defects.

Interactions

Combining herbs with certain drugs may alter their action or produce unwanted side effects. Tell your health care practitioner about any prescription or nonprescription drugs you're taking.

Important points to remember

- Don't take meadowsweet if you're pregnant or breast-feeding.
- Don't use this herb if you have asthma or are allergic to aspirin.
- Don't give meadowsweet to children.
- Be aware that proven antiulcer drugs exist.

Other names for meadowsweet

Other names for meadowsweet include bridewort, dolloff, dropwort, *Filipendula*, fleur d'ulmaire, flores ulmariae, gravel root, meadwort, mede-sweet, queen-of-the-meadow, spierstaude, *Spiraeae flos* (meadowsweet flower), and *S. herba* (meadowsweet herb).

WHAT THE RESEARCH SHOWS

According to the German Commission E (similar to the U.S. Food and Drug Administration), meadowsweet has no known side effects except for people allergic to aspirin. The Commission supports its use in treating the common cold.

American medical experts acknowledge that meadowsweet has potential therapeutic value. Nonetheless, they won't recommend the herb until more studies are done.

Products containing meadowsweet are sold under such names as Arkocaps, Artival, Neutracalm, Rheuma-Tee, Rheumex, Santane, and Spireadosa.

Selected reference

Yanutsh, A.Y., et al. "A Study of the Antiulcerative Action of the Extracts from the Supernatant Part and Roots of *Filipendula ulmaria*," *Farmatsevtychnyi Zhurnal* 37:53-56, 1982.

Milk thistle

Milk thistle preparations are made from the seeds of *Silybum marianum*, a member of the Asteraceae or Compositae family (daisies and thistles). Native to the Mediterranean area, this herb also grows in Europe, North America, South America, and Australia.

The German Federal Institute for Drugs and Medical Devices has approved the use of milk thistle for a condition called toxic liver and as a supportive treatment for chronic inflammatory liver disease and liver cirrhosis.

Why people use this herb

- As an antidote for poisonous mushrooms
- Hepatitis C
- To aid liver function
- To "cleanse" the liver
- To promote recovery after a liver transplant

Common doses

Milk thistle comes as:

- capsules (50, 100, 175, 200, and 505 milligrams)
- tablets (85 milligrams standardized to contain 80% silymarin with the flavonoid silibinin)
- extract.

Some experts recommend the following doses:

- 420 to 800 milligrams taken orally daily as a single dose or divided into two to three equal doses.
- 200 to 400 milligrams of silymarin (calculated as the silibinin component) taken orally daily.

Side effects

Call your health care practitioner if you experience a mild laxative effect after taking a standardized extract. Milk thistle also may stimulate the uterus and trigger menstruation.

Interactions

Combining herbs with certain drugs may alter their action or produce unwanted side effects. Tell your health care practitioner about any prescription or nonprescription drugs you're taking.

Important points to remember

- Don't take milk thistle if you're pregnant or breast-feeding or if you're planning a pregnancy.

- Know that you may experience an allergic reaction to this herb if you're sensitive to plants of the Asteraceae family.
- Consult a liver disease specialist before using milk thistle to treat liver disease.
- Immediately report unusual symptoms to your health care practitioner.

Other names for milk thistle

Other names for milk thistle include *Carduus marianus* L., *Cnicus marianus*, holy thistle, Lady's thistle, Mary thistle, Marian thistle, and St. Mary thistle.

Products containing milk thistle are sold under such names as Beyond Milk Thistle, Milk Thistle Extract, Milk Thistle Phytosol, Milk Thistle Power, NU VEG Milk Thistle Power, and Silymarin.

WHAT THE RESEARCH SHOWS

Recent studies and milk thistle's traditional use in treating liver disorders in Europe suggest the herb may play a role in preventing acute liver damage from toxic substances. Lacking alternatives, medical experts believe milk thistle treatments are warranted in certain people with life-threatening liver disease.

Selected references

Feher, J., et al. "Hepatoprotective Activity of Silmarin (Legalon) Therapy in Patients with Chronic Liver Disease," *Orvosi Hetilap* 130:2723-27, 1989.

Fintelmann, V., and Albert, A. "Nachweis der therapeutischen Wirksamkeit von Legalon bei Toxischen Lebererkrankungen im Doppelblindversuch," *Therapiewoche* 30:5589-94, 1980.

Flora, K., et al. "Milk Thistle (*Silybum marianum*) for the Therapy of Liver Disease," *American Journal of Gastroenterology* 93:139-43, 1998.

Salmi, A., and Sarna, S. "Effect of Silymarin on Chemical, Functional, and Morphological Alterations of the Liver," *Scandinavian Journal of Gastroenterology* 174:517-21, 1982.

Mint

Peppermint and spearmint are the two best known and most widely cultivated members of the fragrant mint family (Labiatae). Peppermint *(Mentha x piperita)* is a hybrid of spearmint *(Mentha spicata)* and watermint *(M. aquatica)*. The essential oils of peppermint and spearmint are extracted from the leaves and flowering tops of these plants. Native to Europe, both plants are widely cultivated in the United States and Canada.

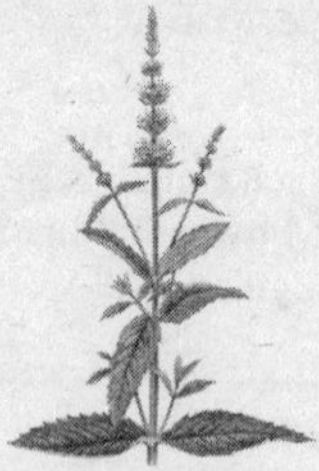

The Food and Drug Administration has demoted the oils from nonprescription drug status due to lack of information about their safety and effectiveness as digestive aids.

Why people use this herb

- Abdominal or intestinal pain
- Bronchitis, laryngitis
- Chest complaints
- Common cold, nasal congestion
- Cough, throat infection
- Diarrhea
- Headache
- Indigestion, intestinal gas
- Irritable bowel syndrome
- Itching
- Mouth sores
- Muscle spasms
- Nausea, motion sickness
- Rheumatism
- Sunburn
- To aid digestion
- Toothache
- Wasp stings

Common doses

Both peppermint and spearmint are available as liquid extracts, tea, oil, and inhalant preparations. Peppermint oil also comes as enteric-coated capsules. Menthol, the main component in peppermint oil, is an ingredient in several pain-relief lotions, anesthetics, and itch-relief preparations. It also comes as a cough suppressant ointment, lozenge, and throat spray. Experts disagree on the spearmint dose, but recommend the following doses for peppermint:

- As *capsules,* 1 to 2 capsules (0.2 milliliter per capsule) taken orally three times daily for irritable bowel syndrome.
- As *spirits* (10% oil and 1% leaf extract), 1 milliliter (20 drops) with water.
- As a *tea,* 1 to 1.5 grams (1 tablespoon) of leaves in 160 milliliters of boiling water. Drink two or three times daily.
- As a *topical preparation,* apply externally three or four times daily.

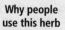

Side effects

Call your health care practitioner if you experience any of these possible side effects of mint:

- allergic symptoms, such as flushing, headache, heartburn, irritated mucous membranes, muscle tremors, and skin rash (from an internal dose)
- skin inflammation with external use.

Mint also can cause:

- throat or airway closure in infants and small children or in adults who drink tea that contains menthol
- relaxation of the lower esophageal sphincter and digestive tract muscles
- worsened symptoms of acid reflux disease and hiatal hernia.

Interactions

Combining herbs with certain drugs may alter their action or produce unwanted side effects. Tell your health care practitioner about any prescription or nonprescription drugs you're taking.

Important points to remember

- Don't use this herb if you're pregnant or breast-feeding.
- Don't give peppermint or spearmint products to infants or small children.
- Don't swallow mint products if you have gastroesophageal reflux (acid reflux) disease.
- Don't put mentholated products on broken skin or use them on your skin under a heating pad.
- Keep in mind that the fatal menthol dose in people is roughly 1,000 milligrams per kilogram of body weight.
- Be aware that menthol can cause allergic reactions in adults and children. Symptoms include hives, skin reddening, and other skin problems.
- Note that applying a mentholated ointment to an infant's nostrils for cold relief may cause a brief period of unconsciousness.
- Know that peppermint oil has caused nervous system poisoning and brain lesions in rats fed up to 100 milligrams per kilogram of body weight daily for 28 days.
- Be aware that medical experts warn against long-term inhalant use of peppermint oil.

Other names for mint

Other names for mint include balm mint, brandy mint, green mint, lamb mint, Our Lady's mint, peppermint, and spearmint.

Products containing mint are sold under such names as Ben-Gay, Rhuli Gel, Robitussin Cough Drops, and Vicks VapoRub.

WHAT THE RESEARCH SHOWS

Menthol, a peppermint component, generally is considered safe and effective when used externally to relieve local pain and itching. Menthol also is approved as an externally applied cough suppressant and an inhalant.

However, medical experts don't recommend using peppermint or spearmint internally except as a flavoring. Although some people claim these extracts have value in treating some digestive disorders, no studies prove that they're safe or effective—especially for children.

Selected references

Jacknowitz, A.I. "External Analgesic Products," in *Handbook of Nonprescription Drugs*, edited by Covington, T.R., et al. Washington, D.C.: American Pharmaceutical Association, 1996.

Murray, M. *The Healing Power of Herbs*. Rocklin, Calif.: Prima Publishing, 1995.

Olsen, P., and Thorup, I. "Neurotoxicity in Rats with Peppermint Oil and Pulegone," *Archives of Toxicology Supplement* 7:408-09, 1984.

Mistletoe

Mistletoe preparations come from the leaves, branches, and berries of European mistletoe, *Viscum album,* and the related species *V. abietis* and *V. austriacum.* These plants, which live as parasites on tree branches, are native to England, Europe, and Asia. North American mistletoes are used mainly as Christmas greens. Also parasitic, they grow on fruit trees, poplars, and oaks.

Why people use this herb

- Arteriosclerosis (hardening of the arteries)
- Cancer
- Depression
- Epilepsy
- Headache
- High blood pressure
- Insomnia
- Irregular heartbeat
- Nervousness
- Sterility
- Tension
- Ulcers
- Urinary disorders

Common doses

Mistletoe comes as dried leaves, capsules, an infusion, liquid extract, tablets, and tincture. Some experts recommend the following doses:

- As *dried leaves,* 2 to 6 grams orally three times daily.
- As *liquid extract* (1:1 solution in 25% alcohol), 1 to 3 milliliters orally three times daily.
- As *tincture* (1:5 solution in 45% alcohol), 0.5 milliliter orally three times daily.

Side effects

Call your health care practitioner if you experience any of these possible side effects of mistletoe:

- change in pupil size
- dehydration
- delirium
- diarrhea
- hallucinations
- mild fever
- nausea
- seizures
- slow pulse
- vomiting.

This herb also can cause:

- coma or cardiac arrest
- gastroenteritis (inflammation of the stomach lining and intestines)

- hepatitis (liver damage)
- high or low blood pressure
- increased white blood cell count.

Interactions

Combining herbs with certain drugs may alter their action or produce unwanted side effects. Don't use mistletoe while taking:

- alcohol and other drugs that slow the nervous system, such as cold and allergy drugs, sedatives, tranquilizers, narcotic pain relievers, barbiturates, seizure drugs, and muscle relaxants
- drugs that lower blood pressure
- drugs to relieve depression called MAO inhibitors (such as Marplan and Nardil)
- drugs used to treat heart conditions.

Important points to remember

- Don't use mistletoe if you're pregnant or breast-feeding. The herb may stimulate the uterus.
- Be aware that all plant parts are toxic.
- If you're considering taking mistletoe for cancer, know that medical experts recommend trying conventional treatments first.
- Keep mistletoe out of children's reach.

Other names for mistletoe

Other names for mistletoe include all heal, bird lime, devil's fuge, golden bough, and *Viscum*.

A product containing mistletoe is sold as Iscador.

WHAT THE RESEARCH SHOWS

Despite mistletoe's known toxic effects, some people still use it as a natural remedy. Certain chemicals in mistletoe have shown antitumor activity, but more studies must be done to evaluate the herb's effectiveness and long-term safety. In the United States, intravenous mistletoe preparations aren't standardized, so researchers probably won't evaluate the herb as a tumor treatment in the near future.

Selected references

Bradley, G.W., et al. "Apparent Response of Small Cell Lung Cancer to an Extract of Mistletoe and Homeopathic Treatment," *Thorax* 44:1047-48, 1989.

Hajto, T., et al. "Increased Secretion of Tumor Necrosis Factors Alpha, Interleukin 1, and Interleukin 6 by Human Mononuclear Cells Exposed to Beta-Galactoside-Specific Lectin from Clinically Applied Mistletoe Extract," *Cancer Research* 50:3322-26, 1990.

Motherwort

Motherwort extracts typically come from the seeds or nutlets found in the dry, thorny flowering heads of *Leonurus cardiaca*. Active components of another plant variety, *L. artemisia*, are extracted from the dried leaves.

Why people use this herb

- Heart conditions such as palpitations
- Menstrual cramps
- To aid childbirth

Members of the mint family (Labiatae), these plants have been transplanted to the United States and Canada from Europe. Some people refer to other species as motherwort.

Common dose

Motherwort comes as dried leaves and extracts. Experts disagree on what dose to take.

Side effects

Call your health care practitioner if you experience these possible side effects of motherwort:

- prolonged bleeding
- skin sensitivity to light.

Interactions

Combining herbs with certain drugs may alter their action or produce unwanted side effects. Don't use motherwort while taking:

- Coumadin
- drugs used to treat liver disease
- heart drugs called beta blockers (such as Inderal)
- Lanoxin
- other heart drugs.

Important points to remember

- Don't take motherwort if you're pregnant.
- Avoid this herb if you have a low platelet count (ask your health care practitioner).
- Avoid direct sunlight when using motherwort.
- Report unusual bleeding or bruising to your health care practitioner.

Other names for motherwort

Other names for motherwort include i-mu-ts'ao, lion's-ear, lion's-tail, lion's-tart, and throwwort.

No known products containing motherwort are available commercially.

> **WHAT THE RESEARCH SHOWS**
>
> Although some studies suggest motherwort may have promising antitumor and antioxidant properties, more studies are needed to support therapeutic claims.

Selected references

Bol'shakova, I.V. "Antioxidant Properties of a Series of Extracts from Medicinal Plants," *Biofizika* 42:480-83, 1997.

Xia, Y.X. "The Inhibitory Effect of Motherwort Extract on Pulsating Myocardial Cells In Vitro," *Journal of Traditional Chinese Medicine* 3:185-88, 1983.

Zou, Q.Z. "Effect of Motherwort on Blood Viscosity," *American Journal of Chinese Medicine* 17:65-70, 1989.

Mugwort

In Chinese traditional medicine, mugwort is used for *moxa* treatments. Small cones of dried mugwort leaves are burned in cups on certain points of the body, many of which coincide with acupuncture points.

Herbalists prepare mugwort from the dried leaves and roots of *Artemisia vulgaris*. This shrubby perennial from the daisy family (Compositae) is native to North America. It sometimes is confused with wormwood *(Artemisia absinthium)*.

Common doses

Mugwort comes as dried leaves and roots, fluid extract, infusion, and tincture. Some experts recommend the following doses:

- For *stress,* 5 milliliters of root tincture taken orally 30 minutes before bedtime.
- For *heavy menstruation,* drink an infusion of 15 grams of dried herb added to 500 milliliters of water, or take up to 2.5 milliliters of the tincture orally three times daily.
- To *stimulate the appetite,* 150 milliliters of boiling water poured over 1 to 2 teaspoons of the dried herb. Let steep for 5 to 10 minutes and strain. Drink two to three cups before meals.
- For *other complaints,* take 1 to 4 milliliters of the tincture orally three times daily.

Why people use this herb

- Anxiety, stress, insomnia
- Asthma
- Bacterial and fungal infections
- Coughing or vomiting up blood
- Diarrhea, cramps, intestinal gas
- Epilepsy
- Fever
- Headache
- Irritability, restlessness
- Menopause symptoms
- Menstrual complaints
- Mild depression
- Muscle spasms
- Persistent vomiting
- Poor circulation
- Rheumatism
- Skin inflammation
- Tapeworms and other worms

Side effects

Call your health care practitioner if you experience any of these possible side effects of mugwort:

- skin inflammation
- symptoms of a severe allergic reaction, such as chest tightness, wheezing, hives, itching, and rash.

Mugwort can strongly stimulate the uterus.

Interactions

Combining herbs with certain drugs may alter their action or produce unwanted side effects. Don't use mugwort while taking blood thinners such as Coumadin.

Important points to remember

- Don't use mugwort if you're pregnant or breast-feeding.
- Avoid this herb if you have a bleeding disorder or acid reflux disease.
- Don't use mugwort if you've ever had an allergic reaction to mugwort or if you're allergic to hazelnuts.
- Be aware that mugwort pollen is a known allergen that contributes to hay fever in some people.

> **WHAT THE RESEARCH SHOWS**
>
> No scientific studies support the long list of therapeutic claims for mugwort. Without persuasive evidence, medical experts won't recommend this herb for any use.

Other names for mugwort

Other names for mugwort include ai ye, felon herb, St. John's plant, *Summitates artemisiae*, and wild wormwood.

No known products containing mugwort are available commercially.

Selected references

Caballero, T., et al. "IgE Crossreactivity Between Mugwort Pollen (*Artemisia vulgaris*) and Hazelnut (*Abellana nux)* in Sera from Patients with Sensitivity to Both Extracts," *Clinical and Experimental Allergy* 27:1203-11, 1997. Abstract.

Garcia Ortiz, J.C., et al. "Allergy to Foods in Patients Monosensitized to *Artemisia* Pollen," *Allergy* 51:927-31, 1996.

Mullein

In the 19th century, people smoked mullein's roots or dried flowers to treat respiratory diseases and asthma symptoms—a practice borrowed from the Mohegan and Penobscot Indians. The unprocessed drug comes from the dried leaves and flowers of *Verbascum thapsus,* a tall biennial of the snapdragon family (Scrophulariaceae). Native to Europe and Asia, the plant grows in the United States. You can spot it easily from its distinctive fuzzy leaves and yellow flower spikes.

Why people use this herb

- As an expectorant
- Asthma
- Bronchitis
- Cough
- Painful urination
- Skin inflammation
- To stimulate earwax production

Common doses

Mullein comes as:

- dried leaf
- capsules (290 or 330 milligrams of leaf)
- flower oil (1 or 2 ounces)
- liquid extract (2 ounces).

Some experts recommend the following doses:

- As *capsules,* two 290-milligram capsules taken orally with two meals daily or as needed.
- As *flower oil,* 5 to 10 drops taken orally.
- As *leaves,* mix 1 cup of boiling water with 1 to 2 teaspoons of dried leaf. Let steep for 10 to 15 minutes. Drink three times daily.

Side effects

Call your health care practitioner if you experience these possible side effects of mullein:

- sedation
- skin inflammation.

Interactions

Combining herbs with certain drugs may alter their action or produce unwanted side effects. Tell your health care practitioner about any prescription or nonprescription drugs you're taking.

Important points to remember

- Don't take this herb if you're pregnant or breast-feeding.
- Don't give mullein to children.

WHAT THE RESEARCH SHOWS

Preliminary studies suggest certain mullein components may fight tumors and inflammation. However, more tests must be done in people before medical experts will recommend the herb.

Other names for mullein

Other names for mullein include Aaron's rod, bunny's ears, candlewick, flannel-leaf, great mullein, and Jacob's-staff.

Products containing mullein are sold under such names as Mullein Flower Oil, Mullein Leaves, and Verbascum Complex.

Selected references

Saracoglu, I., et al. "Studies on Components with Cytotoxic and Cytostatic Activity of Two Turkish Medicinal Plants," *Biological and Pharmaceutical Bulletin* 18:1396-400, 1995.

Zheng, R.L., et al. "Inhibition of the Autooxidation of Linoleic Acid by Phenylpropanoid Glycosides from *Pedicularis* in Micelles," *Chemistry and Physics of Lipids* 65:151-54, 1993.

Mustard

Mustard comes from black and white mustard plants *(Brassica nigra* and *B. alba),* which are native to the southern Mediterranean area. Other *Brassica* species grow in eastern Europe, India, and the Middle East. White mustard is also called *Sinapis alba*.

Mustard's volatile oil, used medicinally, is made by pressing or steam-distilling mustard seeds. Some people grind the seeds for a flour that's made into paste and placed on the body. The German government has approved external application of a white mustard seed poultice to treat respiratory congestion and inflamed joints and soft tissues.

Why people use this herb

- Fluid retention
- Intestinal gas
- Muscle aches and pains
- Respiratory congestion
- Rheumatism and arthritis of the feet
- To induce vomiting

Common doses

Mustard comes as a tea, ground mustard seeds (mustard flour), and mustard oil. Some experts recommend the following doses:

- For a *footbath,* mix 1 tablespoon of mustard seeds with 1 liter of hot water, and soak feet.
- As a *topical treatment* to coat and redden the skin, make a paste by mixing 120 grams (4 ounces) of ground black mustard seeds in warm water. To ease skin irritation from the paste, apply olive oil after removing the paste.

Side effects

Call your health care practitioner if you experience severe irritation of the skin or mucous membranes from contact with mustard.

Important points to remember

- Don't use this herb if you're pregnant or breast-feeding.
- If you have respiratory disease, know that inhaling fumes from mustard may aggravate your condition.
- Never taste or inhale volatile mustard oil in its undiluted form because poisoning may occur.

- If you prepare a medicinal mustard product, wash your hands after working with the herb and avoid contact with the eyes.
- Don't apply mustard preparations to mucous membranes.
- Keep mustard products out of reach of children and pets.

> **WHAT THE RESEARCH SHOWS**
>
> Mustard's unique pungent properties have led some people to use it as an herbal remedy. If not handled properly, though, mustard can cause tissue damage. Although white mustard has been used medicinally in Germany, no studies are available.

Other names for mustard

Other names for mustard include black mustard, brown mustard, California rape, charlock, Chinese mustard, Indian mustard, white mustard, and wild mustard.

Medicinal products containing mustard are sold under such names as Act-On Rub and Musterole.

Selected reference

Choudhury, A.R., et al. "Mustard Oil and Garlic Extract as Inhibitors of Sodium Arsenite-Induced Chromosomal Breaks in Vivo," *Cancer Letters* 121:45-52, 1997.

Myrrh

Myrrh is a mixture of volatile oil, gum, and resin (oleo-gum-resin) from *Commiphora molmol* and other *Commiphora* species. These shrubs, members of the bursera family (Burseraceae), are native to Ethiopia, Somalia, and the Arabian Peninsula.

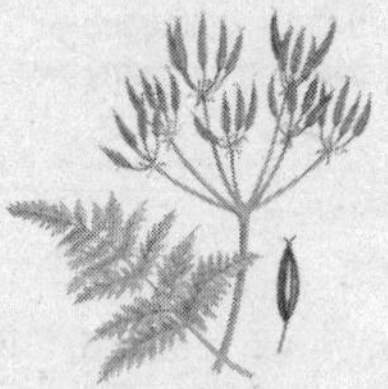

Why people use this herb

- Abrasions
- Bedsores
- Gingivitis (gum disease)
- Hemorrhoids
- HIV and AIDS
- Infections
- Mouth sores
- Respiratory congestion
- Sore throat
- Wounds

The *Federal Register* has recommended against recognizing myrrh tincture as safe and effective. If you see myrrh in a product promoted as an oral health aid, consider it mislabeled.

Common doses

Myrrh is available as:

- capsules (525 and 650 milligrams)
- salves
- mouthwash
- tinctures
- fluid extracts.

Some experts recommend the following doses:

- As a *tea,* 1 to 2 teaspoons of resin in 1 cup of boiling water. Let steep for 10 to 15 minutes. Drink three times daily.
- As a *tincture,* dissolve resin in alcohol. As needed, apply 1 to 4 milliliters externally three times daily.

Side effects

Call your health care practitioner if you experience any of these possible side effects of myrrh:

- diarrhea
- hiccups
- restlessness
- skin inflammation.

Interactions

Combining herbs with certain drugs may alter their action or produce unwanted side effects. Tell your health care practitioner about any prescription or nonprescription drugs you're taking, especially:

- insulin
- oral drugs that lower blood sugar (such as Amaryl, DiaBeta, Diabinese, Glucophage, Glucotrol, Precose, and Rezulin).

Important point to remember

- Don't use myrrh if you're pregnant or breast-feeding.

> **WHAT THE RESEARCH SHOWS**
>
> With little available information on myrrh's effects on people, medical experts don't recommend using it medicinally. To evaluate the herb's potential in treating HIV infection as well as use of a related plant, *Commiphora mukul*, against diabetes, researchers must conduct thorough clinical studies.

Other names for myrrh

Other names for myrrh include African myrrh, Arabian myrrh, bal, bol, bola, gum myrrh, heerabol, Somali myrrh, and Yemen myrrh.

Products containing myrrh are sold under such names as Astring-O-Sol, Myrrh Gum, and Odara. Myrrh also comes in combination products with goldenseal.

Selected references

Al-Awadi, F.M., and Gumaa, K.A. "Studies on the Activity of Individual Plants of an Antidiabetic Plant Mixture," *Acta Diabetologica Latina* 24:37-41, 1987.

Malhotra, S.C., and Ahuja, M.M. "Comparative Hypolipidemic Effectiveness of Gum Guggulu (*Commiphora mukul*) Fraction, Alpha-ethyl-p-chlorophenoxyisobutyrate, and Cica-13437-Su," *Indian Journal of Medical Research* 59:1621-32, 1971.

Tripathi, S.N., et al. "Effect of a Keto-Steroid of *Commiphora mukul* on Hypercholesterolemia and Hyperlipidemia Induced by Neomercazole and Cholesterol Mixture in Chicks," *Indian Journal of Experimental Biology* 13:15-18, 1975.

Myrtle

In some parts of Greece, myrtle is used as a dye. Herbal preparations of myrtle come from the seeds and leaves of *Myrtus communis,* an evergreen shrub native to the Middle East and Mediterranean regions. This plant is distinct from Madagascar myrtle *(Eugenia jambolana)* and common periwinkle *(Vinca minor),* though some people confuse the two plants.

Why people use this herb

- Diabetes
- Digestive disorders
- Repiratory congestion
- Urinary disorders
- Wounds

Common dose

Myrtle comes in extracts. Some experts recommend the following dose:

- As the *essential oil,* 1 to 2 milliliters taken orally daily.

Side effects

Call your health care practitioner if you experience an allergic reaction when using myrtle. This drug also can lower blood sugar.

Interactions

Combining herbs with certain drugs may alter their action or produce unwanted side effects. Tell your health care practitioner about prescription or nonprescription drugs you're taking, especially:

- drugs metabolized by the liver's cytochrome P-450 system, such as certain antibiotics (including Ery-Tab and Nizoral), Coumadin, Inderal, nonsteroidal anti-inflammatory drugs (including Advil and Naprosyn), Theo-Dur, and Tylenol
- insulin
- oral drugs that lower blood sugar (such as Amaryl, DiaBeta, Diabinese, Glucophage, Glucotrol, Precose, and Rezulin).

Important points to remember

- Don't take myrtle if you're pregnant or breast-feeding.
- If you have diabetes, consult your health care practitioner before taking this herb.
- Don't take the essential oil internally except under a health care practitioner's supervision.

Other names for myrtle

Other names for myrtle include bridal myrtle, common myrtle, Dutch myrtle, Jew's myrtle, mirtil, and Roman myrtle.

No known products containing myrtle are available commercially.

> **WHAT THE RESEARCH SHOWS**
>
> Although myrtle shows some promise in treating diabetes in animals, researchers haven't gathered much human data on this use. Medical experts don't recommend using the herb medicinally.

Selected references

Al-Hindawi, M.K., et al. "Anti-inflammatory Activity of Some Iraqi Plants Using Intact Rats," *Journal of Ethnopharmacology* 26:163-68, 1989.

Elfellah, M.S., et al. "Antihyperglycemic Effect of an Extract of *Myrtus communis* in Streptozotocin-Induced Diabetes in Mice," *Journal of Ethnopharmacology* 11:275-81, 1984.

Ortega, M., and Rodenas, S. "*Myrtus communis* L. Phytohemagglutinins as a Clarifying Agent for Lipemic Sera," *Clinica Chimica Acta* 92:135-39, 1979.

Pochinok, V., et al. "Possibility of Control of Resistance to Antibiotics of Pathogenic Staphylococci by the Tincture of *Myrtus communis* Leaves," *Farmatsevtychnyi Zhurnal* 23:72-74, 1968. Abstract.

Nettle

Nettle has left traces throughout history. Archaeologists found Bronze Age burial shrouds made of nettle fabric. Some 19th-century hair-growth preparations contained nettle. Native American women used nettle tea to ease delivery and stop uterine bleeding after childbirth. Nonetheless, the Food and Drug Administration lists nettle as an herb of undefined safety.

Nettle preparations come from leaves, stems, and roots of *Urtica dioica*, a perennial of the nettle family (Urticaceae). One of three nettle species native to Europe, *U. dioica* grows throughout the United States and parts of Canada.

Why people use this herb

- As an expectorant
- Asthma
- Benign prostatic hyperplasia
- Benign prostate tumors (adenomas)
- Cancer
- Cough
- Diabetes
- Eczema (a type of skin inflammation)
- Fluid retention
- Gout
- Heart failure
- High blood pressure
- Muscle spasms
- Nasal allergies
- Nosebleed
- Rheumatism
- To promote hair growth
- To reduce postoperative blood loss, infection, and inflammation
- Tuberculosis
- Urinary, bladder, and kidney disorders
- Urinary tract inflammation
- Uterine bleeding
- Wounds

Common doses

Nettle comes as:

- capsules (150 and 300 milligrams)
- dried leaf and root extract
- tincture.

Some experts recommend the following doses:

- For *nasal allergies,* 150- to 300-milligram capsules taken orally.
- As a *tea,* mix 1 to 2 teaspoons of dried herb in 1 cup of boiling water. Drink up to 2 cups daily.
- As a *tincture,* ¼ to 1 teaspoon of tincture taken up to twice daily.

Side effects

Call your health care practitioner if you experience any of these possible side effects of nettle:

- decreased urine flow
- diarrhea
- hives
- stomach irritation
- swelling.

Nettle also can cause digestive tract irritation.

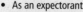

Interactions

Combining herbs with certain drugs may alter their action or produce unwanted side effects. Don't use nettle while taking diuretics.

Important points to remember

- Don't use nettle if you're pregnant or breast-feeding. It may stimulate the uterus.
- Don't give this herb to children under age 2.
- Check with your health care practitioner before giving nettle to older children and before using it yourself if you're over age 65.
- If you take nettle as a diuretic, eat foods high in potassium, such as bananas and fresh vegetables, to replenish body salts lost through increased urination.
- Check with your health care practitioner before you use nettle for benign prostatic hyperplasia or fluid build-up caused by heart failure.
- Know that rubbing nettle against the skin can cause intense burning for 12 hours or even longer. Wash thoroughly with soap and water, use antihistamines and steroid creams, and wear heavy gloves if you must handle the plant again.

Other names for nettle

Other names for nettle include common nettle, greater nettle, and stinging nettle.

Products containing nettle are sold under such names as Nettles Capsules and Nettles Liquid Extract.

Selected references

Lichius, J.J., and Muth, C. "The Inhibiting Effects of *Urtica dioica* Root Extracts on Experimentally Induced Prostatic Hyperplasia in the Mouse," *Planta Medica* 63:307-10, 1997.

Mittman, P., "Randomized, Double-Blind Study of Freeze-Dried *Urtica dioica* in the Treatment of Allergic Rhinitis," *Planta Medica* 56:44-47, 1990.

WHAT THE RESEARCH SHOWS

Despite its traditional use in treating several conditions, nettle has been proven effective only as a diuretic. Researchers consider the herb relatively safe in the amounts recommended, and side effects from oral forms of nettle are rare. More studies must be done to find out if the herb has a role in treating benign prostatic hyperplasia and nasal allergies.

Night-blooming cereus

Night-blooming cereus comes from the stems and flowers of a cactus called *Selenicereus grandiflorus*. This plant is native to tropical and subtropical America, including the West Indies.

Why people use this herb

- Anemia
- Angina pectoris
- Bladder inflammation
- Depression
- Endocarditis (inflammation of the heart's interior lining)
- Fatigue
- Fluid retention
- Graves' disease (overactive thyroid)
- Heart palpitations
- Indigestion
- Irritable bladder
- Kidney congestion
- Myocarditis (inflammation of the heart wall)
- Nervous headache
- Prostate disease
- Rheumatism
- Shortness of breath
- Tobacco poisoning

Common doses

Night-blooming cereus is available as a liquid extract and tincture. Some experts recommend the following doses:

- As a *liquid extract,* 0.7 milliliter taken orally every 4 hours.
- As a *tincture,* 1 to 1.8 milliliters taken orally every 4 hours.

Side effects

Call your health care practitioner if you experience any of these possible side effects of night-blooming cereus:

- burning sensation in the mouth
- diarrhea
- nausea
- vomiting.

Interactions

Combining herbs with certain drugs may alter their action or produce unwanted side effects. Don't use night-blooming cereus while taking:

- digitalis drugs used to treat heart failure or irregular heartbeats
- ACE inhibitors, such as Accupril, Altace, Capoten, Lotensin, Monopril, and Vasotec
- drugs for irregular heartbeats
- heart drugs called beta blockers, such as Inderal
- heart drugs called calcium channel blockers, such as Calan and Procardia.

Important points to remember

- Don't use night-blooming cereus if you're breast-feeding or in the first three months of pregnancy, if you suspect you may be pregnant, or if you're planning a pregnancy.
- If you're taking prescription heart drugs, have your health care practitioner monitor your heart rate and blood pressure.
- Immediately report palpitations, an increased pulse, or blood pressure changes.

> **WHAT THE RESEARCH SHOWS**
>
> Although night-blooming cereus contains a digitalis-like chemical, researchers haven't studied it as a substitute for digitalis drugs (such as Lanoxin) or as a treatment for heart conditions. Medical experts strongly recommend getting medical advice before using this herb for heart problems or while taking prescribed heart drugs.

Other names for night-blooming cereus

Other names for night-blooming cereus include *Cactus grandiflorus*, *Cereus grandiflorus*, large-flowered cactus, queen of the night, sweet-scented cactus, and vanilla cactus.

Products containing night-blooming cereus are sold under such names as Cactus Grandiflorus, Cactus-Hawthorn Compound, Cereus Grandiflorus, and Night-Blooming Cereus.

Selected references

Hapke, H.J. "Pharmacological Effects of Hordenine," *DTW - Deutsche Tierarztliche Wochenschrift* 102:228-32, 1995. Abstract in English.

Wadworth, A.N., and Faulds, D. "Hydroxyethylrutosides: A Review of Pharmacology and Therapeutic Efficacy in Venous Insufficiency and Related Disorders," *Drugs* 44:1013-32, 1992.

Nutmeg

Nutmeg, the dried seed kernel of the nutmeg tree, *Myristica fragrans,* is best known as a spice for foods and drinks and as a fragrance in cosmetics and soaps. Nutmeg trees grow in Sri Lanka, the West Indies, and the Molucca Islands.

Why people use this herb

- Anxiety
- As an aphrodisiac
- Bad breath
- Chronic nervous disorders
- Depression
- Digestive tract disorders
- Indigestion and other stomach problems
- Kidney disorders
- Rheumatism pain
- Toothache
- To stop vomiting

Another spice (mace) is produced from the aril, a netlike substance inside the nutmeg fruit. The aril wraps around the brittle shells containing the nutmeg kernel.

Common doses

Nutmeg comes as:
- capsules (200 milligrams)
- powders
- essential oil.

Some experts recommend the following doses (some of which are in the hazardous range):
- For *nausea* or *gastric upset,* 1 to 2 capsules of nutmeg "kernel" taken orally as a single dose, or 3 to 5 drops of essential oil on a sugar lump or in a teaspoon of honey.
- For *chronic diarrhea,* 4 to 6 tablespoons of powder taken orally daily.
- For *toothache,* rub 1 to 2 drops of essential oil on the gum around the aching tooth until you can get to the dentist.

Side effects

Call your health care practitioner if you experience unusual symptoms when using nutmeg. Excessive doses may cause:
- an unusual sense of well-being
- delusions
- hallucinations.

Consuming nutmeg oil or using doses over 5 grams can cause:

- confusion
- constipation
- dry mouth
- flushing
- nausea
- rapid pulse
- stupor
- vomiting.

This herb also can cause miscarriage, seizures, and even death.

Interactions

Combining herbs with certain drugs may alter their action or produce unwanted side effects. Consult your health care practitioner about any prescription or nonprescription drugs you're taking, especially drugs to stop diarrhea. Don't use nutmeg when taking:

- Clozaril
- Haldol
- Navane
- Zyprexa.

Important points to remember

- Don't use nutmeg if you're pregnant or breast-feeding, if you suspect you're pregnant, or if you're planning a pregnancy. The herb may cause miscarriage.
- If you're being treated for a psychiatric condition, check with your health care practitioner before using nutmeg. It may trigger symptoms of your condition.
- Know that some people abuse or misuse nutmeg.
- If you use nutmeg, avoid driving and other hazardous activities until you know how the herb affects you.
- Don't take large amounts of nutmeg because it may be toxic.
- Keep nutmeg products out of reach of children and pets.
- For treating diarrhea, be aware that medical experts recommend less toxic agents, such as bulk laxatives, milk of magnesia, or casanthranol with docusate sodium.

Other names for nutmeg

Other names for nutmeg include mace, macis, muscadier, muskatbaum, myristica, noz moscada, nuez moscada, and nux moschata.

Products containing nutmeg are sold under such names as Agua del Carmen, Aluminum Free Indigestion, Incontinurina, Klosterfrau Magentonikum, Melisana, Nervospur, and Vicks Vaporub.

WHAT THE RESEARCH SHOWS

Nutmeg has interesting properties, but the risks of toxicity, abuse, and misuse limit its therapeutic use. People have died from eating excessive amounts of nutmeg. With less toxic drugs available for treating diarrhea, medical experts don't recommend nutmeg for that complaint or any other.

Selected references

Abernethy, M.K., and Beckel, L.B. "Acute Nutmeg Intoxication," *American Journal of Emergency Medicine* 10:429-30, 1992.

Barrowman, J.A., et al. "Diarrhea in Thyroid Medullary Carcinoma: Role of Prostaglandins and Therapeutic Effect of Nutmeg," *BMJ* 3:11-12, 1975.

Ram, A., et al. "Hypolipidaemic Effect of *Myristica fragrans* Fruit Extract in Rabbits," *Journal of Ethnopharmacology* 55:49-53, 1996.

Shafran, I., and *McCrone, D.* "Nutmeg and Medullary Carcinoma of Thyroid," *New England Journal of Medicine* 293:1266, 1975. Letter.

Oak

A slow-growing tree of North America, Europe, Asia, and Australia, oak is prized by European herbalists for its astringent bark, leaves, and acorns. The Druids of prehistoric Britain considered oak trees sacred, as did the ancient Greeks and Romans. *Quercus,* the Latin name for the oak tree, probably comes from the Celtic *quer* (fine) and *cuez* (tree).

Historically, the oak tree has served many purposes. Its bark has been used to tan leather and smoke fish. Native Americans ground the acorns into meal. Some people have used an infusion of oak bark to dye wool and yarn. Others have made a coffee substitute from roasted acorns mixed with cream and sugar, which they used to treat tender, enlarged, inflamed neck lymph nodes caused by tuberculosis.

Today, herbalists use bark from young branches and twigs of the white oak *(Quercus alba),* English oak *(Q. robur),* and durmast oak *(Q. petraea)*—members of the beech family (Fagaceae). The bark can measure up to 4 millimeters thick. White oak bark makes a yellowish tea with a slightly bitter, astringent taste.

Herbalists gather oak galls as well. Rich in astringent substances called tannins, galls are bumps that grow on oak stems and leaves, usually in response to damage done by insects and worms. Most often, oak galls result from tiny wasps. A female insect pierces a shoot or young bough of an oak tree and lays her egg in the wound. After hatching from the egg, the young insect produces a fluid that changes the starch in nearby oak cells into sugar, which the larva then

Why people use this herb

- Anal fissures
- As an antiseptic
- Bacterial and viral infections
- Bladder or genital inflammation
- Bleeding gums
- Burns (small)
- Diarrhea
- Eye inflammation
- Foot odor
- For antioxidant effects
- For mind-altering effects
- Hemorrhoids
- Kidney inflammation
- Laryngitis
- Mouth or throat inflammation
- Nasal polyps
- Skin inflammation
- To harden the nipples for breast-feeding
- Tonsillitis
- To prevent cancer
- To protect the liver
- To suppress the immune system
- Vaginal discharge
- Varicose veins
- Weeping eczema and other skin rashes

eats. Plant cells can use this sugar as well, and they grow into a large, protective bump around the developing insect. Once the insect reaches adulthood, it eats its way out of the gall.

Common doses

Oak comes as capsules, decoctions, extracts, ointments, ooze (a tea of oak bark), tincture, unground or powdered oak bark, and oak galls. Also, certain prepared herbal mixtures include oak bark. Some experts recommend the following doses:

- For *diarrhea,* 3 grams of powdered oak bark or a similar preparation taken orally daily or 1 cup of tea taken three times daily. To make the tea, add either 1 gram of finely cut or coarsely powdered herb or 1 to 2 teaspoons of chopped bark to 500 milliliters of water. Boil for 15 minutes, strain and cool the tea, then drink undiluted. If diarrhea lasts more than 3 days, call your health care practitioner.
- As a *bath,* 5 grams of oak per liter of water, or 1 to 3 teaspoons of bark extract added to a partial bath.
- As *capsules,* 2 capsules taken orally with meals three times daily.
- As a *tincture,* 1 to 2 milliliters taken orally three times daily.
- As a *compress, rinse,* or *gargle,* prepare a fresh decoction daily by boiling 20 grams of oak per liter of water for 10 to 15 minutes. Use the strained liquid undiluted. Apply compresses loosely to the affected area so moisture can evaporate freely. Don't use these preparations for more than 3 weeks.

Side effects

Call your health care practitioner if you experience any of these possible side effects of oak:

- constipation
- nausea or vomiting
- stomach upset or abdominal pain.

This herb also can cause:

- death from tannic acid enemas or extended use on the skin
- kidney problems
- liver damage
- respiratory failure.

Interactions

Combining herbs with certain drugs may alter their action or produce unwanted side effects. Don't take oak internally while using:

- atropine
- caffeine
- digoxin
- heavy metal salts, such as iron or gold
- morphine
- nicotine
- quinine.

Important points to remember

- Don't use oak if you're pregnant or breast-feeding.
- Don't use this herb for full-body baths.
- Avoid contact with the eyes. If oak gets in your eye, flush with tepid water for at least 15 minutes.
- Don't put oak on your skin if you have widespread skin damage.
- If you get oak on large areas of damaged or normal skin, wash it off with soap and water.
- Don't take oak galls internally.
- Be aware that barium enemas no longer use tannic acid because of reports of death from liver problems (possibly caused by the tannic acid).

Other names for oak

Other names for oak include British oak, brown oak, common oak, cortex quercus, ecorce de chene, eicherinde, eichenlohe, encina, English oak, gravelier, nutgall, oak apples, oak bark, oak galls, stone oak, and tanner's bark.

Products containing oak are sold under such names as Conchae Compound, Eichenrinden-Extrakt, Entero-Sanol, Hamon No. 14, Kernosan Elixir, Menodoron, Peerless Composition Essence, Pektan N, Silvapin, Tisanes de l'Abbe, Tonsilgon-N, and Traxaton.

WHAT THE RESEARCH SHOWS

Studies show that short-term, external use of oak decoctions can relieve certain skin problems, such as eczema, inflammation, and minor burns. Although some herbalists also claim oak is useful for diarrhea, clinical studies don't support this claim. At least for now, medical experts caution against taking oak internally until it's shown to be safe and effective.

Selected references

Boulton, D.W., et al. "Extensive Binding of the Bioflavonoid Quercetin to Human Plasma Proteins," *Journal of Pharmacy and Pharmacology* 50:243-49, 1998.

Conquer, J.A., et al. "Supplementation With Quercetin Markedly Increases Plasma Quercetin Concentration Without Effect on Selected Risk Factors for Heart Disease in Healthy Subjects," *Journal of Nutrition* 128:593-97, 1998.

Dobelis, I.N., ed. *Magic and Medicine of Plants.* Pleasantville, N.Y.: Reader's Digest Association Inc., 1986.

Murakami, S., et al. "Inhibitory Effect of Tannic Acid on Gastric H^+, K^+, ATPase," *Journal of Natural Products* 55:513-16, 1992.

Oats

Derived from the grains of the *Avena sativa* plant, oats are cultivated mainly in the United States, Russia, Canada, and Germany. Like other grains, they're sometimes contaminated with aflatoxin, a fungal toxin linked to some cancers.

Why people use this herb

- As a sedative
- Gout
- Itching
- Skin irritation
- To reduce blood sugar and insulin levels
- To lower cholesterol
- To treat certain addictions, including cigarette smoking

Common doses

Oats come as:

- tablets (850 or 1,000 milligrams)
- whole grains
- cereals
- wafers (750 milligrams)
- soaps
- gels
- teas
- powders
- lotions
- bath preparations.

Some experts recommend the following doses:

- To *lower cholesterol,* 50 to 100 grams of dietary fiber from oat bran daily.
- For *topical use,* apply once or twice daily.

Side effects

Call your health care practitioner if you experience any of these possible side effects of oats:

- bloating or a feeling of abdominal fullness
- frequent bowel movements
- intestinal gas
- irritation around the genitals and buttocks
- skin irritation from contact with oat flour.

Interactions

Combining herbs with certain drugs may alter their action or produce unwanted side effects. Tell your health care practitioner about any prescription or nonprescription drugs you're taking.

Important points to remember

- Don't use oats if you have celiac disease. Oats contain gluten.
- If you have bowel problems, check with your health care practitioner before using oats.
- If you take oat bran, drink plenty of water to help regulate your bowel movements.
- When bathing in a colloidal oat product, take care not to get it in your eyes or on inflamed skin.
- Keep in mind that oat products can cause intestinal gas and frequent bowel movements.

Other names for oats

Other names for oats include groats, haver, haver-corn, haws, and oatmeal.

Products containing oats are sold under such names as Aveeno Cleansing Bar, Aveeno Colloidal, Aveeno Dry, Aveeno Lotion, Aveeno Oilated Bath, Aveeno Regular Bath, Oats and Honey, Oat Bran, Oat Straw Tea, and Quaker Oat Bran.

WHAT THE RESEARCH SHOWS

Oats provide an important source of dietary fiber, and studies support the use of oats to reduce the risks of heart disease and postoperative constipation. As for herbalists' claims that oatmeal helps heal minor skin irritations, researchers have found little evidence of this effect.

Selected references

Hallfrisch, J., et al. "Diets Containing Soluble Oat Extracts Improve Glucose and Insulin Responses of Moderately Hypercholesterolemic Men and Women," *American Journal of Clinical Nutrition* 61:379-84, 1995.

He, J., et al. "Oats and Buckwheat Intakes and Cardiovascular Disease Risk Factors in an Ethnic Minority of China," *American Journal of Clinical Nutrition* 61:366-72, 1995.

Pick, M.E. "Oat Bran Concentrate Bread Products Improve Long-Term Control of Diabetes: A Pilot Study," *Journal of the American Dietetic Association* 96:1254-61, 1996.

van Horn, L.V., et al. "Serum Lipid Response to Oat Product Intake with a Fat-Modified Diet," *Journal of the American Dietetic Association* 86:759-64, 1986.

Oleander

A popular ornamental shrub native to the Mediterranean region, oleander *(Nerium oleander)* grows widely throughout the southern and southwestern United States and California. Reaching about 20 feet tall, it has long, narrow, pointed leaves and produces small clusters of red, pink, or white blossoms.

Herbalists around the world use oleander's active components, obtained mostly from the leaves. For example, in Curaçao, the sap is applied to warts, added to beverages, and used to treat pinworms, tapeworms, and other worm infections. In Venezuela, people boil the leaves and inhale the steam to treat sinus problems. Some people use oleander leaves as poultices for skin problems and to kill skin parasites or maggots in wounds.

Despite this long history of medicinal use, you should avoid oleander—it's highly poisonous. Swallowing just one leaf could kill a healthy adult. Death typically results from heart failure or respiratory paralysis.

Common dose

Oleander comes as a tincture and leaf extract. Experts disagree on what dose to take. More importantly, the herb is poisonous and shouldn't be taken internally.

Side effects

Call your health care practitioner if you experience any of these possible side effects of oleander:

- abdominal cramps or pain
- appetite loss
- bloody diarrhea
- depression
- dizziness
- drowsiness
- enlarged pupils
- fainting
- fast, slow, or irregular pulse
- nausea
- seizures

Why people use this herb

- Asthma
- Cancer
- Corns
- Heart problems
- Menstrual problems
- Seizures
- Skin problems
- To cause vomiting
- To induce abortion
- To repel insects and parasites
- To stimulate bowel movements

- severe airway irritation (from smoke inhalation)
- skin irritation
- vomiting.

All parts of the oleander plant are toxic. Adults and children have died after eating the flowers, leaves, and nectar and after using oleander twigs as skewers to roast foods. People also have died after using oleander rectally. Smoke from burning oleander wood and water in which the plant has soaked can be toxic.

Interactions

Combining herbs with certain drugs may alter their action or produce unwanted side effects. Don't use oleander while taking digoxin.

Important points to remember

- Don't use oleander in any form because it's extremely poisonous.
- If you decide to use oleander or keep it around, make sure to store it safely away from children, pets, and livestock. Label it clearly so you don't take it accidentally.
- Don't burn oleander branches or leaves, especially in poorly ventilated areas.
- Be aware that someone who ingests oleander will need to have his or her stomach pumped, will receive drugs to cause vomiting and soak up the poison, and may need drugs to help the heart keep working properly.

WHAT THE RESEARCH SHOWS

According to medical experts, oleander is simply too poisonous to take for any purpose. What's more, no scientific studies support its use.

Other names for oleander

Other names for oleander include adelfa, laurier rose, rosa francesa, rosa laurel, and rose bay.

No known products containing oleander are available commercially.

Selected reference

Clark, R.F., et al. "Digoxin-Specific Fab Fragments in the Treatment of Oleander Toxicity in a Canine Model," *Annals of Emergency Medicine* 20:1073-77, 1991.

Oregano

The ancient Greeks crowned newlyweds with oregano and planted the herb on graves. Other ancient civilizations used oregano as a remedy for narcotic poisoning and seizures. Now, it's widely used as a spice and food preservative.

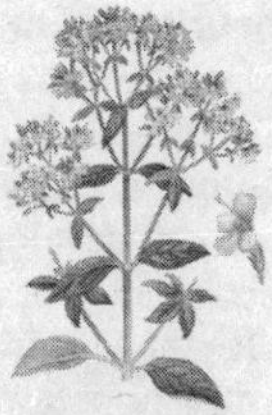

A coarse plant, oregano *(Origanum vulgare)* has sprawling stems, pink or white flowers, and a balsamic aroma. A member of the mint family, it's closely related to the spice marjoram *(O. majorana).*

Why people use this herb

- For antioxidant effects
- Infections
- To induce sweating
- To stimulate menstruation

Common doses

Oregano comes as:
- capsules (450 milligrams)
- oil (0.45 fluid ounces)
- a spice.

Some experts recommend the following doses:
- As a *dietary supplement,* 2 capsules taken orally once or twice daily, preferably with meals.
- As an *oil,* add a few drops to milk or juice.
- For *topical use,* apply oregano oil directly to the affected body area once or twice daily.
- As a *shampoo,* add a small amount of oregano oil to commercial shampoo. Leave it on your hair for a few minutes before rinsing.
- As an *antiseptic cleanser,* add to liquid soaps and use when showering and washing your hands.

Side effects

Call your health care practitioner if you experience any of these possible side effects of oregano:
- difficulty breathing, speaking, or swallowing
- facial swelling
- itching.

The side effects listed above indicate a serious allergic reaction to oregano that demand immediate medical treatment.

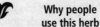

Interactions

Combining herbs with certain drugs may alter their action or produce unwanted side effects. Tell your health care practitioner about any prescription or nonprescription drugs you're taking, especially iron supplements.

Important points to remember

- Don't use oregano if you've had an allergic reaction to it or to other herbs in the same family, such as thyme, hyssop, basil, marjoram, mint, and sage.
- If you develop a rash or skin irritation while using oregano, discontinue it at once.
- If you have iron-deficiency anemia, consult your health care practitioner before using oregano.
- Don't use oregano within 2 hours before or after taking an iron supplement or eating foods high in iron.

Other names for oregano

Other names for oregano include mountain mint, origanum, and wild marjoram.

Products containing oregano are sold under such names as Oil of Oregano, Oregamax, and Oregano.

WHAT THE RESEARCH SHOWS

Oregano shows some antiseptic, antifungal, and antioxidant effects. However, studies on people haven't been done, so medical experts recommend against using oregano for these effects.

Selected references

Benito, M., et al. "Labiatae Allergy: Systemic Reactions Due to Ingestion of Oregano and Thyme," *Annals of Allergy Asthma and Immunology* 76:416-18, 1996.

Brune, M., et al. "Iron Absorption and Phenolic Compounds: Importance of Different Phenolic Structures," *European Journal of Clinical Nutrition* 43:547-58, 1989.

Kanazawa, K., et al. "Specific Desmutagens in Oregano Against a Dietary Carcinogen, Trp-P-2, are Galengin and Quercetin," *Journal of Agricultural and Food Chemistry* 43:404-09, 1995.

Lagouri, V., and Boskou, D., "Nutrient Antioxidants in Oregano," *International Journal of Food Sciences and Nutrition* 47:493-97, 1996.

Oregon grape

Oregon grape comes from the bark of the roots and stems of *Mahonia aquifolium,* a bushy shrub that grows in thickets and pastures in the western United States. The herb gets its name from its use as a food and medicine along the Oregon trail. The shrub's fruits are used in wines and brandies.

Why people use this herb

- Acne
- Arthritis
- As an expectorant
- Bloodstream infection
- Bronchitis
- Diarrhea
- Eczema (a type of skin inflammation)
- Fever
- Fluid retention
- Gallbladder disease
- Hepatitis
- Herpes
- Kidney stones
- Painful urination
- Psoriasis (scaly, raised skin patches)
- Rheumatism
- Stomach upset
- Syphilis
- To stimulate bile production
- Vaginitis

Common doses

Oregon grape comes as:
- capsules (400 milligrams)
- powder
- tincture.

Some experts recommend the following doses:
- As a *tincture,* 2 to 4 milliliters taken orally three times daily.
- As a *powder,* 0.5 to 1 gram taken orally three times daily.

Side effects

Seek medical help immediately if you get sick after taking Oregon grape. Excessive doses of berberine, an alkaloid in this herb, have caused poisoning and death.

Interactions

Combining certain herbs with drugs may alter their action or cause unwanted side effects. Tell your health care practitioner about any prescription or nonprescription drugs you're taking.

Important points to remember

- Don't use Oregon grape if you're pregnant or breast-feeding.
- Don't take this herb if you've experienced an allergy to it or a related plant.
- Avoid getting Oregon grape in your eyes. If you do, flush your eyes well with water.

- Be aware that skin contact with Oregon grape may cause intense pain.
- Don't confuse Oregon grape with the common barberry *(Berberis vulgaris)*.

Other names for Oregon grape

Other names for Oregon grape include holly-leaved barberry and mountain grape.

Products containing Oregon grape are sold under such names as Mountain Grape and Oregon Grape Root.

> **WHAT THE RESEARCH SHOWS**
>
> Studies suggest Oregon grape may be useful in treating psoriasis (scaly, raised skin patches). However, researchers know little about the herb's safety and effectiveness. More studies on people are needed.

Selected references

Bezakova, L., et al. "Lipoxygenase Inhibition and Antioxidant Properties of Bisbenzylisoquinoline Alkaloids Isolated from *Mahonia aquifolium*," *Pharmazie* 51:758-61, 1996.

McCutcheon, A.R., et al. "Antifungal Screening of Medicinal Plants of British Columbian Native Peoples," *Journal of Ethnopharmacology* 44:157-69, 1994.

Misik, V., et al. "Lipoxygenase Inhibition and Antioxidant Properties of Protoberberine and Aporphine Alkaloids Isolated from *Mahonia aquifolium*," *Planta Medica* 61:372-73, 1995.

Müller, K., et al. "The Antipsoriatic *Mahonia aquifolium* and Its Active Components II. Antiproliferative Activity Against Cell Growth of Human Keratinocytes," *Planta Medica* 61:74-75, 1995.

Pansy

Herbalists get active components of pansy from the flowers of *Viola tricolor*, the wild pansy plant.

Why people use this herb

- Bronchitis
- Rheumatism
- Skin cancer
- Whooping cough

Common doses

Pansy is available as an extract. Some experts recommend the following doses:

- As a *tincture*, 2 to 4 milliliters taken orally.
- As a *tea*, drink three times daily.

Side effects

Call your health care practitioner if you experience diarrhea when using pansy.

Interactions

Combining herbs with certain drugs may alter their action or produce unwanted side effects. Tell your health care practitioner about any prescription or nonprescription drugs you're taking, especially aspirin or other products that contain salicylates.

Important points to remember

- Don't use pansy if you're pregnant or breast-feeding.
- Be aware that no evidence supports using pansy for any medical condition.

Other names for pansy

Other names for pansy include field pansy, heartsease, Johnny-jump-up, jupiter flower, ladies' delight, and wild pansy.

No known products containing pansy are available commercially.

Selected reference

Pápay, V., et al. "Study of Chemical Substances of *Viola tricolor* L.," *Acta Pharmaceutica Hungarcia* 157:153-58, 1987.

WHAT THE RESEARCH SHOWS

In one Hungarian study, pansy showed some ability to prevent heart spasms and reduce inflammation. However, without enough available clinical data, medical experts can't support pansy's medicinal use.

Papaya

Used to flavor candies and ice cream, papaya also is found in some facial creams to soften the skin. Some people use it as a meat tenderizer.

Papaya components used for herbal therapy usually come from the leaves, seeds, pulp, and latex of *Carica papaya.* Native to Mexico and Central America, this plant also grows in other tropical areas.

Why people use this herb

- Athletic injuries
- Herniated ("slipped") vertebral disk
- Inflammation
- Pinworm, tapeworm, and other worm infections
- Swelling and bruising after surgery
- To remove dead tissue

Common dose

Papaya comes as:

- tablets (5 milligrams)
- chewable tablets (25 milligrams)
- tea.

Some experts recommend the following dose:

- For *inflammation,* 10 milligrams taken orally four times daily for 7 days.

Side effects

Call your health care practitioner if you experience any of these possible side effects of papaya:

- abdominal pain or discomfort
- paralysis
- skin rash
- slow pulse
- symptoms of an acute allergic reaction, such as difficulty breathing, swallowing, or talking
- yellowish skin.

Injections of chymopapain (an enzyme in papaya) may cause a severe allergic reaction leading to death.

Interactions

Combining herbs with certain drugs may alter their action or produce unwanted side effects. Tell your health care practitioner about any prescription or nonprescription drugs you're taking.

Important points to remember

- Don't use papaya if you're pregnant or breast-feeding.
- Use papaya cautiously if you have a history of allergic reactions or if papaya gives you a skin rash.
- Don't take papaya for a long time because this may increase the risk of severe gastritis (inflammation of the stomach lining) and allergic reactions.
- Be aware that latex in the papaya plant can cause a skin rash.

> **WHAT THE RESEARCH SHOWS**
>
> Studies on people suggest that papaya may help ease inflammation caused by injuries or surgery. Lab tests on mice suggest that the herb also may act against digestive tract bacteria, although no human studies have been done in this area.

Other names for papaya

Other names for papaya include melon tree, papain, and pawpaw.

Products containing papaya are sold under such names as Papaya Enzyme, Papaya Enzyme with Chlorophyll, and Papaya Leaf.

Selected references

Giordani, R., et al. "Fungicidal Activity of Latex Sap from *Carica papaya* and Antifungal Effect of D(+)-Glucosamine on *Candida Albicans* Growth," *Mycoses* 39:103-10, 1996.

Lund, M., and Royer, R. "*Carica papaya* in Head and Neck Surgery," *Archives of Surgery* 98:180-82, 1969.

Pareira

Pareira is the source of curare, a poison that Amazonian and other South American Indians used when hunting. Curare quickly paralyzes an animal hit with a curare-tipped dart or spear. Tubocurarine, the modern medicine made from pareira, is used to relax a patient's muscles during surgery and other medical procedures.

Pareira comes from the roots and stems of *Chondrodendron tomentosum,* a tropical, woody vine found in the rain forests of the upper Amazon, Ecuador, and Panama. To prepare the herb, root and stem sections are cleaned, cut into segments, and dried.

Commercial pareira supplies come mainly from Rio de Janeiro and Bahia, Brazil. Traditional oral and topical use of pareira seems to be less dangerous than getting the poison into the bloodstream. The herb is bitter and slightly sweet.

Why people use this herb

- As an antiseptic
- Chronic urinary tract inflammation
- Constipation (mild)
- Fluid retention
- Generalized swelling
- Gonorrhea
- Jaundice
- Kidney stones
- Rheumatism
- Snakebite
- To induce menstruation
- Vaginal discharge

Common doses

Pareira is available as dried roots and stems and as powders or granules. In homeopathic preparations (such as Pareira Complex), it's typically combined with other plant species.

Some experts recommend the following doses:

- For *snakebites,* drink tea made from roots and apply bruised leaves to the area around the bite.
- For *other disorders,* take 2 to 4 milliliters of fluid extract orally, 10 to 20 grains of solid extract orally, or 1 to 4 fluid ounces of infusion orally.

Side effects

Call your health care practitioner if you experience unusual symptoms while using pareira.

Interactions

Combining herbs with certain drugs may alter their action or produce unwanted side effects. Don't use pareira while taking:

- Amikin
- Garamycin
- Mycifradin
- Nebcin
- Polymyxin B
- Streptomycin
- Xylocaine.

Important points to remember

- Use pareira only under the close supervision of a health care practitioner.
- Don't use this herb if you've had an allergic reaction to pareira, histamines, or tubocurarine during surgery.
- Avoid this herb if you have a liver, kidney, heart, respiratory, or endocrine disorder.
- Keep pareira away from broken skin or mucous membranes.
- Remember that the oral or topical form of pareira isn't the same as the medication used in surgery.
- Don't take pareira orally if you have ulcers in your mouth, stomach, or duodenum or if you have mouth sores or cuts. The chemicals could get into your blood and cause muscle paralysis. Seek immediate medical attention for such symptoms as blurred vision, droopy eyelids, a heavy feeling in your face, and jaw relaxation. The problem may progress to weak neck muscles, inability to raise your head, shallow breathing, and weakness or complete paralysis of your legs, and arms, and spine.

Other names for pareira

Other names for pareira include pareira brava and pareira radix.

A product containing pareira is sold as Pareira Complex.

Selected reference

Osol, A., and Farrar, G.E. *Dispensatory of the United States of America*, 25th ed. Philadelphia: Lippincott Williams & Wilkins, 1955.

WHAT THE RESEARCH SHOWS

The prescription drug tubocurarine (derived from pareira) has a definite role in modern medicine. However, use of pareira as an herb has little supporting evidence. Its potential risks outweigh any possible but unproven therapeutic benefits.

Parsley

The ancient Greeks made funeral wreaths from parsley and sprinkled the herb on dead bodies to help mask the smell of decomposition. Today, parsley serves mainly as a culinary herb and garnish. Small amounts of parsley leaves and oils are used in baked goods, sauces, stews, packaged meats, soups, and other processed foods.

Parsley comes from *Petroselinum crispum,* a wild plant found in parts of the Mediterranean area and cultivated in herb gardens worldwide. Herbalists use the leaves and, less often, the roots, seeds, and oil. Germany, France, Belgium, Hungary, and California are the largest parsley oil producers.

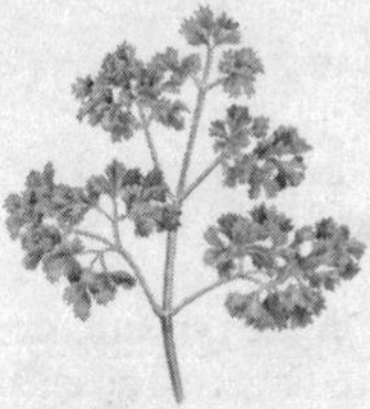

Why people use this herb

- Asthma
- Bladder problems
- Cough
- Fluid retention
- Digestive problems
- Generalized swelling
- High blood pressure
- Infections
- Intestinal gas
- Kidney problems
- Liver problems
- Muscle spasms
- Plague
- Rheumatism
- To stimulate menstruation

Common doses

Parsley comes as:

- capsules (430, 450, and 455 milligrams)
- liquid extract (1 ounce made from 1:1 in 25% alcohol)
- tea.

Some experts recommend the following doses:

- As a *tea,* 1 to 2 grams of the leaf or root steeped for 10 minutes in 1 cup of hot water. Drink two or three times daily.
- As a *liquid extract,* 2 to 4 milliliters taken orally three times daily.

Side effects

Call your health care practitioner if you experience any of these possible side effects of parsley:

- change in pulse rate
- sensitivity to sunlight
- skin rash.

Parsley oil can cause:

- congested blood vessels in the lungs
- digestive tract bleeding

- kidney damage
- liver problems
- low blood pressure
- smooth muscle contractions in the bladder, uterus, or intestine.

Interactions

Combining herbs with certain drugs may alter their action or produce unwanted side effects. Tell your health care practitioner about any prescription or nonprescription drugs you're taking, especially drugs that reduce blood pressure.

Don't use parsley while taking:
- antidepressants
- cough medicines that contain dextromethorphan
- Lithobid
- narcotic pain killers.

Important points to remember

- Don't use parsley (especially parsley oil) if you're pregnant or breast-feeding.
- Avoid this herb if you have multiple health problems.
- If you have heart problems, low blood pressure, kidney failure, a peptic ulcer, or liver disease, consult your health care practitioner before using parsley.
- Know that parsley sometimes is labeled *Apium petroselinum, Carum petroselinum,* or *Petroselinum sativum.*
- Be aware that little clinical evidence supports medicinal parsley use.

Other names for parsley

Other names for parsley include common parsley and garden parsley.

Products containing parsley are sold under such names as Insure Herbal, Parsley Herb, and Parsley Leaves.

WHAT THE RESEARCH SHOWS

Although parsley has shown some useful effects in animals, no studies on people have been done. Consequently, medical experts advise against eating more parsley than the amounts normally found in food.

Selected references

Buchanan, R.L. "Toxicity of Spices Containing Methylenedioxybenzene Derivatives: A Review," *Journal of Food Safety* 1:275-93, 1978.

Gershbein, L.L. "Regeneration of Rat Liver in the Presence of Essential Oils and Their Components," *Food and Cosmetic Toxicology* 15:171-81, 1977.

Petkov, V. "Plants with Hypotensive, Antiatheromatous and Coronarodilating Action," *American Journal of Chinese Medicine* 7:197-236, 1979.

Ziyyat, A., et al. "Phytotherapy of Hypertension and Diabetes in Oriental Morocco," *Journal of Ethnopharmacology* 58:45-54, 1997.

Parsley piert

A small, hairy annual reaching a height of about 4 inches, parsley piert *(Aphanes arvensis)* grows in Europe, North Africa, and North America. The herb's above-ground parts are harvested when the flower blooms in the summer and can be used fresh or dried.

Common doses

Parsley piert comes as:

- liquid extract (1:1 in 25% alcohol)
- tincture (1:5 in 45% alcohol)
- dried herb.

Some experts recommend the following doses:

- As *dried herb,* 2 to 4 grams taken orally.
- As a *liquid extract,* 2 to 4 milliliters taken orally three times daily.
- As a *tincture,* 2 to 10 milliliters taken orally three times daily.
- As a *tea,* mix a handful of the herb in 1 pint of boiling water, and drink 3 or 4 cups daily.

Why people use this herb

- Bladder inflammation
- Bladder stones
- Kidney problems
- Recurrent urinary tract infections
- Swelling caused by kidney or liver problems
- Urinary problems

Side effects

Call your health care practitioner if you experience unusual symptoms while using parsley piert.

Interactions

Combining herbs with certain drugs may alter their action or produce unwanted side effects. Tell your health care practitioner about any prescription or nonprescription drugs you're taking.

Important points to remember

- Don't use parsley piert if you're pregnant or breast-feeding.
- Know that medicinal use of parsley piert has no scientific basis.

Other names for parsley piert

Other names for parsley piert include field lady's mantle, parsley breakstone, and parsley piercestone.

A product containing parsley piert is sold as Parsley Piert.

WHAT THE RESEARCH SHOWS

Scientists have little chemical or clinical information on parsley piert. Medical experts say you shouldn't use this herb until they know more about its safety and effectiveness.

Selected reference

Newall, C.A., et al. *Herbal Medicines: A Guide for Healthcare Professionals.* London: Pharmaceutical Press, 1996.

Passion flower

Passion flower is a component in some European sedative drug mixtures. The Council of Europe lists the herb as a natural food flavoring, and in 1978 a passion flower chewing gum was patented in Romania.

Active components of the herb come from dried flowers and fruits of *Passiflora incarnata,* a perennial climbing vine found in tropical and subtropical areas of the Americas. Passion flower is collected almost entirely for export around the world.

Common doses

Available in several homeopathic remedies, passion flower comes as:

- liquid extract (1:1 in 25% alcohol)
- tincture (1:8 in 45% alcohol, or containing 0.7% flavonoids)
- crude extract
- dried herb.

Why people use this herb

- For calming effects

Some experts recommend the following doses:

- For *Parkinson's disease,* 10 to 30 drops of 0.7% flavonoids taken orally three times daily.
- As *dried herb,* 0.25 to 1 gram taken orally three times daily.
- As a *liquid extract,* 0.5 to 1 milliliter taken orally three times daily.
- As a *tea,* 4 to 8 grams (3 to 6 teaspoons) taken orally in equal doses throughout the day.
- As a *tincture,* 0.5 to 2 milliliters taken orally three times daily.

Side effects

Call your health care practitioner if you experience unusual symptoms while using passion flower.

Interactions

Combining herbs with certain drugs may alter their action or produce unwanted side effects. Tell your health care practitioner about any prescription or nonprescription drugs you're taking, especially:

- drugs that depress the central nervous system, such as alcohol, cold and allergy medicines, sedatives, tranquilizers, narcotic pain relievers, barbiturates, seizure drugs, and muscle relaxants
- drugs used to relieve depression called MAO inhibitors, such as Marplan or Nardil.

Important points to remember

- Don't use passion flower if you're pregnant or breast-feeding.
- Tell your health care practitioner if you are planning a pregnancy or suspect you're pregnant.
- Be aware that this herb may make you feel relaxed or sleepy.
- Don't confuse the passion flower used in herbal therapy with its close relative, the cultivated blue passion flower *(P. caerulea)*, which isn't used as an herb.

WHAT THE RESEARCH SHOWS

Although studies don't show that passion flower is dangerous, they don't show that it's effective in treating any medical condition. Thus, medical experts don't recommend this herb.

Other names for passion flower

Other names for passion flower include apricot vine, granadilla, Jamaican honeysuckle, maypop, passion fruit, and water lemon.

No known products containing passion flower are available commercially.

Selected references

Aoyagi, N., et al. "Studies on *Passiflora incarnata* Dry Extract. I. Isolation of Maltol and Pharmacological Action of Maltol and Ethylmaltol," *Chemical and Pharmaceutical Bulletin* 22:1008-13, 1974.

Hegnauer, R. *Chemotaxonomie der Planzen*, Vol 5: 295. Cited in Tyler, V., *The Honest Herbal,* 3rd ed. Binghamton, N.Y.: Pharmaceutical Products Press, 1993, p. 238.

Kimura, R., et al. "Central Depressant Effects of Maltol Analogs in Mice," *Chemical and Pharmaceutical Bulletin* 28:2570-79, 1980.

Ramstad, E. *Modern Pharmacognosy*. London: McGraw Hill, 1959.

Pau d'arco

South American Indians used the hard, durable wood of the pau d'arco tree *(Tabebuia impetiginosa, T. avellanedae,* or *Tecoma curialis)* to make bows for hunting. A flowering evergreen that belongs to the Bignonia family, the tree is native to Florida, the West Indies, Mexico, Central America, and South America.

Some pau d'arco species have been part of Latin American and Caribbean folk medicine for many years. The Portuguese, who first colonized Brazil, gave the tree its name. (Pau d'arco means "bow stick.")

Pau d'arco herbal products come from the tree bark. Researchers have extensively investigated lapachol and xyloidone, compounds in the herb, for antibacterial activity. However, many commercial pau d'arco products don't contain lapachol.

Common doses

Pau d'arco comes as:

- capsules (460 milligrams)
- tablets
- skin salve
- extract
- tea.

Some experts recommend the following doses:

- As *capsules,* 1 to 2 capsules taken orally twice daily at meals with water or as a tea, or 3 to 4 capsules taken orally three times daily for no more than 7 days.
- As *lapachol* (unspecified product), 1 to 2 grams taken daily.
- As *lapachol tea,* boil 15 to 20 grams of bark in 16 ounces of water for 10 minutes, to make a tea with a lapachol content of about 3%.

Why people use this herb

- AIDS
- Allergies
- Anemia
- As an aphrodisiac
- Backache
- Bed-wetting
- Boils
- Cancer
- Common cold
- Diabetes
- Dysentery
- External wounds
- Gonorrhea
- Headache
- Hernia
- Incontinence
- Infection
- Inflammation
- Liver disease
- Lupus
- Painful or difficult urination
- Rheumatism
- Smoker's cough
- Snakebite
- Sore throat
- Syphilis
- Toothache
- To "purify" the blood
- Ulcers
- Warts

Side effects

Call your health care practitioner if you experience any of these possible side effects of pau d'arco:

- nausea
- pinkish urine
- unusual or excessive bleeding
- vomiting.

Interactions

Combining herbs with certain drugs may alter their action or produce unwanted side effects. Don't use pau d'arco while taking blood thinners.

Important points to remember

- Don't use this herb if you're pregnant or breast-feeding.
- Avoid pau d'arco if you have a blood clotting disorder, such as hemophilia, severe liver disease, von Willebrand's disease, or thrombocytopenia.
- Be aware that some packages don't state how much pau d'arco they contain.
- Know that medical experts caution against using this herb instead of conventional medical treatment.

WHAT THE RESEARCH SHOWS

Researchers have studied only some of pau d'arco's chemical components—and found no evidence that they have benefits in treating any medical condition. Knowing that some chemicals in this herb could be toxic and that scientific data don't support herbalists' claims, most medical experts don't recommend using this herb.

Other names for pau d'arco

Other names for pau d'arco include ipe roxo, ipe, ipes, la pacho, lapacho colorado, lapacho, lapachol, lapacho morado, purple lapacho, red lapacho, roxo, taheebo, tajibo, trumpet bush, and trumpet tree.

Products containing pau d'arco are sold under such names as Advance Defense System Tablets, Brazilian Herbal Tea, Candistroy, Cat's Claw Defense Complex, Cellguard Coq 10 Nac, Healthgard With Echinacea, Immuno-Nourish, Pau D'arco, Pau D'arco Inner Bark,

Ultra Multiple Vitamin, Wellness Formula Vitamin, Wellness Multiple Max Daily, and Women's Ut Formula.

Selected references

Block, J.B., et al. "Early Clinical Studies with Lapachol (NSC-11905)," *Cancer Chemotherapy Reports* Part 2. 4:27-28, 1974.

Dinnen, R.D., and Ebisuzaki, K. "Search for Novel Anticancer Agents: A Differentiation-Based Assay and Analysis of a Folklore Product," *Anticancer Research* 17:1027-34, 1997.

Guiraud, P., et al. "Comparison of Antibacterial and Antifungal Activities of Lapachol and B-Lapachone," *Planta Medica* 60:373-74, 1994.

Peach

Many parts of the peach tree *(Prunus persica)* have been used for herbal therapy, including the leaves, bark, and seeds or kernels of the fruit. Typically, the bark is harvested from young trees in the spring, whereas leaves are gathered in summer. Both the bark and leaves are dried after harvest.

The fleshy, succulent fruit of the peach tree contains a hard, deeply wrinkled stone or pit surrounding a seed or kernel. Crushed seeds are marketed as health foods, cancer remedies, and vitamin supplements—even though they contain potentially harmful chemicals. An oil called persic oil can be expressed from the kernels. A substance called laetrile (also known as amygdalin or vitamin B-17) can be obtained from the kernels of peaches, apricots, plums, cherries, nectarines, apples, and almonds. Laetrile has been touted as a cancer prevention and cure. Unfortunately, extensive testing by the National Cancer Institute failed to show an anticancer effect. Laetrile has since been banned by the Food and Drug Administration because of the risk of cyanide poisoning.

Why people use this herb

- Constipation
- Cough
- Bad breath
- Blisters
- Boils
- Bronchitis
- Bruises
- Burns
- Dysentery
- Earache
- Eczema (a type of skin inflammation)
- Fluid retention
- Generalized swelling
- Headache
- Hemorrhage
- High blood pressure
- Lockjaw
- Menstrual pain
- Minor wounds
- Nervousness
- Pain
- Pinworm, tapeworm, and other worm infections
- Pneumonia
- Scurvy
- Shingles
- Skin irritation or inflammation
- Sore throat
- Stomach upset
- Warts

Common dose

Peach is available as persic oil, peach kernel oil, bark, leaves, and seeds. None of these preparations contain standardized amounts of active ingredient. Some experts recommend the following dose:

- As a *tea*, place 0.5 ounce of dried bark or 1 ounce of dried leaves in 16 ounces of boiling water, and steep for 15 minutes. Drink three times daily.

Side effects

Call your health care practitioner if you experience any of these possible side effects of peach:

- allergic reactions to the skin of the fruit
- symptoms of cyanide poisoning, including severe vomiting and stomach pain followed by fainting, drowsiness, and possibly seizures and coma.

Several people have died after eating peach pits. The seeds, leaves, flowers, and bark of the peach tree contain cyanogenic glycosides, which cause cyanide poisoning and can be lethal in fairly small amounts. A single gram of peach seeds contains about 2.6 milligrams of hydrocyanic acid. An adult who consumes 50 to 60 milligrams (about 20 grams of peach seeds) may die.

Interactions

Combining herbs with certain drugs may alter their action or produce unwanted side effects. Tell your health care practitioner about any prescription or nonprescription drugs you're taking.

Important points to remember

- Don't use peach as an herbal therapy if you're pregnant or breast-feeding.
- Wear gloves when handling peaches if you're allergic to the skin of the fruit.
- Keep peach pits and seeds away from children and pets.
- Don't eat peach pits or kernels because you could be poisoned.
- Know that chronic consumption of cyanogenic glycosides can cause vision problems, deafness, trouble walking, spastic muscles, and nerve damage in the feet and hands.

WHAT THE RESEARCH SHOWS

No clinical evidence supports the use of peach bark or leaves. More importantly, plenty of clinical data show the dangers of consuming peach pits, which can cause cyanide poisoning and death. Because of this risk and lack of evidence that peach pits prevent or cure cancer, medical experts warn against using them medicinally.

Other names for peach

Other names for peach include amygdalin, *Amygdalus persica,* laetrile, *Persica vulgaris,* and vitamin B-17.

Products containing peach are sold under such names as Laetrile and Vitamin B-17.

Selected references

Holzbecher, M.D., et al. "The Cyanide Content of Laetrile Preparations, Apricot, Peach, and Apple Seeds," *Clinical Toxicology* 22:341-47, 1984.

Mishra, A.K., and Dubey, N.K., "Fungitoxic Properties of *Prunus persica* Oil," *Hindustan Antibiotics Bulletin* 32:91-93, 1990. Abstract.

Moertel, C.G., et al. "A Clinical Trial of Amygdalin (Laetrile) in the Treatment of Human Cancer," *New England Journal of Medicine* 306:201-06, 1982.

Pennyroyal

In ancient times, people hung pennyroyal near convalescents to hasten their recovery. Pennyroyal garlands worn around the head were thought to cure dizziness and headache. The use of pennyroyal to induce abortion dates back to ancient Rome at the time of Pliny the Elder (23 to 79 A.D.).

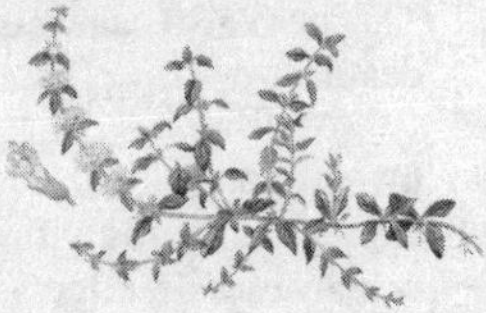

Active components come from the dried leaves and flowers of American pennyroyal *(Hedeoma pulegioides)* and European pennyroyal *(Mentha pulegium)*. Both plants, which belong to the mint family (Labiatae), have a strong, pungent odor similar to spearmint.

Pennyroyal's scientific name stems from the Latin term for flea, "pulex," which refers to the plant's use as an insect repellent. Some people rub pennyroyal leaves on their clothes and skin for this effect. The oil, which smells like citronella, has been used to scent soaps and detergents and as an insect repellent.

Why people use this herb

- Chest congestion
- Common cold
- Fever
- Flu
- Premenstrual syndrome
- Sharp intestinal pain
- To induce abortion
- Toothache
- To stimulate menstruation
- Tumors
- Uterine fibroids and hardening

Common doses

Pennyroyal comes as an oil, dried leaves, and flowers. Some experts recommend the following doses:

- As an *oil,* apply 1 to 8 drops to the skin as an insect repellent or as aromatherapy.
- As a *tea,* steep 1 to 2 teaspoons of dried pennyroyal leaves in 1 cup of boiling water for 10 to 15 minutes, or mix 1 tablespoon of dried herb in 1 cup of warm water. Drink up to 2 cups daily.

Side effects

Call your health care practitioner if you experience any of these possible side effects of pennyroyal:

- abdominal cramps
- confusion
- dizziness

- hallucinations
- lethargy
- malaise
- nausea
- seizures
- vomiting
- vomiting of blood.

This herb also can cause liver or kidney failure, weakness, coma, and death.

Interactions

Combining herbs with certain drugs may alter their action or produce unwanted side effects. Tell your health care practitioner about any prescription or nonprescription drugs you're taking, especially:

- Biaxin
- Cordarone
- Diflucan
- Ery-Tab
- Nizoral
- Prilosec
- Sporanox
- Tagamet
- Zithromax.

Important points to remember

- Don't use pennyroyal if you're pregnant or breast-feeding.
- Don't give this herb to children.
- Don't take pennyroyal if you have seizures, kidney problems, or liver problems.
- Don't consume pennyroyal oil internally. Less than 1 teaspoonful can cause seizures and as little as 1 tablespoon can cause death.
- Be aware that using pennyroyal to induce abortion could be fatal.
- Keep pennyroyal out of reach of children and pets.
- If you wish to take pennyroyal despite the risks, never exceed recommended doses and don't take the herb for more than 1 week.
- Stop using pennyroyal right away if you develop unusual symptoms.
- Know that although some herbalists continue to promote pennyroyal oils and teas for several ailments, these products can be harmful and shouldn't be ingested except under the close supervision of an experienced health care practitioner.

WHAT THE RESEARCH SHOWS

Studies show that pennyroyal can be harmful. No research proves that it's effective in treating any medical condition. Naturally, medical experts caution against using this herb.

Other names for pennyroyal

Other names for pennyroyal include American pennyroyal, European pennyroyal, mosquito plant, and squawmint.

Products containing pennyroyal are sold under such names as Aloe Herbal Horse Spray, Miracle Coat Spray-On Dog Shampoo, Pennyroyal, and Pennyroyal Essential Oil.

Selected references

Anderson, I.B., et al. "Pennyroyal Toxicity: Measurement of Toxic Metabolite Levels in Two Cases and Review of the Literature," *Annals of Internal Medicine* 124:726-34, 1996.

Sullivan, J.B., et al. "Pennyroyal Oil Poisoning and Hepatotoxicity," *JAMA* 242:2873-74, 1979.

Pepper, black

The most widely used spice in the world, black pepper has been used medicinally since the time of Hippocrates. In India, it's found in nearly every medicinal preparation. Black pepper also is used as an insecticide, in perfumes, as a brandy flavoring, and as a spice in foods, drinks, and desserts.

Why people use this herb

- Abdominal pain
- Arthritis
- Common cold
- Constipation
- Diabetes
- Diarrhea
- Digestive problems
- Dysentery
- Flu
- Fluid retention
- Heartburn
- Inadequate stomach juices
- Indigestion
- Intestinal gas
- Mental exhaustion
- Nicotine craving
- Obesity
- Pain
- Poor appetite
- Poor memory
- Poor spirits
- Respiratory phlegm and mucus
- Rheumatism
- Runny nose
- Sharp intestinal pain
- Sprains
- Stiffness
- Tumors
- Ulcers
- Weakness caused by cholera, coma, or vertigo

Piper nigrum, the black pepper plant, is a woody vine that can grow to 20 feet high. Originating in Southeast Asia, it was first cultivated by Indian colonists in Indonesia and has since been transplanted to equatorial areas, such as Brazil, Malaysia, Sumatra, and China.

Slow drying of the unripe fruit (berries) creates black pepper. (Quick drying of the unripe fruit produces green pepper; drying the ripe fruit after washing it down to the seed core yields white pepper.) Once dried, the pepper can be ground to varying grades of coarseness. Other plant parts, such as the essential oils, roots, and ethanol extracts, also can be used. These may be ground into a powder and mixed with other types of peppers.

Peppers once were named according to the port from which they were shipped—a system that hinted at the product's grade and potency. For example, Malabar pepper indicated the best peppercorns in India. Tellicherry, also from India, was a particularly bold version of Malabar pepper. These days, all Indian pepper is labeled Malabar.

Common dose

Black pepper is available as a powder ground to various grades of coarseness. Experts disagree on what dose to take.

Side effects

Call your health care practitioner if you experience unusual symptoms while taking black pepper.

Several children have died after eating a handful of black pepper.

Interactions

Combining herbs with certain drugs may alter their action or produce unwanted side effects. Tell your health care practitioner about any prescription or nonprescription drugs you're taking, especially:

- Coumadin
- drugs metabolized by the liver's cytochrome P-450 system, such as certain antibiotics (including Ery-Tab and Nizoral), Coumadin, Inderal, nonsteroidal anti-inflammatory drugs (for instance, Advil and Naprosyn), Theo-Dur, and Tylenol
- smoking cessation aids.

Important points to remember

- Use black pepper cautiously if you're pregnant or breast-feeding.
- Be aware that moderate doses of black pepper are harmless. The Food and Drug Administration considers this herb generally safe.
- Know that although black pepper may be useful as a smoking cessation aid, its full effects aren't known. If you want help in quitting smoking, consult your health care practitioner about standard smoking cessation treatment.

WHAT THE RESEARCH SHOWS

Most herbalists' claims for black pepper lack supporting evidence. However, animal studies suggest the spice might aid smoking cessation and make drugs more available in the body. Results of human studies are needed, though, before medical experts can recommend black pepper for these or other uses.

Other names for black pepper

Other names for black pepper include biber, filfil, hu-chiao, lada, kosho, krishnadi, pepe, peper, pfeffer, phi noi, pimenta, pjerets, poivre, the master spice, and the king of spices.

Products containing black pepper are sold under such names as Curry Powder, Galat Dagga, Garam Masala, Lowrey, McCormick, Panch Phoron, Quatre Epices, Ras El Hanout, Sambaar Podi, and Trikatu.

Selected references

Bano, G., et al. "Effect of piperine on Bioavailability and Pharmacokinetics of Propranolol and Theophylline in Healthy Volunteers," *European Journal of Clinical Pharmacology* 41:615-17, 1991.

Mujumdar, A.M., et al. "Anti-inflammatory Activity of Piperine," *Japanese Journal of Medical Science and Biology* 43:95-100, 1990.

Rose., J.E., and Behm., F.M. "Inhalation of Vapor from Black Pepper Extract Reduces Smoking Withdrawal Symptoms," *Drug and Alcohol Dependence* 34:225-92, 1994.

Peyote

The Native American Church uses peyote as a sacramental rite. Both peyote and mescaline, the chief active ingredient of the peyote cactus, are schedule I controlled substances. This means that in the federal government's view, they have no known medicinal value and a high abuse potential. (Native American Church members can't be prosecuted for using peyote or mescaline because it's part of their religion.)

Peyote comes from the dried tops or whole plants of *Lophophora williamsii*, a small cactus native to Mexico and southern Texas. Mescaline has been synthesized in laboratories as well.

Common doses

Peyote comes as:

- basic pan peyote (a chloroform extract of ground peyote)
- buttons (45 milligrams)
- mescaline hydrochloride or sulfate (375 milligrams of hydrochloride salt equals 500 milligrams of the sulfate salt)
- soluble peyote (hydrochloride extract of basic pan peyote used for injection)
- tincture (70% alcohol extract).

Mescaline doses of 5 milligrams per kilogram of body weight produce physical effects and hallucinations.

Side effects

Call your health care practitioner if you experience any of these possible side effects of peyote:

- abnormal eye movements
- anxiety
- enlarged pupils
- increased reflexes
- light sensitivity
- mood swings

Why people use this herb

- Alcoholism
- Angina
- Arthritis
- As part of religious ceremonies
- Backache
- Burns
- Corns
- Fever
- For a calming effect
- For a narcotic effect
- Headache
- Infections
- Paralysis
- Rheumatism
- Snakebite
- Sunstroke
- Throat irritation
- To cause hallucinations
- To induce intoxication

- nausea
- paranoia
- rapid pulse
- slow pulse
- sweating
- tremors
- trouble walking
- uncontrolled muscle contractions
- visual hallucinations
- vomiting.

Mescaline doses over 20 milligrams per kilogram of body weight may cause low blood pressure, slow pulse, and respiratory depression.

Interactions

Combining herbs with certain drugs may alter their action or produce unwanted side effects. Don't use peyote while taking drugs that act on the central nervous system, such as:

- alcohol
- marijuana
- narcotic pain relievers
- psychedelic drugs.

Important points to remember

- Don't use peyote or mescaline if you're pregnant or breast-feeding.
- Avoid peyote if you have a central nervous system disorder.
- Remember that although peyote doesn't seem to cause physical addiction, no one knows if it causes psychological dependence.
- Be aware that injuries and death are less likely to result from peyote itself than from the altered perception caused by high doses.
- Keep in mind that if you develop a severe mental reaction to peyote, a physician may need to prescribe a mild tranquilizer.
- Know that the peyote sometimes is mixed with phencyclidine (commonly called PCP or angel dust) and other illegal drugs that could be harmful.

Other names for peyote

Other names for peyote include anhalonium, big chief, buttons, cactus, mesc, mescal, mescal buttons, mescaline, mexc, moon, pan peyote, and peyote button.

No known products containing peyote are available commercially.

WHAT THE RESEARCH SHOWS

Peyote has no known valid medicinal use. Also, it's illegal.

Selected references

Ghansah, E., et al. "Effects of Mescaline and Some of Its Analogs on Cholinergic Neuromuscular Transmission," *Neuropharmacology* 32:169-74, 1993.

Giannini, A.J., et al. "Contemporary Drugs of Abuse," *American Family Physician* 33:207-16, 1986.

Monte, A.P., et al. "Dihydrobenzofuran Analogues of Hallucinogens. 4. Mescaline Derivatives," *Journal of Medicinal Chemistry* 40:2997-3008, 1997.

Pill-bearing spurge

Pill-bearing spurge *(Euphorbia pilulifera)* is an annual herb that's native to India and Australia. In the United States, it grows from Texas to Arizona. The crude drug comes from the dried plant. Other names for the plant are *E. hirta* and *E. capitata.*

Why people use this herb

- Asthma
- Bronchitis
- Cough
- Diarrhea
- Dysentery
- Eye problems
- Gonorrhea
- Hay fever
- Intestinal ameba infection
- Snakebite
- Thrush (yeast infection in the mouth)

Common doses

Pill-bearing spurge comes as capsules, dried plant (powder), liquid extract, tablets, and tincture. Some experts recommend the following doses:

- As *dried plant,* 120 to 300 milligrams taken orally or by infusion (orally) three times daily.
- As a *liquid extract* (1:1 in 45% alcohol*),* 0.12 to 0.3 milliliter taken orally three times daily.
- As a *tincture* (1:5 in 60% alcohol), 0.6 to 2 milliliters taken orally three times daily.

Side effects

Call your health care practitioner if you experience any of these possible side effects of pill-bearing spurge:

- overdose symptoms, such as increased salivation, tiny pupils, throat closure, slow pulse, intestinal contractions, and frequent urination
- skin rash
- stomach irritation
- vomiting.

Interactions

Combining herbs with certain drugs may alter their action or produce unwanted side effects. Tell your health care practitioner about any prescription or nonprescription drugs you're taking, especially:

- ACE inhibitors, such as Capoten and Vasotec
- Antabuse
- anticholinergics such as atropine
- Antilirium

- Aricept
- barbiturates
- blood thinners such as Coumadin
- cholinesterase inhibitors such as Antilirium
- Ery-Tab
- muscarinic agonists, such as arecoline, methacholine, and muscarine
- Sandimmune
- Tensilon.

Important points to remember

- Don't use pill-bearing spurge if you're pregnant or breast-feeding.
- If you have a bleeding disorder, use this herb carefully, if at all.
- Stop using pill-bearing spurge at once if you start sweating, salivating, or vomiting; if your eyes start tearing; or if your pulse slows.
- Know that handling products that contain pill-bearing spurge may cause allergies and skin reactions.
- If you take Antabuse, don't use forms of pill-bearing spurge that contain alcohol.

Other names for pill-bearing spurge

Other names for pill-bearing spurge include asthma weed, catshair, euphorbia, garden spurge, milkweed, queensland asthmaweed, and snake weed.

Products containing pill-bearing spurge are sold under such names as As-Comp, Ephedra Plus, Euphorbia, *Euphorbia hirta,* and Sinus and Catarrh Complex.

WHAT THE RESEARCH SHOWS

Studies on animals suggest pill-bearing spurge has some ability to treat certain infections and reduce pain, fever, inflammation, nervousness, and anxiety. No research has been done on people to support these early results. However, one study showed that pill-bearing spurge is neither safe nor effective in treating asthma. Because of the risk of drug interactions, most medical experts urge anyone who takes prescription medications to use this herb cautiously, if at all.

Selected references

Galvez, J., et al. "Antidiarrheic Activity of *Euphorbia hirta* Extract and Isolation of an Active Flavonoid Constituent," *Planta Medica* 59:333-36, 1993.

Lanhers, M.C., et al. "Analgesic, Antipyretic, and Anti-inflammatory Properties of *Euphorbia hirta,*" *Planta Medica* 57:225-31, 1991.

Watt, J.M., and Breyer-Brandwijk, M.G. *The Medicinal and Poisonous Plants of Southern and Eastern Africa,* 2nd ed. Edinburgh and London: E and S Livingston LTD., 1962.

Pineapple

Pineapple's active components—chiefly the enzyme bromelain—come from the juice and fruiting portion of the pineapple plant *(Ananas comosus)*. A member of the bromeliad family (Bromeliaceae), this plant originated in South America and now is cultivated widely in tropical regions, especially Hawaii and Thailand.

Bromelain was once used to treat burns and stings, but its effectiveness was never proven and its popularity for that purpose waned. The food industry still uses it as a meat tenderizer.

Common dose

Pineapple is available as juice, syrup, candy, whole fruit, and extracts. Experts disagree on what dose to take.

Side effects

Call your health care practitioner if you experience any of these possible side effects of excessive amounts of pineapple juice:

- diarrhea
- nausea
- skin rash
- sores at the corners of the mouth
- uterine contractions
- vomiting.

Why people use this herb

- Constipation
- Jaundice
- Localized inflammation and swelling
- Obesity
- To prevent ulcers
- Wounds

Interactions

Combining herbs with certain drugs may alter their action or produce unwanted side effects. Don't use pineapple while taking:

- ACE inhibitors, such as Capoten or Vasotec
- blood thinners such as Coumadin.

Important points to remember

- Don't consume large amounts of pineapple if you're pregnant or breast-feeding. Be aware that drinking large amounts of juice during pregnancy may promote uterine contractions.
- Know that drinking large amounts of juice may cause stomach distress.

Other names for pineapple

Other names for pineapple include ananas, golden rocket, and smooth cayenne pineapple.

A product containing pineapple is sold as Ananase.

> **WHAT THE RESEARCH SHOWS**
>
> Pineapple is a good source of bromelain, an enzyme with useful properties. But researchers don't have enough data to support therapeutic use of the pineapple plant. Medical experts caution against consuming pineapple in amounts greater than those normally found in food.

Selected references

Helser, M.A., et al. "Influence of Fruit and Vegetable Juices on the Endogenous Formation of N-Nitrosoproline and N-Nitrosthiozolidine-4-Carboxylic Acid In Humans on Controlled Diets," *Carcinogenesis* 13:2277, 1992.

Lotz-Winter, H. "On the Pharmacology of Bromelain: An Update with Special Regard to Animal Studies on Dose-Dependent Effects," *Planta Medica* 56:249, 1990.

Rowan, A.D., et al. "Debridement of Experimental Full-Thickness Skin Burns of Rats with Enzyme Fractions Derived from Pineapple Stem," *Burns* 16:243, 1990.

Pipsissewa

Pipsissewa comes from the dried leaves of the creeping perennial *Chimaphila umbellata*. This herb, which belongs to the heath family (Ericaceae), originated in Eurasia and northern North America.

Common dose

Pipsissewa comes as a crude extract. Experts disagree on what dose to take.

Side effects

Call your health care practitioner if you experience any of these possible side effects of pipsissewa:

- diarrhea
- nausea
- skin eruptions
- upset stomach
- vomiting.

Why people use this herb

- Diarrhea
- Fluid loss
- Fluid retention
- Nervous disorders
- Seizures
- Sores
- To cause sweating
- To ease muscle spasms
- Ulcers

Interactions

Combining herbs with certain drugs may alter their action or produce unwanted side effects. Tell your health care practitioner about any prescription or nonprescription drugs you're taking, especially iron supplements.

Don't take pipsissewa within 2 hours of consuming iron-rich foods, such as meat, poultry, fish, whole or enriched grains, citrus fruits, and leafy green vegetables.

Important points to remember

- Don't use pipsissewa if you're pregnant or breast-feeding.
- Use pipsissewa cautiously, if at all, if you have iron deficiency or a digestive tract disorder (such as ulcerative colitis, esophageal reflux disease, a stomach or duodenal ulcer, or a malabsorption disorder).
- Stop taking this herb at once if you develop unusual symptoms.

Other names for pipsissewa

Other names for pipsissewa include ground holly, prince's-pine, spotted wintergreen, and wintergreen.

WHAT THE RESEARCH SHOWS

No research results are available to establish safe doses or support the therapeutic use of this herb. Medical experts don't recommend consuming it.

No known products containing pipsissewa are available commercially.

Selected reference

Segelman, A.B., and Farnsworth, N.R. "Biological and Phytochemical Evaluation of Plants. IV. A New Rapid Procedure For the Simultaneous Determination of Saponins and Tannins," *Lloydia* 32:5695, 1969.

Plantains

Plantains include several plants from the buckwheat family (Polygonaceae). Active ingredients come from the leaves of *Plantago lanceolata* and *P. major* and from the seeds and husks of *P. psyllium* and *P. ovata*. Products from these plants are distributed worldwide. The best known is psyllium.

Common dose

Plantains are available as psyllium supplied as seeds, powder, or tablets. They also come as:

- liquid extract (1:1 in 25% alcohol)
- tincture (1:5 in 45% alcohol) of the leaves of other plantain species.

Some experts recommend the following dose:

- As a *laxative,* 7.5 grams of plantain seeds taken orally with 12 to 16 ounces of water.

Why people use this herb

- Burns
- Cancer
- Chronic bronchitis
- Chronic diarrhea
- Constipation
- Cough
- Dysentery
- Fluid retention
- High cholesterol
- Immune system problems
- Poison ivy
- Skin and mucous membrane inflammation
- Throat irritation
- Urinary tract disorders
- Wounds

Side effects

Call your health care practitioner if you experience any of these possible side effects of plantains:

- abdominal bloating
- allergic reaction
- diarrhea
- intestinal gas
- skin rash.

This herb also can cause:

- intestinal obstruction
- low blood pressure.

Anaphylaxis, a life-threatening allergic reaction, has occurred in people not previously allergic to psyllium who were exposed to plantains at work.

Interactions

Combining herbs with certain drugs may alter their action or produce unwanted side effects. Don't use plantains while taking:

- digoxin
- heart drugs called beta blockers (such as Inderal) or calcium channel blockers (such as Calan or Procardia)
- Lithobid
- Tegretol.

Important points to remember

- Don't use plantains if you're pregnant or breast-feeding.
- Avoid plantains if you've had an intestinal obstruction.
- Use plantains carefully, if at all, if you're allergic to weed pollens or are exposed to plantains at work.
- If you get a rash while using plantains, stop taking them at once and call your health care practitioner.
- Keep in mind that there are better, more standard forms of bulk laxatives than plantains.
- Take plantains several hours before or after other medications—not at the same time.
- Know that the Food and Drug Administration recently found that some plantains are contaminated with cardiac glycosides (chemicals that can affect heart contractions).

Other names for plantains

Other names for plantains include blond plantago, broadleaf plantain, buckhorn, cart tract plant, common plantain, English plantain, flea seed, French psyllium, greater plantain, Indian plantago, lanten, narrowleaf plantago seed, plantain, plantain seed, psyllium, ribwort, ripple grass, snakeweed, Spanish psyllium, tract plant, way-bread, white man's foot, wild plantain, and wild saso.

Products containing plantains are sold under such names as Effer-Syllium, Hydrocil, Konsyl, Metamucil, and Perdeim.

WHAT THE RESEARCH SHOWS

Although psyllium, a plantain product, shows some ability to reduce cholesterol, the clinical jury is still out. Until more research results are available, medical experts can't say that plantains have a valid therapeutic use.

Selected references

Lantner R.R., et al. "Anaphylaxis Following Ingestion of a Psyllium-Containing Cereal," *JAMA* 264:2534-36, 1990.

Murai, M., et al. "Phenylethanoids in the Herb of *Plantago lanceolata* and Inhibitory Effect on Arachidonic Acid-Induced Mouse Ear Edema," *Planta Medica* 61:479-80, 1995.

Pokeweed

Pokeweed has long been used as an edible green vegetable, but only the young shoots are safe to eat—and only after boiling. A weedy, perennial shrub, pokeweed *(Phytolacca americana)* grows throughout eastern North America. Active components come from the plant's roots, stems, leaves, and berries.

Why people use this herb

- Breast abscess or inflammation
- Cough
- Itching
- Laryngitis
- Mumps
- Rheumatism
- Swollen lymph nodes
- To induce vomiting
- To promote bowel movements
- Tonsillitis

Common doses

Pokeweed comes as an extract (1:1 in 45% alcohol) and a tincture. Some experts recommend the following doses:

- To *induce vomiting,* 60 to 300 milligrams of dried root.
- As an *extract,* 0.1 to 0.5 milliliter taken orally.

Side effects

Call your health care practitioner if you experience any of these possible side effects of pokeweed:

- blurred vision
- confusion
- diarrhea
- dizziness
- drooling
- eye irritation
- fainting
- fast pulse
- headache
- incontinence
- nausea
- seizures
- skin rash (from touching the plant)
- sneezing
- sore throat
- sweating
- tremors
- vomiting
- weakness.

This herb also can cause:
- blood disorders
- coma
- low blood pressure
- respiratory problems.

Several children have died from heart problems after taking pokeweed.

Interactions

Combining herbs with certain drugs may alter their action or produce unwanted side effects. Don't use pokeweed when taking:
- Antabuse
- drugs that depress the nervous system, such as alcohol, cold and allergy drugs, sedatives, tranquilizers, narcotic pain relievers, barbiturates, seizure drugs, and muscle relaxants
- fertility drugs
- oral contraceptives.

Important points to remember

- Don't use pokeweed if you're pregnant or breast-feeding.
- Tell your health care practitioner if you are planning a pregnancy or suspect you're pregnant.
- Use pokeweed cautiously, if at all, if you have a history of allergic reactions or skin inflammation after contact with certain substances.
- Don't drive or perform other dangerous activities until you know how pokeweed affects you.
- If you're taking Antabuse, don't use a pokeweed form that contains alcohol.
- Keep pokeweed and its preparations away from children and pets.
- Keep in mind that this herb is toxic and can be dangerous.
- Wear gloves if you must handle the plant, especially if you have cuts or abrasions on your hands.

Other names for pokeweed

Other names for pokeweed include cancer jalap, cancer root, changras, coakum, crowberry, garget, pigeonberry, pocon, pokeberry, poke salad, pokeweed root, redink plant, redwood, scoke, txiu kub nyug, and Virginia poke.

No known products containing pokeweed are available commercially.

WHAT THE RESEARCH SHOWS

All parts of the pokeweed plant seem to be toxic. Although early studies suggest a pokeweed protein may help treat certain types of cancer (leukemias and osteosarcomas), it's too early to know for sure.

Selected references

Anderson, P.M., et al. "In Vitro and In Vivo Cytotoxicity of an Anti-osteosarcoma Immunotoxin Containing Pokeweed Antiviral Protein," *Cancer Research* 55:1321-27, 1995.

Fernald, M.L., and Kinsey, A.C. *Edible Wild Plants of Eastern North America.* New York: Harper & Brothers, 1958.

Hamilton, R.J., and Shih, R.D. "Mobitz Type I Heart Block After Pokeweed Ingestion," *Veterinary and Human Toxicology* 37:66-67, 1995.

Jansen, B., et al. "Establishment of a Human T(4;11) Leukemia in Severe Combined Immunodeficient Mice and Successful Treatment Using Anti-CD19 (B43)-Pokeweed Antiviral Protein Immunotoxin," *Cancer Research* 52:406-12, 1992.

Myers, D.E., et al. "Large Scale Manufacturing of TXU (Anti-CD7)-Pokeweed Antiviral Protein (PAP) Immunoconjugate for Clinical Trials," *Leukemia and Lymphoma* 27:275-302, 1997.

Roberge, R., et al. "The Root of Evil: Pokeweed Intoxication," *Annals of Emergency Medicine* 15:470-73, 1986.

Pomegranate

A shrub that originated in northwestern India, the pomegranate plant *(Punica granatum)* now grows in many tropical areas. Active herbal components come from the bark, roots, stems, and fruit.

Common dose

Pomegranate comes as crude herb or extract. Experts disagree on what dose to take.

Side effects

Call your health care practitioner if you experience any of these possible side effects of pomegranate:

- allergic reactions, such as skin rash
- nausea
- vomiting.

Why people use this herb

- Diarrhea
- Pinworms, tapeworms, and other worm infections

This herb also can cause liver damage.

Pomegranate seeds and peels may increase the risk of some cancers because dried pomegranate peel contains high amounts of aflatoxin B-1, a known carcinogen. Scientists have discovered that women in northern Iran have the highest esophageal cancer rate in the world, possibly because they eat a local food called majum or majoweh during pregnancy. It contains crushed sour pomegranate seeds, black pepper, dried raisins, and sometimes garlic—a harsh mixture that seems to injure the esophagus. (Other local practices, such as eating foods at higher-than-normal temperatures, preserving food by sun-drying, and eating few fruits and vegetables, also may be factors).

Interactions

Combining herbs with certain drugs may alter their action or produce unwanted side effects. Tell your health care practitioner about any prescription or nonprescription drugs you're taking.

Important points to remember

- Don't use pomegranate if you're pregnant or breast-feeding.
- Avoid this herb if you have asthma or have a history of allergic reactions.

- If you have liver problems, use pomegranate cautiously, if at all. Your health care practitioner may recommend periodic liver function tests.
- Be aware that continued use of pomegranate may increase your risk for certain cancers.

WHAT THE RESEARCH SHOWS

In the test tube, pomegranate has acted against some causes of diarrhea, including certain fungi, viruses, and intestinal worms. Few studies have been done in people, though, and scientists suspect pomegranate may be linked to certain cancers. Medical experts say you shouldn't take the herb internally until more information is available.

Other names for pomegranate

Other names for pomegranate include granatum.

No known products containing pomegranate are available commercially.

Selected references

Ghadirian, P. "Food habits of the People of the Caspian Littoral of Iran in Relation to Esophageal Cancer," *Nutrition and Cancer* 9:147-57, 1987.

Navarro, V., et al. "Antimicrobial Evaluation of Some Plants Used in Mexican Traditional Medicine for the Treatment of Infectious Diseases," *Journal of Ethnopharmacology* 53:143-47, 1996.

Segura, J.J., et al. "Growth Inhibition of *Entamoeba histolytica* and *E. invadens* Produced by Pomegranate Root," *Archivos de Investigacion Medica* 21:235-39, 1990.

Selim, M.I., et al. "Aflatoxin B-1 in Common Egyptian Foods," *Journal of AOAC International* 79:1124-29, 1996.

Poplar

Herbalists use bark from the white poplar *(Populus alba)*, quaking aspen *(P. tremuloides)*, and black poplar *(P. nigra)* as well as liquid produced by poplar leaf buds. In fact, honeybees collect this liquid from buds, especially those from poplar trees. Getting the liquid on your skin, though, can cause a severe rash.

Common doses

Poplar comes as dried powdered bark or liquid extract (1:1 in 25% alcohol). Some experts recommend the following doses:

- As *a liquid extract,* 1 to 5 milliliters taken orally three times daily.
- As *powdered bark,* 1 to 5 grams taken orally or by decoction three times daily.

Why people use this herb

- Bladder inflammation
- Common cold
- Diarrhea
- Inflammation
- Liver disorders
- Rheumatism
- Stomach problems

Side effects

Call your health care practitioner if you experience any of these possible side effects of poplar:

- asthma
- itching
- ringing in the ear
- skin rash
- stomach upset.

This herb also can cause digestive tract bleeding, kidney problems, and liver damage.

Interactions

Combining herbs with certain drugs may alter their action or produce unwanted side effects. Don't use poplar if you're taking:

- antiplatelet drugs, such as Ticlid
- aspirin or other products that contain salicylates.
- blood thinners, such as Coumadin

Important points to remember

- Don't use poplar if you're pregnant or breast-feeding.
- Use poplar cautiously, if at all, if you're allergic to plants, aspirin, or other drugs that contain salicylates or if you have digestive tract bleeding, nasal polyps, bronchial asthma, kidney disease, or peptic ulcer disease.

- Know that taking poplar orally can raise your risk of digestive tract bleeding if you have peptic ulcer disease or if you're taking a blood thinner or antiplatelet drug.
- Don't use poplar if you have a viral illness because you could develop a serious disease called Reye's syndrome. For the same reason, don't give this herb to a child with a viral illness.
- Don't use poplar while taking drugs that contain aspirin or salicylates.

WHAT THE RESEARCH SHOWS

With so little available animal and human data, medicinal use of poplar can't be recommended.

Other names for poplar

Other names for poplar include American aspen, black poplar, quaking aspen, and white poplar.

No known products containing poplar are available commercially.

Selected references

Amoros, M., et al. "Comparison of the Anti-Herpes Simplex Virus Activities of Propolis and 3-methyl-but-2-enyl Caffeate," *Journal of Natural Products* 57:644-47, 1994.

Hausen, B.M., et al. "Propolis Allergy. (I) Origin, Properties, Usage, and Literature Review," *Contact Dermatitis* 17:163-70, 1987.

Hausen, B.M., et al. "Propolis Allergy. (II) The Sensitizing Properties of 1,1,-dimethylallyl Caffeic Acid Ester," *Contact Dermatitis* 17:171-77, 1987.

Prickly ash

In folk medicine, prickly ash is known as the "toothache tree" because chewing the bark supposedly relieves toothache pain. However, experts suspect that ingesting parts of prickly ash trees has sickened or killed sheep and cattle in Indiana and Georgia.

Herbal products containing prickly ash come from the bark of the northern prickly ash *(Zanthoxylum americanum)* and the southern prickly ash *(Z. clava-herculis)* trees. Both belong to the rue (citrus) family (Rutaceae) and are native to the United States.

Common doses

Prickly ash comes as:

- tincture (1:5 in 45% alcohol)
- berry liquid extract (1:1 in 25% alcohol)
- bark.

Some experts recommend the following doses:

- As a *tincture,* up to 5 milliliters taken orally three times daily.
- As a *decoction,* 15 grams of bark in 600 milliliters of water taken orally in equal doses three times daily.

Why people use this herb

- Fever
- Intestinal gas
- Rheumatism
- To induce sweating
- To promote circulation
- To stimulate the digestive tract

Side effects

Call your health care practitioner if you experience any of these possible side effects of prickly ash:

- bruising
- heavy bleeding
- increased sensitivity to sunlight.

Interactions

Combining herbs with certain drugs may alter their action or produce unwanted side effects. Don't use prickly ash while taking:

- Antabuse
- aspirin or another drug containing salicylates
- blood thinners.

Important points to remember

- Don't use prickly ash if you're pregnant or breast-feeding.
- Tell your health care practitioner if you are planning a pregnancy or suspect you're pregnant.
- Don't use prickly ash if you're allergic to it or to other plants.
- If you're taking Antabuse, don't use a prickly ash product that contains alcohol.
- If you notice unexplained bruising, bleeding, or other unusual symptoms, stop using prickly ash at once and call your health care practitioner.

> **WHAT THE RESEARCH SHOWS**
>
> Clinical information doesn't support the use of prickly ash, so medical experts don't recommend it for any condition.

Other names for prickly ash

Other names for prickly ash include angelica tree, Hercules' club, northern prickly ash, southern prickly ash, suterberry, and toothache tree.

No known products containing prickly ash are available commercially.

Selected reference

Newall, C.A., et al., eds. *Herbal Medicines: A Guide for Health Care Professionals.* London: Pharmaceutical Press, 1996.

Primrose, evening

Evening primrose *(Oenothera biennis)* recently made headlines as a possible remedy for premenstrual syndrome. A biennial, it is cultivated or grows wild in parts of North America and Europe. The oil, extracted from the seeds, can be used as an herbal preparation or as a vegetable with a peppery flavor.

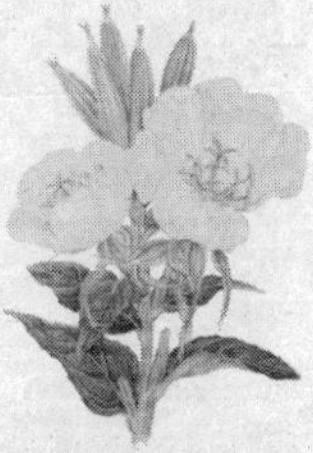

Common doses

Evening primrose comes as:

- capsules (50, 500, and 1,300 milligrams)
- gelcaps (500 and 1,300 milligrams).

Some experts recommend the following doses (based on a standardized gamma linoleic acid content of 8%):

- For *eczema (a type of skin inflammation) in an adult,* 320 milligrams to 8 grams taken orally daily for 3 months.
- For *eczema in children ages 1 to 12,* 160 milligrams to 4 grams taken orally daily for 3 months.
- For *mastalgia,* 3 to 4 grams taken orally daily.

For other disorders, experts disagree on what dose to take.

Side effects

Call your health care practitioner if you experience any of these possible side effects of evening primrose:

- headache
- inflammation
- nausea
- skin rash.

This herb also can cause:

- blood clots
- immune system suppression.

Why people use this herb

- Allergic skin reactions
- Asthma
- Breast pain
- Cough from asthma
- Eczema (a type of skin inflammation)
- High cholesterol
- Multiple sclerosis
- Nerve pain caused by diabetes
- Nervousness
- Pain
- Premenstrual syndrome
- Psoriasis (scaly, raised skin patches)
- Raynaud's disease (a type of circulation disorder)
- Rheumatoid arthritis
- Sjögren's syndrome (a connective tissue disease)
- Whooping cough
- Wounds

Using evening primrose oil makes you more prone to seizures, especially if you have schizophrenia or take a medication that lowers your seizure threshold, such as Compazine, Mellaril, Navane, Permitil, Phenergan, Prolixin, Serentil, Stelazine, Thorazine, or Trilafon.

Interactions

Combining herbs with certain drugs may alter their action or produce unwanted side effects. Don't use evening primrose while taking:

- Compazine
- Mellaril
- Navane
- Permitil
- Phenergan
- Prolixin
- Serentil
- Stelazine
- Thorazine
- Trilafon.

Important points to remember

- Don't use evening primrose oil if you're pregnant or breast-feeding.
- Use evening primrose oil cautiously, if at all, if you have a history of seizures or take a drug that makes seizures more likely.
- Give this herb to a hyperactive child *only* under close supervision of a primary health care practitioner.

Other names for evening primrose

Other names for evening primrose include king's-cure-all.

Products containing evening primrose are sold under such names as Efamol, Epogram, Evening Primrose Oil, Mega Primrose Oil, My Favorite Evening Primrose Oil, and Primrose Power.

Selected reference

Kleijnen, J. "Evening Primrose Oil," *BMJ* 309:824-25, 1994.

WHAT THE RESEARCH SHOWS

In theory, the chemicals in evening primrose oil may have a therapeutic effect on the way the body metabolizes fatty acids. Clinical trials on people and animals are underway, but the results aren't conclusive for any medical claims made for this herb. More studies must be done to confirm the therapeutic value of evening primrose oil.

Pulsatilla

Pulsatilla has a long history in many cultures. The Greeks believed that Anemos, god of the winds, sent the plant's flowers to herald his coming in early spring. The English called pulsatilla plants *windflowers* because they seemed to be blown open by the wind. The French called pulsatilla *pasque flower*, a reference to Easter. The Chinese considered pulsatilla a bad omen and called it the flower of death. Still other cultures viewed it as a charm against disease.

Active components come from dried leaves, stems, and flowers of pulsatilla *(Anemone pulsatilla)*, also called anemone. When this perennial plant flowers, some parts of it open wide in the sunshine but close and fold over when evening approaches or rain threatens. This folded flower has been likened to a tiny tent. Legend has it that fairies used these tents for shelter from the elements.

Pulsatilla has been used medicinally for centuries. The Roman physician Dioscorides (40 to 90 A.D.) used it to treat eye problems. Native Americans used a poultice of crushed, fresh leaves to treat rheumatism and neuralgia. They also inhaled the dried, pulverized leaves for headache and took a decoction of the root for respiratory problems.

Why people use this herb

- Cataracts
- Circulatory problems
- Common cold
- Cough
- Digestive problems
- Earache
- Fluid retention
- Genitourinary tract spasms
- Glaucoma
- Gynecologic disorders
- Iris inflammation
- Middle ear infection in children
- Migraine
- Nervousness
- Pain
- Respiratory phlegm and mucus
- Restlessness
- Retinal disease
- Scleritis (inflammation of a part of the eye)
- Sharp stabbing pain
- Skin inflammation or infection
- Sleep disorders
- To stimulate menstruation

Common doses

Pulsatilla comes as dried herb, liquid extract, tincture, and in homeopathic remedies. Some experts recommend the following doses:

- As *dried herb,* 0.1 to 0.3 gram in an infusion taken orally three times daily. Or half a teaspoon of dried herb added to 1 cup of boiling water, steeped for 10 to 15 minutes, and taken orally three times daily.

- As a *liquid extract* (1:1 in 25% alcohol), 0.1 to 0.3 milliliter taken orally three times daily.
- As a *tincture* (1:10 in 25% alcohol), 0.5 to 3 milliliters taken orally three times daily.

Side effects

Call your health care practitioner if you experience any of these possible side effects of pulsatilla:

- bloody urine
- burning of the throat and tongue (if chewed)
- stomach upset
- vomiting.

This herb also may cause:

- irritation of the kidney and urinary tract
- proteins in the urine
- severe skin or mucous membrane irritation from contact with fresh plant parts.

Interactions

Combining herbs with certain drugs may alter their action or produce unwanted side effects. Tell your health care practitioner about any prescription or nonprescription drugs you're taking.

Important points to remember

- Don't use pulsatilla if you're pregnant or breast-feeding.
- Don't use or handle fresh plant parts.
- Call your health care practitioner immediately if you experience painful urination or see blood in your urine.
- Be aware that pulsatilla is a poison. In animals, it has caused vision problems, blindness, nose and throat irritation, sneezing, paralysis, seizures, dizziness, mouth and throat sores, vomiting, abdominal pain, diarrhea, excessive salivation, kidney damage, blisters, pigment changes, and urinary problems.

Other names for pulsatilla

Other names for pulsatilla include crowfoot, Easter flower, kubjelle, meadow anemone, pasque flower, prairie anemone, *Pulsatillae herba*, smell fox, stor, and windflower.

Products containing pulsatilla are sold under such names as Ana-Sed, Biocarde, Calmo, Cicaderma, Cirflo, Eviprostat, Eviprostat N,

Hemoluol, Histo-Fluine P, Mensuosedyl, Nytol Herbal, Premantaid, Pulsatilla Med Complex, Viburnum Complex, and Yeast-X.

WHAT THE RESEARCH SHOWS

Until clinical studies document that pulsatilla is safe and effective in people, medical experts can't recommend this herb for medicinal uses. The potential for side effects outweighs known therapeutic benefits.

Selected references

Dobelis, I.N., ed. *Magic and Medicine of Plants*. Pleasantville, N.Y.: Reader's Digest Association, Inc., 1986.

Friese, K.H., et al. "The Homeopathic Treatment of Otitis Media in Children–Comparisons with Conventional Therapy," *International Journal of Clinical Pharmacology Therapy* 35:296-301, 1997.

Pumpkin

In many cultures, people eat small amounts of pumpkin seed daily to prevent worm infections. In Bulgaria, Turkey, and Ukraine, some people eat a handful of pumpkin seeds every day to treat benign prostate enlargement.

Pumpkin comes from *Cucurbita pepo,* a plant cultivated for medicinal, nutritional, and other practical uses. It's used most often for medicinal products in the United States. Roasted seeds commonly are sold as snacks.

Common dose

Pumpkin comes as seeds (whole or crushed), seed extract or oil, tablets, and tea. Some experts recommend the following dose:

- *To prevent or eliminate worm infestations,* 60 to 500 grams of pumpkin seeds taken in equal doses as a tea or an emulsion of the crushed seeds, placed in powdered sugar and either milk or water.

Why people use this herb

- Benign prostate enlargement
- Intestinal worms and parasites such as tapeworms

Side effects

Call your health care practitioner if you experience unusual symptoms while using pumpkin.

Interactions

Combining herbs with certain drugs may alter their action or produce unwanted side effects. Tell your health care practitioner about any prescription or nonprescription drugs you're taking, especially diuretics.

Important points to remember

- Don't use pumpkin if you're pregnant or breast-feeding.
- Avoid this herb if you have prostate enlargement of unknown cause.
- Know that because of its diuretic effect, pumpkin could alter your body salt levels. Call your health care practitioner if you experience nausea, cramps, weakness, tremors, or tingling.
- Be aware that although pumpkin has been used to treat intestinal worm infections, this use requires large doses. What's more, the

herb may be ineffective. Most experts recommend more reliable and effective treatments for such infections.

- If you have symptoms of a prostate problem, such as trouble starting your urine stream, see a qualified health care practitioner for a full evaluation.

WHAT THE RESEARCH SHOWS

Several small studies suggest possible benefits from pumpkin seeds, seed extracts, and oils (except in cases of enlarged prostate, where the herb had no effect). However, pumpkin products vary widely in their active ingredients and may contain amounts too small to be effective. Medical experts say you should check the label for toxic ingredients before using a pumpkin product.

Other names for pumpkin

Other names for pumpkin include cucurbita, pumpkinseed oil, and vegetable marrow.

Products containing pumpkin are sold under such names as Action Super Saw Palmetto Plus, Hain Pumpkin Seed Oil Caps, Max Nutrition System, Mega Men Men's Vitapak, Men's Multiple Formula, Proleve 40, Prost-Answer Alcohol-Free, Pumpkin Seed Shield, Saw Palmetto Formula, Saw Palmetto Pygeum Plus, and Ultimate Oil.

Selected references

Bracher, F. "Phytotherapy of Benign Prostatic Hyperplasia," *Urologe Ausgabe A* 36:10-17, 1997. In German; abstract used.

Carbin, B.E., et al. "Treatment of Benign Prostatic Hyperplasia with Phytosterols," *British Journal of Urology* 6:639-41, 1990.

Mihranian, V.H., and Abou-Chaar, C.I. "Extraction, Detection and Estimation of Cucurbitin in Cucurbita Seeds," *Lloydia* 31:23-29, 1968.

Queen Anne's lace

Queen Anne's lace was named for its lacy, intricately patterned white flowers. However, some people refer to Queen Anne's lace *(Daucus carota)* as mother's die, thanks to the superstition that your mother will die if you bring the plant into your home. Herbalists obtain active ingredients from the leaves, roots, and seeds.

Why people use this herb

- As an aphrodisiac
- Cancer
- Dysentery
- Fluid retention
- Gout
- Heart disease
- Kidney disease
- Menstrual problems
- Night blindness
- Stomach upset
- To induce abortion
- To lower blood sugar
- Ulcers
- Uterine pain
- Worm infections

Queen Anne's lace grows wild in many parts of North America. It can be used as a dye, a fragrance, and a flavoring agent.

Common dose

Queen Anne's lace comes as a crude extract and teas. Experts disagree on what dose to take.

Side effects

Call your health care practitioner if you experience any of these possible side effects of Queen Anne's lace:

- increased sensitivity to sunlight
- increased urination
- skin inflammation (especially from contact with wet leaves).

This herb also can cause:

- an extremely slow pulse
- low blood pressure
- nervous system depression, leading to excessive drowsiness or sleepiness, slow breathing, and reduced mental alertness.

Interactions

Combining herbs with certain drugs may alter their action or produce unwanted side effects. Tell your health care practitioner about any prescription or nonprescription drugs you're taking, especially:

- drugs that lower blood pressure
- drugs used to control the heart rate, such as digoxin
- drugs used to reduce anxiety
- muscle relaxants or other drugs that affect muscle function

- pain killers
- sedatives.

Important points to remember

- Don't use Queen Anne's lace if you're pregnant or breast-feeding.
- Tell your health care practitioner if you plan to get pregnant or suspect you're pregnant.
- Don't drive or perform other dangerous activities until you know how Queen Anne's lace affects you.
- If this herb makes you unusually sensitive to sunlight, apply sunblock and wear a hat, sunglasses, and protective clothing when you go outside.
- Keep in mind that skin contact with the leaves of Queen Anne's lace could cause a rash.
- Know that you may develop neurologic problems if you take large amounts of this plant's seeds.
- Don't confuse the cultivated carrot *(D. carota carota)* with the Queen Anne's lace subspecies used in herbal therapy *(D. carota sativas).*
- Take care not to mistake poisonous wild plants, such as water hemlock *(Cicuta maculata),* poison hemlock *(Conium maculatum),* and fool's parsley *(Aethusa cynapium)* for Queen Anne's lace.

Other names for Queen Anne's lace

Other names for Queen Anne's lace include bee's nest, bird's nest, devil's plague, mother's die, oil of carrot, wild carrot, and wild carrot seed.

No known products containing Queen Anne's lace are available commercially.

WHAT THE RESEARCH SHOWS

Studies on animals suggest that Queen Anne's lace may be good for the liver, may help reduce spasms, and may aid the treatment of fungal infections. The herb also may alter the body's response to its own steroids, such as cortisol, estrogen, and testosterone.

However, no studies on people have been done to support these or any other claims. More research is needed before medical experts can recommend Queen Anne's lace for medicinal use.

Selected references

Bishayee, A., et al. "Hepatoprotective Activity of Carrot (*Daucus carota* L.) Against Carbon Tetrachloride Intoxication in Mouse Liver," *Journal of Ethnopharmacology* 47:69-74, 1995.

Farnsworth, N.R., et al. "Potential Value of Plants as Sources of New Antifertility Agents I," *Journal of Pharmaceutical Sciences* 64:535-98, 1975.

Quince

A popular ornamental plant, Japanese quince *(Cydonia japonica)* grows all over the world. The fruit and seeds of its relative, *C. oblonga*, are used to prepare medicinal products. Other quince varieties have no role in herbal therapy.

Common dose

Quince comes as fruit syrup, decoctum cydoniae, B.P. (decoction from seeds), and a mucilage of quince seeds. Experts disagree on how much to use for external purposes. For internal use, some experts recommend the following dose:

- *For diarrhea, dysentery, gonorrhea, or thrush,* drink "large quantities" of decoctum cydoniae (2 drams of quince seed boiled in 1 pint of water for 10 minutes).

Why people use this herb

- Cancer
- Canker sores
- Diarrhea
- Dysentery
- Gonorrhea
- Gum problems
- Sore throat
- Thrush

Side effects

Call your health care practitioner if you experience unusual symptoms while using quince, especially preparations made from seeds.

Interactions

Combining herbs with certain drugs may alter their action or produce unwanted side effects. Tell your health care practitioner about any prescription or nonprescription drugs you're taking.

Important points to remember

- Don't use quince if you're pregnant or breast-feeding.
- Keep quince out of reach of children and pets.
- If you're considering taking quince for a digestive problem, be aware that other treatments of known safety and effectiveness are available.

Other names for quince

Other names for quince include common quince, *Cydonia vulgaris*, golden apple, and *Pyrus cydonia*.

No known products containing quince are available commercially.

WHAT THE RESEARCH SHOWS

Preparations made from quince or its seed coats may provide minor relief from diarrhea and sore throat. However, the laetrile component of quince—once thought to be a potential cancer treatment—is toxic and ineffective. Medical experts warn against using quince as a cancer treatment.

Selected references

Guevara, J.M., et al. "The In Vitro Action of Plants on *Vibrio cholerae*," *Revista de Gastroenterologia de Peru* 14:27-31, 1994.

Moertel, C.G., et al. "A Clinical Trial of Amygdalin (Laetrile) in the Treatment of Human Cancer," *New England Journal of Medicine* 306:201-06, 1982.

Ragwort

A member of the daisy (Compositae) family, ragwort (Senecio jacobae) is native to North America. Herbalists use its leaves, seeds, and flowers. Some South Africans eat parts of certain Senecio species.

Common doses

Ragwort comes as fresh and dried herb. Some experts recommend the following doses *for external use only*:

- As a *poultice,* apply the bruised, fresh plant directly on the affected area.
- As *dried herb,* soak the herb in warm water and then apply.
- As a *gargle,* soak the plant in warm water. Then strain the water and gargle with it.

Side effects

Call your health care practitioner if you experience any of these possible side effects of ragwort:

- coughing
- nausea or vomiting
- shortness of breath
- symptoms of liver problems, such as jaundice, fatigue, fever, and abdominal pain.

Why people use this herb

- Bee stings
- Burns
- Cancerous ulcers
- Menstrual problems
- Rheumatism
- Throat and mouth ulcers

When ingested, ragwort changes into several chemicals that damage the liver. People and animals have died from liver failure caused by these chemicals.

Interactions

Combining herbs with certain drugs may alter their action or produce unwanted side effects. Tell your health care practitioner about any prescription or nonprescription drugs you're taking.

Important points to remember

- Don't use ragwort if you're pregnant or breast-feeding.
- Avoid this herb if you have liver problems. Even if you don't have such problems, your health care practitioner may recommend periodic liver function tests while you're taking ragwort.

WHAT THE RESEARCH SHOWS

Ragwort is a well-documented poison in both animals and humans. Medical experts caution against using it for any medicinal purpose.

Other names for ragwort

Other names for ragwort include cankerwort, cocashweed, coughweed, dog standard, false valerian, golden ragwort, golden senecio, liferoot, ragweed, St. James wort, staggerwort, stammerwort, stinking nanny, squaw weed, and squawroot.

No known products containing ragwort are available commercially.

Selected reference

Dooren, B., et al. "Composition of Essential Oils of Some *Senecio* Species," *Planta Medica* 42:385-89, 1981.

Raspberry

The red raspberry comes from the *Rubus idaeus* plant. As the name implies, its berries usually are red (sometimes yellow). Most other raspberry species are called blackberries.

Herbalists use the plant's leaves, berries, and sometimes the root for medicinal purposes. Raspberry syrup is commonly used to mask the taste of bitter drugs.

Common doses

Raspberry is available as:

- capsules (384 or 400 milligrams)
- liquid (1 or 2 ounces).

Some experts recommend the following doses:

- As *dried red raspberry leaf powder* or *tablets*, 4 to 8 grams taken orally three times daily.
- As a *liquid extract* (1 gram of leaf per milliliter of 25% alcohol), 4 to 8 milliliters taken orally three times daily.

Why people use this herb

- Canker sores
- Cough
- Fluid retention
- Gallstones
- Infections
- Inflamed tonsils
- Inflammation
- Kidney stones
- Sore throat
- Urinary problems
- Wounds

Side effects

Call your health care practitioner if you experience unusual symptoms while using raspberry.

Interactions

Combining herbs with certain drugs may alter their action or produce unwanted side effects. Tell your health care practitioner about any prescription or nonprescription drugs you're taking, especially drugs that reduce blood sugar.

Don't use raspberry extract while taking Antabuse.

Important points to remember

- If you're pregnant, use caution when taking raspberry leaves or preparations made from them. They could trigger labor.
- If you are planning a pregnancy or suspect you're pregnant, tell your health care practitioner—and don't consume more than moderate amounts of raspberry.

- If you have diabetes, monitor your blood sugar carefully while using this herb.
- If you take Antabuse, don't use raspberry forms that contain alcohol.

WHAT THE RESEARCH SHOWS

Raspberry seems to be harmless when consumed as a food. However, researchers haven't identified medicinal uses for this plant.

Other names for raspberry

Other names for raspberry include black raspberry *(Rubus occidentalis),* blackberry *(R. fruticosus, R. frondosus, R. hispidus, R. macropetalus),* bramble, bramble of Mount Ida, hindberry, raspbis, red raspberry *(R. idaeus),* and Rubus.

A product containing raspberry is sold as Red Raspberry Leaves.

Selected reference

Briggs, C.J., and Briggs, K. "Raspberry," *Canadian Pharmaceutical Journal* 130:41-43, 1997.

Rauwolfia

More than 100 species of rauwolfia grow in India, Thailand, South America, Asia, and Africa. Of these, one species, *Rauvolfia serpentina*, is known for its medicinal properties.

In the body, rauwolfia forms several chemicals called alkaloids. One such alkaloid, reserpine, lowers blood pressure and eases certain mental problems. Doctors in Spain and some other European countries still prescribe reserpine. In the United States, its use has dropped sharply because of its side effects and the availability of effective alternative drugs.

Why people use this herb

- Diarrhea
- Dysentery
- Fever
- High blood pressure
- Mental illness
- To calm noisy infants

Common doses

Rauwolfia comes as:

- tablets (50 milligrams, sold as Raudixin)
- crude root
- tea
- liquid extract
- powdered extract
- reserpine (used for injection).

Some experts recommend the following doses:

- For *high blood pressure,* daily doses of 200 milligrams of Raudixin, 4 milligrams of Rauwiloid, or 0.25 milligram of reserpine taken orally. The average daily dose of the raw herb is 600 milligrams.

Side effects

Call your health care practitioner if you experience unusual symptoms when using rauwolfia. High doses may cause:

- decreased sex drive
- depression and thoughts of suicide
- diarrhea
- difficulty walking
- digestive problems
- generalized swelling
- hallucinations
- increased appetite
- low blood pressure symptoms, such as dizziness
- nasal congestion

- nightmares
- peptic ulcer
- slow pulse
- tremors
- weight gain.

Some reports have tried to link breast cancer with rauwolfia derivatives. This link hasn't been verified, but the issue remains controversial.

Interactions

Combining herbs with certain drugs may alter their action or produce unwanted side effects. Tell your health care practitioner about any prescription or nonprescription drugs you're taking, especially:

- adrenergics, such as Alupent, Aramine, Brethine, Bronkosol, Dobutrex, Intropin, Isuprel, Levophed, Maxair, Medihaler-Iso, Neo-Synephrine Primatene Mist, Proventil, Tornalate, or Yutopar
- drugs that reduce blood pressure
- drugs that slow the heart rate
- nitrates, such as nitroglycerin
- nonsteroidal anti-inflammatory drugs such as Advil
- tricyclic antidepressants.

Don't use rauwolfia or reserpine if you're taking:

- drugs that slow the central nervous system, such as alcohol, barbiturates, cold and allergy drugs, sedatives, tranquilizers, narcotic pain relievers, seizure drugs, and muscle relaxants
- Larodopa.

Important points to remember

- Don't use rauwolfia if you have a peptic ulcer or ulcerative colitis.
- Avoid this herb if you have a history of depression or a high risk for depression.
- Use rauwolfia cautiously if you are pregnant or have had breast cancer.
- Don't drive or perform other dangerous activities until you know how rauwolfia affects you.
- Have your blood pressure checked routinely while using rauwolfia.
- Stop using rauwolfia at least 2 weeks before electroconvulsive therapy.
- Remember that other drugs with fewer side effects are available for rauwolfia's purported uses, such as high blood pressure and mental illness.

Other names for rauwolfia

Other names for rauwolfia include Indian snakeroot, *Rauvolfia,* and snakeroot.

Products containing rauwolfia are sold under such names as Harmonyl (deserpidine, U.K.), Raudixin, Rauwiloid (alseroxylon fraction), and Serpasil (reserpine).

> **WHAT THE RESEARCH SHOWS**
>
> Rauwolfia alkaloids, including reserpine, are useful in treating high blood pressure and psychoses. But because reserpine also has unpleasant side effects, medical experts recommend using other safe and effective drugs instead.

Selected references

Armstrong, B., et al. "Rauwolfia Derivatives and Breast Cancer in Hypertensive Women," *Lancet* 2:8-12, 1976.

Capella D., et al. "Utilization of Antihypertensive Drugs in Certain European Countries," *European Journal of Clinical Pharmacology* 25:431-35, 1983.

O'Fallon, W.M., et al. "Rauwolfia Derivatives and Breast Cancer. A Case/Control Study in Olmsted County, Minnesota," *Lancet* 2:292-96, 1975.

Pfeifer H.J., et al. "Clinical Toxicity of Reserpine in Hospitalized Patients: A Report from the Boston Collaborative Drug Surveillance Program," *American Journal of Medicine* 271:269-76, 1976.

Schyve, P.M., et al. "Neuroleptic-Induced Prolactin Level Elevation and Breast Cancer; An Emerging Clinical Issue," *Archives of General Psychiatry* 35:1291-1301, 1978.

Red clover

Trifolium pratense, **or red clover, was naturalized in the United States from its native Europe. Herbalists use the plant's aerial parts—namely, the rose-colored flower head.**

Why people use this herb

- Chronic skin diseases
- Estrogen replacement after menopause
- Whooping cough

Common doses

Red clover comes as:

- tablets (100 milligrams)
- capsules (200, 354, 375, and 430 milligrams)
- liquid (1 and 2 ounces)
- tea
- raw sprouts.

Some experts recommend the following doses:

- For *skin diseases,* apply a compress twice daily.
- As a *tincture,* 2 to 6 milliliters taken orally three times daily.
- As an *infusion,* pour hot water over 1 to 3 teaspoons of dried herb, let stand for 10 to 15 minutes, and take orally three times daily.

Side effects

Call your health care practitioner if you experience any of these possible side effects of red clover:

- breast tenderness and enlargement
- menstrual changes
- weight gain or redistribution.

This herb also may cause infertility and growth disorders and may foster growth of estrogen-related tumors.

Interactions

Combining herbs with certain drugs may alter their action or produce unwanted side effects. Tell your health care practitioner about any prescription or nonprescription drugs you're taking, especially:

- blood thinners such as Coumadin
- drugs that affect platelets such as aspirin
- oral contraceptives.

Important points to remember

- Don't use red clover if you're pregnant, breast-feeding, or planning a pregnancy.
- Avoid this herb if you've had an estrogen-responsive tumor (ask your health care practitioner).
- Use red clover cautiously, if at all, if you have a bleeding disorder or take a blood thinner.
- Report bruises and abnormal bleeding to your health care practitioner right away.
- When you have a Pap test, tell the health care practitioner that you're taking red clover.
- Know that because red clover hasn't been studied much in people, conventional estrogen products may be a better choice for estrogen replacement.

Other names for red clover

Other names for red clover include beebread, cow clover, meadow clover, Missouri milk vetch, purple clover, trefoil, and wild clover.

Products containing red clover are sold under such names as Red Clover Blossoms, Red Clover Cleanser, Red Clover Combo, Red Clover Plus, and Red Clover Tops.

Selected references

Cassady, J.M., et al. "Use of a Mammalian Cell Culture Benzo(a)pyrene Metabolism Assay for the Detection of Potential Anticarcinogens from Natural Products: Inhibition of Metabolism by Biochanin A, an Isoflavone from *Trifolium pratense* L," *Cancer Research* 48:6257-61, 1988.

Hoffman, P.C., et al. "Performance of Lactating Dairy Cows Fed Red Clover or Alfalfa Silage," *Journal of Dairy Science* 80: 3308-15, 1997.

Wilcox, G., et al. "Estrogenic Effects of Plant Foods in Postmenopausal Women," *BMJ* 301:905-06, 1990.

Zava, D.T., et al. "Estrogen and Progestin Bioactivity of Foods, Herbs, and Spices," *Proceedings of the Society for Experimental Biology and Medicine* 217:369-78, 1998.

WHAT THE RESEARCH SHOWS

Although herbalists claim many uses for red clover, no studies on people have been done. Medical experts advise against taking red clover because the herb's safety and effectiveness haven't been documented and because safe, effective estrogen products exist.

Red poppy

As the name implies, red poppy *(Papaver rhoeas)* produces bright red flowers. A member of the Papaveraceae family, this annual is native to Europe, North Africa, and temperate areas of Asia. It also grows in North and South America.

Why people use this herb

- Cough
- Nervousness
- Pain

Common dose

Red poppy comes as capsules. Experts disagree on what dose to take.

Side effects

Call your health care practitioner if you experience any of these possible side effects of red poppy:

- central nervous system depression, such as excessive drowsiness or sleepiness, slow breathing, and reduced alertness
- skin rash from contact with the plant.

Interactions

Combining herbs with certain drugs may alter their action or produce unwanted side effects. Don't use red poppy while taking:

- central nervous system depressants, such as alcohol, cold and allergy drugs, sedatives, tranquilizers, narcotic pain relievers, barbiturates, seizure drugs, or muscle relaxants
- pain killers.

Important points to remember

- Don't use red poppy if you're pregnant or breast-feeding.
- Avoid this herb if you're allergic to morphine or codeine because it may contain these and other potentially poisonous alkaloids. Be aware that no one knows how much of these alkaloids are in red poppy, so it's impossible to estimate a dangerous red poppy dose.
- Use red poppy cautiously if you have a history of allergic skin inflammation.
- Don't drive or perform other dangerous activities until you know how red poppy affects you.

WHAT THE RESEARCH SHOWS

Unlike the opium poppy, the red poppy hasn't been studied much, so we have little information on it. The herb's components are poorly understood and the amounts of these components haven't been measured. Because red poppy hasn't been proven therapeutically useful and because its safety is unknown, medical experts say you should avoid it.

Other names for red poppy

Other names for red poppy include corn poppy, corn rose, field poppy, flanders poppy, and *Papaver rhoeas*.

No known products containing red poppy are available commercially.

Selected reference

Gamboa, P.M., et al. "Allergic Contact Urticaria from Poppy Flowers *(Papaver rhoeas)*," *Contact Dermatitis* 37:140-41, 1997.

Rhatany

Herbalists use both internal and external preparations of rhatany *(Krameria triandra)* for medicinal purposes. Active ingredients come from the dried root.

Common doses

Rhatany comes as a tincture, mouthwash, lozenges, powder, syrup, and solution. Some experts recommend the following doses:

- As a *decoction,* 1 gram of herb in 1 cup of water or 5 to 10 drops of tincture in a glass of water taken orally.
- For *topical use,* apply two to three times daily.

Why people use this herb

- Bleeding from the bladder or bowel
- Bleeding or irritated gums
- Canker sores
- Diarrhea
- Dysentery
- Periodontal disease
- Skin or mucous membrane irritation
- Throat inflammation
- Urinary incontinence

Side effects

Call your health care practitioner if you experience unusual symptoms while taking rhatany. This herb may cause liver damage.

Interactions

Combining herbs with certain drugs may alter their action or produce unwanted side effects. Don't use rhatany while taking Antabuse; some rhatany forms contain alcohol and could cause a reaction.

Important points to remember

- Don't use rhatany if you've had an allergic reaction to it or any of its components.
- Avoid highly astringent rhatany products. The Food and Drug Administration has deemed only two astringents (aluminum acetate and witch hazel) safe and effective for treating minor skin irritations. It doesn't consider rhatany to be safe or effective for wound healing.
- Know that rhatany products that contain tannic acid probably aren't effective and could be dangerous if the tannic acid is absorbed through the digestive tract or mucous membranes.

- Be aware that your health care practitioner may recommend periodic liver function tests while you're taking rhatany. If you develop symptoms of a liver problem, such as jaundice, fatigue, and fever, tell your health care practitioner right away.
- If you take Antabuse, don't use rhatany tincture because it contains alcohol.

Other names for rhatany

Other names for rhatany include krameria root, mapato, Peruvian rhatany, pumacuchu, raiz para los dientes, ratanhiawurzel, red rhatany, and rhatanhia.

Products containing rhatany are sold under such names as Echtrosept-GT, Encialina, Gengivario, Parodontax, and Repha-OS.

WHAT THE RESEARCH SHOWS

Well-controlled clinical trials supporting rhatany's safety and effectiveness are lacking. According to medical experts, it's best to avoid internal or external use of the herb.

Selected references

Flynn, A.A. "Oral Health Products," in *Handbook of Nonprescription Drugs*, 9th ed. Edited by Covington, T.R., et al. Washington, D.C.: United Book Press, Inc., 1996.

Swinyard, E.A., and Pathak, M.A. "Locally Acting Drugs," in *Goodman and Gilman's: The Pharmacological Basis of Therapeutics,* 7th ed. Edited by Goodman, L.S., et al. New York: Macmillan Publishing Company, 1985.

West, D.P., and Nowakowski, P.A. "Dermatitis," in *Handbook of Nonprescription Drugs,* 9th ed. Edited by Covington, T.R., et al. Washington, D.C.: United Book Press, Inc., 1996.

Rose hips

Rose hips are the dried fruits of rose plants (usually *Rosa canina).* Roses originated in Europe and Asia and now grow throughout North America.

Rose hips contain more vitamin C per milligram than raw broccoli and many citrus fruits. However, processing may destroy more than half the vitamin C. For this reason, you may need to take more than 100 grams of actual rose hips to obtain 1,200 milligrams of vitamin C. (Many products containing rose hips are supplemented with synthetic vitamin C.)

Why people use this herb

- Constipation
- To bolster the immune system
- To strengthen the capillaries
- Wound healing

Common dose

Rose hips comes as capsules, tablets, syrup, tincture, teas, cream, and extracts in combination with vitamin preparations. Experts disagree on what dose to take.

Side effects

Call your health care practitioner if you experience any of these possible side effects of rose hips:

- allergic reaction
- diarrhea.

Interactions

Combining herbs with certain drugs may alter their action or produce unwanted side effects. Tell your health care practitioner about any prescription or nonprescription drugs you're taking.

Important points to remember

- Don't use rose hips if you're pregnant or breast-feeding.
- Use rose hips cautiously, if at all, if you have a history of allergic reactions to plants or other substances.
- If you have diabetes, be aware that high vitamin C doses can interfere with home glucose tests.
- Use rose hips made only by reliable manufacturers. Otherwise, the rose hips themselves may contribute only a minor portion of the vitamin C.

> **WHAT THE RESEARCH SHOWS**
>
> Although rose hips are high in vitamin C, you must ingest large amounts to obtain as much of the vitamin as is found in most tablets. Most medical experts believe that the use of rose hips isn't necessary.

Other names for rose hips

Other names for rose hips include dog rose fruit, dog brier fruit, hipberries, and wild brier berries.

Products containing rose hips are sold under such names as Rose Hips and Vitamin C with Rose Hips.

Selected references

Akhmadieva, A.Kh., et al. "The Protective Action of a Natural Preparation of Anthocyan (Pelargonidin-3,5-diglucoside)," *Radiobiologia* 33:433-35, 1993.

Brand, J.C., et al. "An Outstanding Food Source of Vitamin C," *Lancet* 16:873, 1982. Letter.

Kwaselow, A., et al. "Rose Hips: A New Occupational Allergen," *Journal of Allergy and Clinical Immunology* 85:704-08, 1990.

Yesilada, E., et al. "Inhibitory Effects of Turkish Folk Remedies on Inflammatory Cytokines: Interleukin-1alpha, Interleukin-1beta, and Tumor Necrosis Factor," *Journal of Ethnopharmacology* 58:59-73, 1997.

Rosemary

Widely used for cooking and in cosmetic preparations, rosemary *(Rosemarinus officinalis)* is native to the Mediterranean region and grows in milder North American areas. Herbalists get medicinal components from the plant's leaves, twigs, and flowering tops.

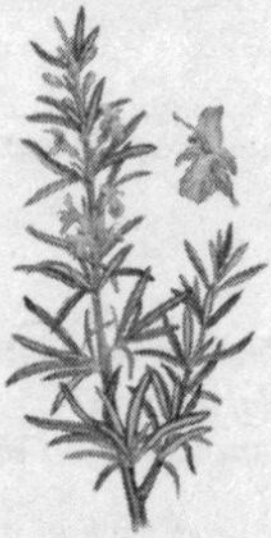

The German government has approved internal rosemary use for treatment of indigestion and as a supportive treatment for rheumatism and related disorders. It has approved the herb for external use by people with circulation problems.

Why people use this herb

- Chronic circulation problems
- Hair loss
- Indigestion
- Intestinal gas
- Low blood pressure
- Rheumatism
- Smooth-muscle spasms
- To cause sweating
- To induce abortion
- To stimulate menstruation

Common doses

Rosemary comes as a volatile oil, an infusion, and a tea. It's also added to bath and toiletry products. Some experts recommend the following doses:

- As a *liquid extract* (1:1 in 45% alcohol), 1 to 4 milliliters taken orally three times daily.
- As a *tea,* use 1 to 4 grams of the leaf, and drink three times daily.
- For *external use,* apply the essential oil as an ointment.

Side effects

Call your health care practitioner if you experience any of these possible side effects of rosemary:

- increased sensitivity to sunlight
- reddened skin
- skin inflammation
- stomach upset.

This herb also may cause:

- fertility problems (by preventing implantation of the fertilized egg in the uterus)
- kidney damage.

Interactions

Combining herbs with certain drugs may alter their action or produce unwanted side effects. Don't use rosemary while taking Antabuse because some herb forms contain alcohol and could cause a reaction.

Important points to remember

- Don't use rosemary if you're pregnant, breast-feeding, or trying to get pregnant.
- Use this herb cautiously if you've ever had an allergic reaction to a plant.
- Don't take undiluted rosemary oil internally because its safety is unproven.
- If you take Antabuse, don't use rosemary extract that contains alcohol.

WHAT THE RESEARCH SHOWS

Several components of rosemary oil have shown therapeutic effects in animals, but human studies aren't available. Future research is likely to focus on rosemary's possible use in cancer chemotherapy and in treating such acute conditions as adult respiratory distress syndrome and septic shock. Until results of these studies are known, medical experts can't vouch for rosemary's therapeutic value.

Other names for rosemary

Other names for rosemary include compass plant, incensor, and old man.

A product containing rosemary is sold as Rosemary Oil.

Selected references

Huang, M.T., et al. "Inhibition of Skin Tumorigenesis by Rosemary and Its Constituents Carnosol and Ursolic Acid," *Cancer Research* 54:701-08, 1994.

Oxford, E.A., et al. "Mechanisms Involved in the Chemoprotective Effects of Rosemary Extract Studied in Human Liver and Bronchial Cells," *Cancer Letters* 114:275-81, 1997.

Rue

Native to the Mediterranean region, rue *(Ruta graveolens)* is cultivated in Europe, America, Asia, and Africa. Herbalists use the leaves and roots of this malodorous plant.

Why people use this herb

- Arthritis
- Bruises
- Digestive problems
- Earache
- Eye strain
- Generalized swelling
- Insect bites
- Joint disorders
- Lack of menstruation
- Menstrual pain
- Muscle disorders
- Nervousness
- Pinworms, tapeworms, and other worm infections
- Severe stabbing pain
- Snakebite
- Spasms
- Sports injuries
- Sprains and strains
- To induce abortion
- To promote lactation in breast-feeding women

Common doses

Rue comes as crude herb, capsules, extracts, and creams. Some experts recommend the following doses:

- For *earache,* a few drops of infused oil on a cotton plug placed over the ear.
- As an *extract,* 0.25 to 1 teaspoon taken orally with food and water three times daily.
- As *capsules,* 1 capsule taken orally with food and water three times daily.
- As *cream,* apply as needed.

Side effects

Call your health care practitioner if you experience any of these possible side effects of rue:

- allergic skin reactions, such as redness, blisters, and increased pigmentation (with topical use)
- increased sensitivity to sunlight.

This herb also can cause:

- increased risk of miscarriage
- low blood pressure.

Interactions

Combining herbs with certain drugs may alter their action or produce unwanted side effects. Tell your health care practitioner about any prescription or nonprescription drugs you're taking, especially:

- digoxin
- Dobutrex
- drugs that lower blood pressure.

Don't use rue while taking a fertility drug because the herb could counteract it.

Important points to remember

- Don't use rue if you're pregnant or breast-feeding. Be aware that rue may increase the risk of miscarriage.
- Tell your health care practitioner if you plan to get pregnant or suspect you're pregnant.
- Use rue cautiously if you have a history of heart failure or irregular heartbeats or if you're taking a drug to lower your blood pressure.
- Keep in mind that large doses of rue can be dangerous.
- If you develop an allergic skin reaction while taking rue, stop taking it right away and call your health care practitioner.

Other names for rue

Other names for rue include herb-of-grace, herbygrass, *Ruta,* rutae herba, and Vinruta.

Products containing rue are sold under such names as Joint and Muscle Relief Cream and Rue.

Selected references

Atta, A.H., and Alkofahi, A. "Anti-nociceptive and Anti-inflammatory Effects of Some Jordanian Medicinal Plant Extracts," *Journal of Ethnopharmacology* 60:117-24, 1998.

Bethge, E.W., et al. "Effects of Some Potassium Channel Blockers on the Ionic Currents in Myelinated Nerve," *General Physiology and Biophysics* 10:225-44, 1991.

Chui, K.W., and Fung, A.Y. "The Cardiovascular Effects of Green Beans *(Phaseolus aureus),* Common Rue *(Ruta graveolens)*, and Kelp *(Laminaria japonica)* in Rats," *General Pharmacology* 29:859-62, 1997.

Ghandi, M., et al. "Post-coital Antifertility Action of *Ruta graveolens* in Female Rats and Hamsters," *Journal of Ethnopharmacology* 34:49-59, 1991.

WHAT THE RESEARCH SHOWS

Preliminary animal tests suggest that rue has many interesting effects. However, too few tests on people have been done to permit conclusions about the herb's therapeutic value. The high risk of skin rash from direct contact with the plant greatly limits its topical use. In Germany, rue is considered ineffective and unsafe. At present, medical experts can't recommend it.

Safflower

Safflower *(Carthamus tinctorius)* originated in the Middle East. It's now grown throughout the United States and Europe for its edible oil, which comes from the seeds.

Why people use this herb

- Constipation
- Fever
- High cholesterol
- Menstrual disorders

Common doses

Safflower comes as:

- tea
- extracts
- capsules (390 milligrams)
- liquid (8.5 ounces).

Some experts recommend the following doses:

- As the *fresh flower,* 1 to 2 tablespoons taken orally three times daily.
- As *dried flower,* 2 to 3 grams taken orally three times daily.
- As an *extract,* 3 grams of dried flower in 15 milliliters of alcohol and 15 milliliters of water taken orally three times daily.

Side effects

Call your health care practitioner if you experience unusual symptoms while using safflower.

Interactions

Combining herbs with certain drugs may alter their action or produce unwanted side effects. Tell your health care practitioner about any prescription or nonprescription drugs you're taking, especially those that affect your immune system, such as Imuran, Prograf, and Sandimmune.

Don't use safflower at the same time you receive a vaccination.

Important points to remember

- Don't use excessive safflower if you're pregnant or breast-feeding.
- Use this herb cautiously, if at all, if you have burns, a blood infection, an organ transplant, or another condition that suppresses your immune system.
- Don't get vaccinations while using safflower.
- Don't rely on safflower to lower your cholesterol. Other medications are more effective.

WHAT THE RESEARCH SHOWS

No clinical evidence backs the use of safflower tea to induce sweating or bowel movements. A diet high in safflower oil does lower cholesterol, although it doesn't seem to reduce the risk of death from heart disease. For this reason, medical experts suggest that people use safflower oil only as a secondary treatment along with proven therapies.

Other names for safflower

Other names for safflower include American saffron, azafran, bastard saffron, benibana, dyer's-saffron, and false saffron.

Products containing safflower are sold under such names as Safflower Oil and Saffron.

Selected references

Shi, M., et al. "Stimulating Action of *Carthamus tinctorius* L., *Angelica sinensis*, (Oliv) Diels and *Leonurus sibiricus* L. on the Uterus," *Chung-Kuo Chung Yao Tsa Chih China Journal of Chinese Materia Medica* 20:173-75,192, 1995.

Wardlaw, G.M., et al. "Serum Lipid and Apolipoprotein Concentrations in Healthy Men on Diets Enriched in Either Canola Oil or Safflower Oil," *American Journal of Clinical Nutrition* 54:104, 1991.

Saffron

Saffron comes from the dried flowers of *Crocus sativus*, a plant that's native to southern Europe and Asia Minor. In Germany, a combination of saffron, quinine, and opium has received a patent for inhibiting premature ejaculation.

Why people use this herb

- As an aphrodisiac
- Cough
- Dry skin
- Nervousness
- To induce sweating

Common dose

Saffron is available as crude powder that you can mix with food or brew as a tea. Experts disagree on what dose to take.

Side effects

Call your health care practitioner if you experience unusual symptoms when using saffron. Doses above 5 grams may cause:

- facial flushing
- heavy menstrual bleeding
- miscarriage
- nosebleeds
- slow pulse
- vertigo
- vomiting.

Interactions

Combining herbs with certain drugs may alter their action or produce unwanted side effects. Tell your health care practitioner about any prescription or nonprescription drugs you're taking.

Important points to remember

- Don't use this herb if you're pregnant or breast-feeding.
- To minimize the risk of side effects, don't take more than 5 grams of saffron daily.
- If you develop unusual symptoms while using saffron, tell your health care practitioner at once.

Other names for saffron

Other names for saffron include Indian saffron and true saffron.

No known medicinal products containing saffron are available commercially.

WHAT THE RESEARCH SHOWS

Although saffron has been used safely to flavor and color foods for many years, its medicinal value remains unproven. Until enough studies on people are done, medical experts can't recommend saffron for preventing or treating cancer or heart conditions.

Selected references

Escribano, J., et al. "Crocin, Safranal, and Picrocrocin from Saffron (*Crocus sativus* L.) Inhibit the Growth of Human Cancer Cells In Vitro," *Cancer Letters* 100:23-30, 1996.

Grisolia, S. "Hypoxia, Saffron and Cardiovascular Disease," *Lancet* 7871:41, 1974.

Sage

Sage comes in many varieties. Herbalists use *Salvia officinalis,* a perennial plant with violet-blue flowers. This herb originated in southern Europe and is now cultivated in North America. It has been used for many years as a food flavoring and as a fragrance in soaps and perfumes.

Common doses

Sage comes as dried and fresh leaves, fresh flowering parts, and oils extracted from flowers and stems. Some experts recommend the following doses:

- For *sore throat,* 1 to 4 grams of leaf used as a gargle three times daily.
- For *menstrual disorders,* 1 to 4 milliliters of leaf extract (1:1 in 45% alcohol) taken orally three times daily.

Why people use this herb

- Diarrhea
- Excessive or untimely breast milk flow
- For antioxidant effects
- Gastritis (inflammation of the stomach lining)
- Gingivitis (red, swollen, bleeding gums)
- Menstrual pain
- Muscle spasms
- Sore throat

Side effects

Call your health care practitioner if you experience any of these possible side effects of sage:

- mouth sores
- seizures
- skin irritation.

Interactions

Combining herbs with certain drugs may alter their action or produce unwanted side effects. Tell your health care practitioner about any prescription or nonprescription drugs you're taking, especially:

- drugs that lower blood sugar
- insulin.

Don't use sage while taking:

- Antabuse
- drugs to control seizures.

Important points to remember

- Don't use sage if you're pregnant, diabetic, or taking a drug to control seizures.

- If you're taking Antabuse, don't use a form of sage that contains alcohol.

WHAT THE RESEARCH SHOWS

Lacking enough clinical data, medical experts can't recommend medicinal use of sage at this time. Also, animal studies suggest sage could be harmful. Specifically, it could increase the risk of seizures in people prone to them and may make it harder for diabetic patients to control their blood sugar.

Other names for sage

Other names for sage include dalmatian, garden sage, meadow sage, scarlet sage, and tree sage.

No known medicinal products containing sage are available commercially.

Selected references

Cabo, J., et al. "Accion hipoglucemiante de prepardos fitoterapicos que contienen especies del genero salvia," *Ars Pharmaceutica* 26:239-49, 1985.

Todorov, S., et al. "Experimental Pharmacological Study of Three Species from Genus *Salvia*," *Acta Physiologica et Pharmacologica Bulgarica* 10:13-20, 1984.

St. John's wort

St. John's wort comes from the flowering tops of the perennial plant *Hypericum perforatum* L. The flower's red-staining oil accounts for the herb's peculiar name. According to legend, St. John's wort arose from the blood of John the Baptist after his beheading.

St. John's wort is native to Europe and Asia. European colonists brought the plant to the United States. St. John's wort oil is prepared by extracting the flowers with olive oil.

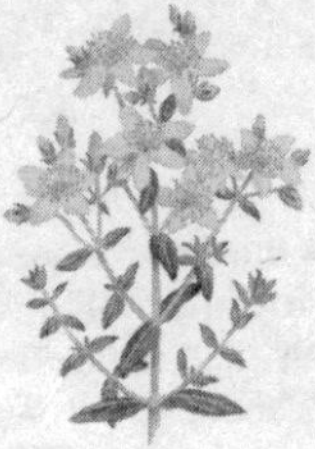

Why people use this herb

- Anxiety
- Bed-wetting
- Bronchial inflammation
- Burns
- Cancer
- Depression (mild to moderate)
- Hemorrhoids
- Insect bites and stings
- Insomnia
- Kidney disease
- Scabies
- Stomach pain from ulcers
- Underactive thyroid
- Wound healing

Common doses

St. John's wort comes as regular capsules, under-the-tongue capsules, creams, and liquid tincture. Solid dosage forms come as 100, 300, 500 milligrams (standardized to 0.3% hypericin) and 250 milligrams (standardized to 0.14% hypericin). Some experts recommend the following doses:

- For *depression,* 300 milligrams of extract preparations standardized to 0.3% hypericin taken orally three times daily for 4 to 6 weeks. Or steep 2 to 4 grams of tea in 1 to 2 cups of water for about 10 minutes, and drink daily for 4 to 6 weeks.
- For *burns* and *skin lesions,* apply cream topically.

Side effects

Call your health care practitioner if you experience any of these possible side effects of St. John's wort:

- allergic reaction
- constipation
- dizziness
- dry mouth
- restlessness
- sensitivity to sunlight
- stomach upset
- trouble sleeping.

Interactions

Combining herbs with certain drugs may alter their action or produce unwanted side effects. Tell your health care practitioner about any prescription or nonprescription drugs you're taking, especially:

- alcohol and other drugs that slow the nervous system, such as cold and allergy drugs, flu medicines, decongestants, and narcotic pain relievers
- amphetamines
- antidepressants called MAO inhibitors (such as Nardil and Parnate)
- antidepressants called selective serotonin reuptake inhibitors (such as Paxil and Prozac)
- Desyrel
- tricyclic antidepressants.

Important points to remember

- Don't take St. John's wort if you've had an allergic reaction to it or its components.
- Don't take this herb if you're pregnant or breast-feeding.
- Before using St. John's wort for depression, consult your health care practitioner. Depending on the severity of your depression, he or she may recommend conventional therapy instead.
- When using St. John's wort, avoid foods and beverages that contain tyramine, such as Chianti wine, beer, aged cheese, chicken livers, chocolate, bananas, and meat tenderizers. Also avoid sun exposure.
- Buy this herb only from a reputable source.
- Be aware that the strength and quality of herbal products may vary among manufacturers.

Other names for St. John's wort

Other names for St. John's wort include amber, amber touch-and-heal, chassediable, devil's scourge, goatweed, God's wonder plant, grace of God, *Hypericum*, Klamath weed, mellepertuis, rosin rose, and witches' herb.

Products containing St. John's wort are sold under such names as Hypercalm, Hypericum, Kira, Mood Support, Nutri Zac, St. John's Wort, and Tension Tamer.

Selected references

Bombardelli, E., et al. "*Hypericum perforatum,*" *Fitoterapia* 66:43-68, 1995.

Golsch, S., et al. "Reversible Increase in Photosensitivity to UV-B caused by St. John's Wort Extract," *Hautarzt* 48:249-52, 1997.

Gordon, J.B. "SSRIs and St. John's Wort: Possible Toxicity?" *American Family Physician* 57:950-53, 1998.

Linde, K., et al. "St. John's Wort for Depression: An Overview and Meta-Analysis of Randomized Clinical Trials," *BMJ* 313:253-58, 1996.

Volz, H.P. "Controlled Clinical Trials of Hypericum Extracts in Depressed Patients—An Overview," *Pharmacopsychiatry* 30(Suppl):72-76, 1997.

Vorbach, E.U. "Efficacy and Tolerability of St. John's Wort Extract LI 160 Versus Imipramine in Patients with Severe Depressive Episodes According to ICD-10," *Pharmacopsychiatry* 30(Suppl):81-85, 1997.

WHAT THE RESEARCH SHOWS

Some research suggests St. John's wort has value in treating mild to moderate forms of depression. From the many case reports and clinical trials that studied the herb's effectiveness and safety, researchers conclude it's probably as effective as standard antidepressants—with fewer side effects. However, an expert government advisory panel found insufficient evidence to support its use in mild to moderate depression.

In a few years, we'll know more. In spring 1998, the National Institutes of Health began a 3-year clinical study to determine if St. John's wort is effective in treating major depression. Patients are divided into three groups. One group is taking St. John's wort. The second is taking a type of antidepressant called a selective serotonin reuptake inhibitor (commonly called an SSRI). The third group is receiving a placebo. Patients don't know which of the three substances they're receiving.

Researchers also have been studying St. John's wort for the possible treatment of HIV infection and as a topical agent in light therapy for psoriasis (scaly, raised skin patches), warts, and Kaposi's sarcoma.

Santonica

Santonica comes from the flowers and seeds of *Artemesia cina,* a member of the Compositae family that grows in most parts of Asia. Russia exported the crude powder to the United States during World War II, until the United States could produce its own domestic supply. The *National Formulary* and the *British Pharmacopeia* listed santonica until the 1950s.

Common dose

Santonica comes as powder (dried powdered santonin), tablets, and oral lozenges. Some experts recommend the following dose:

- As *powder, tablets,* or *oral lozenges,* 2 to 5 grains in varying doses.

Side effects

Call your health care practitioner if you experience any of these possible side effects of santonica:

- headache
- nausea
- seizures
- vision problems, including changes in color vision
- vomiting.

Why people use this herb

- Pinworms, tapeworms, and other worm infections
- Whooping cough

People have died from santonica poisoning.

Interactions

Combining herbs with certain drugs may alter their action or produce unwanted side effects. Don't use santonica while taking while taking a drug to control seizures; santonica may make the drug less effective.

Important points to remember

- Don't use santonica if you're pregnant or breast-feeding.
- Tell your health care practitioner if you plan to get pregnant or suspect you're pregnant.
- Use this herb cautiously if you've had seizures.
- Don't drive or perform other dangerous activities until you know how santonica affects you.
- Keep santonica away from children and pets.
- Don't take this herb without medical supervision.

WHAT THE RESEARCH SHOWS

Although santonica can help treat worm infections, established modern drugs are probably less toxic and more effective against more types of worms.

Other names for santonica

Other names for santonica include levant wormseed, sea wormwood, semen cinae, semen sanctum, and wormseed.

No known products containing santonica are available commercially.

Selected references

Hocking, G.M. *A Dictionary of Natural Products*. Medford, N.J.: Plexus Publishing, Inc., 1997.

Pratt, R., and Youngken, H.W. *Pharmacognosy: The Study of Natural Drug Substances and Certain Allied Products,* 3rd ed. Philadelphia: Lippincott Williams & Wilkins, 1951.

Sarsaparilla

In the Old West of the United States, sarsaparilla was the cowboys' drink of choice. The *U.S. Pharmacopoeia* listed this herb as a syphilis treatment from 1820 to 1910—a use that stretches back to the 16th century. Today, we know sarsaparilla isn't effective against syphilis—yet its reputation as a medicinal herb remains intact. Currently, the Food and Drug Administration accepts sarsaparilla only as a flavoring agent.

Sarsaparilla comes from the dried roots and rhizomes of various *Smilax* species *(S. aristochiifolia, S. regelii, S. febrifuga, S. ornata)*. The plant is cultivated in Mexico, Jamaica, and South America.

Why people use this herb

- Fluid retention
- Kidney disease
- Rheumatism
- Skin diseases such as psoriasis (scaly, raised skin patches)
- To enhance athletic performance
- To induce sweating

Common dose

Sarsaparilla comes as:

- capsules (455 milligrams)
- tablets
- tea
- dried root powder
- liquid extract
- solid root extract.

Some experts recommend the following dose:

- For *psoriasis,* 1 to 4 grams of dried root, 8 to 30 milliliters of concentrated sarsaparilla compound decoction, or 8 to 15 milliliters of liquid extract taken orally three times daily.

Side effects

Call your health care practitioner if you experience any of these possible side effects of sarsaparilla:

- asthma (from inhaling the root dust)
- diarrhea
- stomach upset.

This herb also can cause:

- blood cell damage
- kidney damage.

Interactions

Combining herbs with certain drugs may alter their action or produce unwanted side effects. Tell your health care practitioner about any prescription or nonprescription drugs you're taking, especially:

- any drug taken orally
- diuretics
- drugs called hypnotics.

Don't use sarsaparilla while taking digoxin.

Important points to remember

- Don't use sarsaparilla if you're pregnant or breast-feeding.
- If you have asthma, don't inhale dust or particles from sarsaparilla root.
- Use sarsaparilla cautiously if you take a diuretic.

Other names for sarsaparilla

Other names for sarsaparilla include Ecuadorian sarsaparilla, Honduran sarsaparilla, Jamaican sarsaparilla, Mexican sarsaparilla, salsaparilha, salsepareille, sarsa, sarsaparilla root, and *Smilax*.

Products containing sarsaparilla are sold under such names as Sarsaparilla and Sarsaparilla Root Extract.

WHAT THE RESEARCH SHOWS

Researchers have tested sarsaparilla's ability to treat psoriasis (scaly, raised skin patches) and enhance athletic performance. In the best-known study, psoriasis patients received either sarsaponin (a major sarsaparilla component) or a placebo. Those who received sarsaponin had fewer symptoms and flare-ups. However, flaws in the study design prevented firm conclusions about sarsaparilla's effectiveness against psoriasis.

Because sarsaparilla contains steroids, some people have used it to boost athletic performance. However, research shows that the herb's steroids aren't anabolic, meaning they probably don't do much for athletes. No study results are available to support sarsaparilla's use as a diuretic or digestive aid.

Selected references

Caceres, A., et al. "Plants Used in Guatemala for the Treatment of Dermatophytic Infections," *Journal of Ethnopharmacology* 31:263-76, 1991.

Rollier, R. "Treatment of Lepromatous Leprosy by a Combination of DDS and Sarsaparilla *(Smilax ornata)*," *International Journal of Leprosy* 27:328-40, 1959.

Thermon, F.M. "The Treatment of Psoriasis with a Sarsaparilla Compound," *New England Journal of Medicine* 227:128-33, 1942.

Sassafras

The sassafras tree, *Sassafras albidum* is native to eastern North America. Oil and teas are extracted from its roots and bark. The Food and Drug Administration (FDA) has banned the volatile oil and safrole (the herb's main component) as food additives or flavor-enhancing agents. However, the FDA has approved a safrole-free sassafras extract for food use.

Why people use this herb

- Fluid retention
- General ill health and malnutrition
- Gout
- Intestinal blockage
- Rheumatic pain
- Skin conditions
- Syphilis
- To enhance performance
- To promote sweating
- Venereal disease

Common doses

Sassafras comes as crude bark, liquid extract, oil, tea, and powder. Some experts recommend the following doses for skin conditions and venereal diseases:

- As *bark*, 2 to 4 grams taken orally by infusion three times daily.
- As a *tea*, 0.25 teaspoon of powder added to 1 cup of boiling water and infused for 15 minutes.
- As an *oil*, apply topically.
- As an *extract* (1:1 in 25% alcohol), 2 to 4 milliliters taken orally three times daily.

Side effects

Call your health care practitioner if you experience any of these possible side effects of sassafras:

- drooping eyelids
- hallucinations
- hot flashes
- skin rash
- spasms
- stupor
- sweating
- symptoms of central nervous system depression, such as excessive drowsiness or sleepiness, slow breathing, and reduced mental alertness
- trouble walking
- unusual sensitivity to touch
- vomiting.

This herb also can cause:

- abnormally low body temperature
- heart and blood vessel collapse
- liver cancer
- miscarriage
- paralysis.

One teaspoon of sassafras oil can kill an adult. A few drops can kill a child.

Interactions

Combining herbs with certain drugs may alter their action or produce unwanted side effects. Tell your health care practitioner about any prescription or nonprescription drugs you're taking.

Important points to remember

- Don't use sassafras if you're pregnant or breast-feeding.
- Don't use sassafras internally or externally for more than 2 weeks.
- Be aware that your health care practitioner may recommend periodic liver function tests if you're taking sassafras.
- Don't drive or perform other dangerous activities until you know how sassafras affects you.
- Keep in mind that sassafras has known cancer-causing effects.
- Know that consuming sassafras can reduce your body's ability to eliminate other drugs you're taking.

Other names for sassafras

Other names for sassafras include ague tree, bois de sassafras, cinnamon wood, fenchelholz, lignum floridum, lignum sassafras, root bark, saloop, sassafrasholz, and saxifras.

No known products containing sassafras are available commercially.

WHAT THE RESEARCH SHOWS

Despite its long history of use as a flavoring agent and a treatment for skin and rheumatic conditions, sassafras is toxic and may promote cancer development. It also may interfere with many prescription drugs. Medical experts warn against using it for any purpose.

Selected references

Borchert, P., et al. "The Metabolism of the Naturally Occurring Hepatocarcinogen Safrole to 1'-hydroxysafrole and the Electrophilic Reactivity of 1'-acetoxysafrole," *Cancer Research* 33:575-89, 1973.

Craig, J.O. "Poisoning by the Volatile Oils in Childhood," *Archives of Disease in Childhood* 28:475-83, 1953.

Opdyke, D.L.J. "Safrole," *Food and Cosmetics Toxicology* 12:983-86, 1974.

Saw palmetto

Saw palmetto's active ingredients come from brownish black berries of the American dwarf palm (*Serenoa repens* or *Sabal serrulata).* The berries contain about 1.5% oil. From 1906 to 1950, the *U.S. Pharmacopoeia* and the *National Formulary* listed saw palmetto tea as a treatment for genital and urinary tract ailments.

Common dose

Saw palmetto comes as tablets, capsules, teas, berries (fresh or dried), and liquid extract. Some experts recommend the following dose:

- For *benign prostate enlargement,* 320 milligrams daily taken orally in two equal doses, continued for 3 months. Or 1 to 2 grams of fresh berries or 0.5 to 1 gram of dried berries in decoction taken orally three times daily.

Side effects

Call your health care practitioner if you experience any of these possible side effects of saw palmetto:

- abdominal pain
- back pain
- constipation
- decreased sex drive
- diarrhea
- headache
- impotence
- nausea
- painful urination
- urine retention.

Why people use this herb

- Benign prostate enlargement
- Decreased breast size
- Decreased sex drive
- Decreased sperm production
- Fluid retention
- Genital and urinary problems

This herb also can cause high blood pressure.

Interactions

Combining herbs with certain drugs may alter their action or produce unwanted side effects. Tell your health care practitioner about any prescription or nonprescription drugs you're taking.

Important points to remember

- Don't use saw palmetto if you're pregnant, breast-feeding, or a female of child-bearing age.

- Avoid this herb unless you've been officially diagnosed with benign prostate enlargement—and then use it only on the advice of your health care practitioner.
- Before starting saw palmetto therapy, have your prostate-specific antigen (PSA) level measured.
- Be aware that saw palmetto doesn't seem to change the prostate's size.
- Use saw palmetto cautiously for any condition other than benign prostate enlargement.
- To minimize stomach upset, take saw palmetto with your morning and evening meals.

Other names for saw palmetto

Other names for saw palmetto include American dwarf palm tree, cabbage palm, IDS 89, LSESR, and sabal.

Products containing saw palmetto are sold under such names as Permixon, Propalmex, and Strogen.

Selected references

Carraro, J.C., et al. "Comparison of Phytotherapy (Permixon) with Finasteride in the Treatment of Benign Prostate Hyperplasia: A Randomized International Study of 1,098 Patients," *Prostate* 29:231-40, 1996.

Champault, G., et al. "A Double-Blind Trial of an Extract of the Plant *Serenoa repens* in Benign Prostatic Hyperplasia," *British Journal of Clinical Pharmacology* 18:461-62, 1984.

Plosker, G.L., and Brogden, R.N. "*Serenoa repens* (Permixon). A Review of Its Pharmacology and Therapeutic Efficacy in Benign Prostatic Hyperplasia," *Drugs and Aging* 9:379-95, 1996.

Weisser, H., et al. "Effects of the *Sabal serrulata* Extract IDS 89 and Its Subfractions on 5 Alpha-Reductase Activity in Human Benign Prostatic Hyperplasia," *Prostate* 28:300-06, 1996.

WHAT THE RESEARCH SHOWS

Many test tube, animal, and human studies have found that saw palmetto (especially its component known as LSESR) treats benign prostate enlargement as effectively as a commonly prescribed drug. Current studies focus on comparing how saw palmetto and the prescription drug work. Nonetheless, even though LSESR seems safe and effective, medical experts need to see the results of the comparative research before they can fully recommend saw palmetto.

Scented geranium

Scented geranium (Pelargonium) is the largest subfamily of the geranium family. Although geraniums grow on all continents, the Pelargonium subfamily grows mainly in South Africa. In the United States, scented geranium is a common house plant.

Common dose

Scented geranium comes as potpourri, essential oil, and tea flavoring. The essential oil may be used to make tablets and creams. Experts disagree on what dose to take.

Why people use this herb

- As a pesticide
- Viral infections

Side effects

Call your health care practitioner if you experience any of these possible side effects of scented geranium:

- allergic reactions
- skin inflammation from touching the plant.

Interactions

Combining herbs with certain drugs may alter their action or produce unwanted side effects. Tell your health care practitioner about any prescription or nonprescription drugs you're taking.

Important points to remember

- Don't use scented geranium if you're pregnant or breast-feeding.
- Use this herb cautiously if you've had allergic reactions to various substances.
- Be aware that scented geranium can be used as a natural pesticide in gardens.

Other names for scented geranium

Scented geranium has no other names.

No known products containing scented geranium are available commercially.

WHAT THE RESEARCH SHOWS

Most data on scented geranium's medicinal uses come from other countries and involve test tube and animal studies. Researchers simply don't have enough information to know if this herb is safe or effective for use in people.

Selected references

Gegova, G., et al. "Combined Effect of Selected Antiviral Substances of Natural and Synthetic Origin. II. Anti-influenza Activity of a Combination of a Polyphenolic Complex Isolated from *Geranium sanguineum* L. and rimantadine in vivo," *Acta Microbiologica Bulgarica* 30:37-40, 1993.

Ivancheva, S., et al. "Polyphenols from Bulgarian Medicinal Plants with Anti-infectious Activity," *Basic Life Sciences* 59:717-28, 1992.

Serkedjieva, J. "Antiinfective Activity of a Plant Preparation from *Geranium sanguineum* L.," *Pharmazie* 52:799-802, 1997.

Schisandra

The Chinese name for schisandra, wu-wei-zu, means *five-flavored herb*—a reference to schisandra's sweet, sour, pungent, bitter, and salty taste. *Schisandra chinesis* is native to China, Russia, and Korea. Active ingredients are extracted from the plant's fruit, stems, or kernel.

Why people use this herb

- Eye problems
- Kidney disorders
- Liver disorders
- Lung disorders
- Stress
- To prevent liver damage

Common dose

Schisandra comes as:

- capsules (100 milligrams)
- dried fruit
- extract
- liquid.

Some experts recommend the following dose:

- As an *extract,* 100 milligrams taken orally twice daily.

Side effects

Call your health care practitioner if you experience unusual symptoms while using schisandra.

Interactions

Combining herbs with certain drugs may alter their action or produce unwanted side effects. Tell your health care practitioner about any prescription or nonprescription drugs you're taking.

Important points to remember

- Don't use schisandra if you're pregnant or breast-feeding.
- Know that schisandra may interact with drugs processed mainly by the liver. Tell your health care practitioner about any drugs you're taking, even nonprescription ones.
- Be aware that little information about this herb's safety and effectiveness exists.

Other names for schisandra

Other names for schisandra include gomishi, omicha, schizandra, tjn-101, and wu-wei-zu.

WHAT THE RESEARCH SHOWS

Although animal studies suggest schisandra helps protect the liver, no studies on people have been done. We don't know much about the herb's ability to treat lung and kidney conditions, how much of it to use, or what harmful effects it might cause. Until we know more, medical experts believe it's best to steer clear of schisandra for medicinal use.

Products containing schisandra are sold under such names as Schisandra Extract and Sheng-mai-san.

Selected references

Ko, K.M., et al. "Effect of a Lignan-Enriched Fructus Schisandrae Extract on Hepatic Glutathione Status in Rats: Protection Against Carbon Tetrachloride Toxicity," *Planta Medica* 61:134-37, 1995.

Li, P.C., et al. "*Schisandra chinensis*-Dependent Myocardial Protective Action of Sheng-Mai-San in Rats," *American Journal of Chinese Medicine* 24:255-62, 1996.

Sun, H.D., et al. "Nigranoic Acid, A Triterpenoid from *Schisandra sphaerandra* that Inhibits HIV-1 Reverse Transcriptase," *Journal of Natural Products* 59:525-27, 1996.

Sea holly

Sea holly *(Eryngium maritimum)* typically grows along seashores in temperate regions. Active components come from the dried roots.

Common dose

Sea holly comes as dried roots, extract, and tincture. Some experts recommend the following dose:

- As a *diuretic,* take a decoction (tea) or tincture three times daily.

Side effects

Call your health care practitioner if you experience unusual symptoms while using sea holly.

Interactions

Combining herbs with certain drugs may alter their action or produce unwanted side effects. Tell your health care practitioner about any prescription or nonprescription drugs you're taking, especially diuretics. Sea holly could increase the diuretic's effect on your body's chemical balance.

Important points to remember

- Don't use sea holly if you're pregnant or breast-feeding.
- Avoid this herb if you're taking a diuretic.
- Know that long-term use of sea holly can cause an imbalance in body fluids and chemicals.

Why people use this herb

- Bladder inflammation
- Fluid retention
- Kidney stones
- Prostate enlargement or inflammation
- Urethral inflammation and other urologic conditions

Other names for sea holly

Other names for sea holly include eryngo, sea holme, and sea hulver.

No known products containing sea holly are available commercially.

WHAT THE RESEARCH SHOWS

According to medical experts, too little evidence is available to warrant using sea holly as a remedy.

Selected references

Hiller, K., et al. "Saponins of *Eryngium maritimum* L. 25. Contents of Various Saniculoideae," *Pharmazie* 31:53, 1976.

Lisciani, R., et al. "Anti-inflammatory Activity of *Eryngium maritimim* L. Rhizome Extracts in Intact Rats," *Journal of Ethnopharmacology* 12:263-70, 1984.

Self-heal

Prunella vulgaris **is a perennial weed commonly found in fields, grassy areas, and woods of North America, Asia, and Europe. Herbalists use various parts of the plant for medicinal purposes. For many years, self-heal was thought to cure a disorder called quinsy (inflamed tonsils). In fact, the herb's original name, *Brunella vulgaris*, comes from *bruen*, the German word for quinsy.**

Common dose

Self-heal comes as liquid and fresh plant. Experts disagree on what dose to take but emphasize that the product's formulation may be an important aspect of treatment. Aqueous extracts seem to have the strongest antiviral activity.

Some experts recommend the following dose:

- To make a gargle, mix 1 gram of the fresh plant in boiling water and let cool before using.

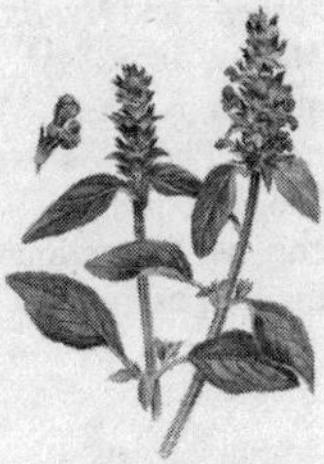

Side effects

Call your health care practitioner if you experience unusual symptoms while using self-heal.

Interactions

Combining herbs with certain drugs may alter their action or produce unwanted side effects. Tell your health care practitioner about any prescription or nonprescription drugs you're taking.

Important points to remember

- Avoid this herb if you're pregnant or breast-feeding.
- Although studies suggest self-heal helps suppress HIV activity, experts advise against using this herb in place of conventional therapy for HIV infection.

Why people use this herb

- Boils
- Cancer
- Diarrhea
- Dysentery
- Hemorrhage
- Hepatitis
- Intestinal gas
- Jaundice
- Lung inflammation and fluid buildup
- Sharp intestinal pain
- Sore throat
- Stomach upset
- Tuberculosis

WHAT THE RESEARCH SHOWS

In test tube studies, self-heal has shown some action against HIV and certain cancers. The herb seems promising, but more studies must be done on animals and people before we'll know if it's truly useful.

Other names for self-heal

Other names for self-heal include all heal, brunella, consuelda menor, hsia ku ts'ao, *Prunella incisa, Prunella querette,* sicklewort, and xia ku cao.

No known products containing self-heal are available commercially.

Selected references

Lee, K.H., et al. "The Cytotoxic Principles of *Prunella vulgaris*, *Psychotrial serpens*, and *Hyptis capitata:* Ursolic Acid and Related Derivatives," *Planta Medica* 54:308-11, 1988.

Yamasaki, K., et al. "Anti-HIV-1 Activity of Labiatae Plants, Especially Aromatic Plants," *International Conference on AIDS* 11:65, 1996. Abstract Mo.A.1062.

Zheng, M. "Experimental Study of 472 Herbs with Antiviral Action Against the Herpes Simplex Virus," *Chung His I Chieh Ho Tsa Chih* 10:39-41, 1990.

Senega

For centuries, senega has been used as an expectorant (to expel mucus from the lungs). The *National Formulary* listed it as an official drug until 1960.

Medicinal senega comes from the dried root and rootstock of *Polygala senega*, a perennial plant native to southern Canada and the United States. Senega is made commercially in Canada and Japan.

Common dose

Senega comes as:

- syrups (various concentrations)
- lozenges
- teas
- tinctures
- dried powdered root
- extract.

Some experts recommend the following dose:

- For *respiratory conditions*, 2 tablespoons of syrup taken orally every 4 hours as needed, 2.5 to 5 milliliters of tincture taken orally, 0.3 to 1 milliliter of extract taken orally, or 0.5 to 1 gram of dried root taken orally three times daily.

Why people use this herb

- Asthma
- Chronic bronchitis
- Cough
- Croup
- Eczema (a type of skin inflammation)
- Graft rejection
- Inflammation
- Multiple sclerosis
- Pneumonia
- Psoriasis (scaly, raised skin patches)
- Rattlesnake bites
- Sore throat
- To cause sweating
- To induce vomiting
- To stimulate saliva production

Side effects

Call your health care practitioner if you experience any of these possible side effects of senega:

- abdominal pain
- anxiety
- diarrhea
- mental dullness
- mouth and throat irritation
- nausea
- stomach upset
- vertigo

- vision disturbances
- vomiting.

This herb also may damage blood cells.

Interactions

Combining herbs with certain drugs may alter their action or produce unwanted side effects. Don't use senega while taking:

- blood thinners
- drugs to control diabetes
- drugs that slow the central nervous system, such as alcohol, cold and allergy drugs, sedatives, tranquilizers, narcotic pain relievers, barbiturates, seizure drugs, and muscle relaxants.

Important points to remember

- Don't use senega if you're pregnant or breast-feeding.
- Avoid this herb if you're allergic to aspirin or other drugs that contain salicylates.
- If you have diabetes, monitor your blood sugar closely while using senega.

Other names for senega

Other names for senega include milkwort, mountain flax, northern senega, polygala root, rattlesnake root, seneca, seneca root, seneca snakeroot, senega root, and senega snakeroot.

Products containing senega are sold under such names as Enhance and SN-X Vegitabs.

Selected references

Carretero, M.E., et al. "Etudes Pharmacodymiques Preliminaires de Polygala Microphylla (L.), sur le Systeme Nerveux Central," *Planta Medica Phytotherapy* 20:148-54, 1986.

Johnson, I.T., et al. "Influence of Saponins on Gut Permeability and Active Nutrient Transport In Vitro," *Journal of Nutrition* 116:2270-77, 1986.

WHAT THE RESEARCH SHOWS

This herb has three strikes against it: lack of data showing its effectiveness, evidence that it can cause significant side effects, and the availability of established effective expectorants. In short, medical experts see little reason to use senega—and plenty of reasons not to—at least for now.

Senna

A well-known ingredient in many nonprescription laxatives, senna comes from the leaves and pods (fruits) of many *Cassia* species, especially *C. acutifolia, C. augustifolia,* and *C. senna*.

Why people use this herb

- Burns
- Constipation
- Fever
- Intestinal worm infections
- Psoriasis (scaly, raised skin patches)
- Skin eruptions
- To induce bowel movements
- Tumors

Common doses

Senna comes as:

- tablets (187 milligrams)
- capsules (10, 25, and 470 milligrams)
- syrup (which also contains coriander)
- tea
- granules
- suppositories
- fluid extract.

Some experts recommend the following doses:

- For *constipation in an adult,* 2 tablets taken orally at bedtime (a maximum of 8 tablets daily).
- For *constipation in a child weighing more than 60 pounds,* 1 tablet taken orally at bedtime (a maximum of 4 tablets daily).

To make a tea or an infusion, place 100 grams of senna leaves and 5 grams of sliced ginger or coriander in 1 liter of distilled boiling water.

Side effects

Call your health care practitioner if you experience any of these possible side effects of senna:

- diarrhea
- intestinal cramps or gripping pains
- rash
- severe weight loss.

This herb also can cause:

- finger clubbing (rounded swelling of the fingertips and nails)
- fluid and chemical imbalances
- jaw tightness.

Interactions

Combining herbs with certain drugs may alter their action or produce unwanted side effects. Don't use senna while taking:

- heart drugs called calcium channel blockers, such as Calan and Procardia
- Indocin.

Important points to remember

- Don't use senna if you have an inflammatory condition of the digestive tract, hemorrhoids, or a prolapsed rectum.
- Don't use this herb to force a daily bowel movement.
- If you take senna to relieve constipation, help it work by drinking more fluids and eating more fiber-rich foods, such as whole-grain breads, grains, fruits, and vegetables.
- Stop taking senna as soon as your constipation clears up. Don't take it or any other stimulant laxative longer than 1 week.
- Stop using senna if you experience intense abdominal pains or nausea.
- Remember that senna supplements differ in potency.
- Know that senna may discolor your urine.

Other names for senna

Other names for senna include Aden senna, *Cassia acutifolia, Cassia augustifolia, Cassia senna,* Mecca senna, nubian senna, and tinnevally senna.

Products containing senna are sold under such names as Senekot, Senexon, Senokot-S, Senolax, and Senna Leaves.

Selected references

Beubler. E., and Kollar, G. "Prostaglandin-Mediated Action of Sennosides," *Pharmacology* 36(Suppl.1):85-91, 1988.

Dreessen, M., and Lemli, J. "Qualitative and Quantitative Interactions Between the Sennosides and Some Human Intestinal Bacteria," *Pharmaceutica Acta Helvetiae* 57:350-52, 1982.

Morton, J.F. *Major Medicinal Plants—Botany, Culture and Uses*. Springfield, Ill.: Charles C. Thomas, Bannerstone House, 1977.

Prior, J., and White, I. "Tetany and Clubbing in Patients Who Ingested Large Quantities of Senna," *Lancet* 2:947, 1978.

WHAT THE RESEARCH SHOWS

Senna seems to be safe and effective in treating constipation, but overuse can lead to many harmful effects. Medical experts say you should use it only occasionally and only for short periods.

Shepherd's purse

Shepherd's purse comes from the leaves and stems of *Capsella bursapastoris*. A member of the mustard family, this white-flowered, weedy annual has flat, heart-shaped pods.

Common doses

Shepherd's purse comes as dried herb and liquid extract. Some experts recommend the following doses:

- As *fluid extract,* 1 teaspoon of extract in 8 ounces of water taken orally four times daily.
- As *dried plant,* 1 ounce of dried plant in 12 ounces of boiling water, cooled and taken orally three times daily.

Side effects

Call your health care practitioner if you experience any of these possible side effects of shepherd's purse:

- enlarged pupils
- neck swelling (thyroid enlargement)
- trouble walking
- unusual drowsiness or sleepiness.

This herb also can cause:

- low blood pressure
- respiratory paralysis and possible death
- underactive thyroid.

Why people use this herb

- Bleeding disorders
- Bloody urine
- Diarrhea
- Heavy menstrual bleeding
- Vomiting of blood

Interactions

Combining herbs with certain drugs may alter their action or produce unwanted side effects. Don't use shepherd's purse while taking:

- digoxin
- drugs that lower blood pressure
- heart drugs called beta blockers (such as Inderal) or calcium channel blockers (such as Calan or Procardia)
- sedatives or hypnotics, such as Ambien, Ativan, Dalmane, Doriden, Halcion, Luminal, Nembutol, Placydil, Restoril, or Seconal.

Important points to remember

- Don't use shepherd's purse if you're pregnant or breast-feeding.
- Use this herb cautiously, if at all, if you have heart or lung disease. Consider using a proven treatment instead of this herb.

- Use shepherd's purse cautiously if you take a drug that alters your heart rate or depresses your nervous system.

Other names for shepherd's purse

Other names for shepherd's purse include capsella, caseweed, mother's-heart, and shovelweed.

No known products containing shepherd's purse are available commercially.

WHAT THE RESEARCH SHOWS

Most of what we know about shepherd's purse comes from test tube and animal studies. Until studies on people are completed, medical experts don't recommend this herb for medicinal purposes.

Selected references

Kuroda, K., and Takagi. K. "Studies on *Capsella bursa-pastoris* II. Diuretic, Anti-inflammatory and Anti-ulcer Action of Ethanol Extracts of the Herb," *Archives Internationales de Pharmacodynamie et de Therapie* 178:392-99, 1969.

Moskalenko, S.A. "Preliminary Screening of Far-Eastern Ethnomedicinal Plants for Antibacterial Activity," *Journal of Ethnopharmacology* 15:231-59, 1986.

Skullcap

Skullcap comes from the leaves and roots of two perennials, *Scutellaria laterifolia* and *S. baicalensis,* that are native to temperate regions of North America. Although usually taken orally, skullcap can be injected into a muscle or vein.

Common doses

Skullcap comes as:

- capsules (425 and 429 milligrams)
- liquid extract (1 and 2 ounces).

Some experts recommend the following doses:

- As *dried herb,* 1 to 2 grams taken orally as tea three times daily.
- As a *liquid extract* (1:1 in 25% alcohol), 2 to 4 milliliters taken orally three times daily.
- As a *tincture* (1:5 in 45% alcohol), 1 to 2 milliliters taken orally three times daily.

Why people use this herb

- Blood clots in the brain
- Inflammation
- Movement disorders
- Seizures
- Spasticity
- Stroke
- To enhance cancer chemotherapy
- To lower cholesterol
- Viral infections

Side effects

Call your health care practitioner if you experience any of these possible side effects of skullcap:

- confusion
- giddiness
- seizures
- stupor
- twitching.

This herb also can cause irregular heartbeats and liver damage.

Interactions

Combining herbs with certain drugs may alter their action or produce unwanted side effects. Don't use skullcap while taking:

- Antabuse
- drugs that suppress the immune system, such as Imuran, Prograf, and Sandimmune.

Important points to remember

- Don't use this herb if you're pregnant or breast-feeding.
- Know that your health care practitioner may recommend periodic liver function tests while you're taking skullcap.
- Don't use large doses of skullcap—they could be toxic.
- Keep in mind that even commercial skullcap sources have been contaminated with other herbs, one of which *(Teucrium)* may damage the liver.

WHAT THE RESEARCH SHOWS

Research suggests skullcap may enhance cancer chemotherapy. One study of lung cancer patients found that adding skullcap to their chemotherapy boosted their immune systems. Another showed that the herb helped to support patients' circulatory and immune systems during chemotherapy. These findings deserve vigorous follow-up studies. In the meantime, medical experts are taking a wait-and-see attitude toward all medicinal uses of skullcap.

Other names for skullcap

Other names for skullcap include helmet flower, hoodwort, and scullcap.

Products containing skullcap are sold under such names as Scullcap Herb and Skullcap.

Selected references

Chung, C.P., et al. "Pharmacological Effects of Methanolic Extract from the Root of *Scutellaria baicalensis* and Its Flavonoids on Human Fibroblast," *Planta Medica* 61:150-53, 1995.

Goldberg, V.E., et al. "Dry Extract of *Scutellaria baicalensis* as a Hemostimulant in Antineoplastic Chemotherapy in Patients with Lung Cancer," *Eksperimentalnaia I Klinicheskaia Farmakologiia* 60:28-30, 1997.

Smolianinov, D.A., et al. "Effect of *Scutellaria baicalensis* Extract on the Immunologic Status of Patients with Lung Cancer Receiving Antineoplastic Chemotherapy," *Eksperimentalnaia I Klinicheskaia Farmakologiia* 69:49-51, 1997.

Skunk cabbage

The Micmac Indians crushed the leaves of skunk cabbage *(Symplocarpus foetidus)* and inhaled the pungent oils to treat headache. Skunk cabbage was named both for the unpleasant smell of its bruised leaves and for the leaves' appearance.

Today, herbalists obtain active ingredients from the plant's rhizome (underground stem) and roots. The root is bitter and acrid and, like the bruised leaves, has a disagreeable odor.

Common doses

Skunk cabbage comes as powdered root, liquid extract, and tincture. Some experts recommend the following doses for treating coughs:

- As an *extract* (1:1 in 25% alcohol), 0.5 to 1 milliliter taken orally three times daily.
- As a *tincture* (1:10 in 25% alcohol), 2 to 4 milliliters taken orally three times daily.
- As *powdered root,* 0.5 to 1 gram mixed with honey taken orally three times daily.

Why people use this herb

- Asthma
- Bronchitis
- Fluid retention
- Headache
- Irritable, tight cough
- Nervousness
- Tightness in the chest
- Whooping cough

Side effects

Call your health care practitioner if you experience any of these possible side effects of skunk cabbage:

- dizziness
- drowsiness
- headache
- irritation or burning of the mouth's mucous membranes
- itchy, reddened, or inflamed skin
- nausea
- vertigo
- vomiting.

This herb also can cause kidney damage.

Interactions
Combining herbs with certain drugs may alter their action or produce unwanted side effects. Tell your health care practitioner about any prescription or nonprescription drugs you're taking.

Important points to remember
- Don't use skunk cabbage if you're pregnant or breast-feeding.
- Avoid this herb if you've had a kidney stone.
- If you're taking skunk cabbage to treat asthma or bronchitis, consider using effective conventional treatments instead.

WHAT THE RESEARCH SHOWS

Researchers know nothing about the chemicals in skunk cabbage or the chemicals' medicinal effects. Nor do they know whether the herb is a safe or effective treatment for any health problem. Medical experts warn against using skunk cabbage until they have such information.

Other names for skunk cabbage
Other names for skunk cabbage include *Dracontium foetidum*, meadow cabbage, pole-cat cabbage, and skunkweed.

No known products containing skunk cabbage are available commercially.

Selected reference
Konyukhov, V.P., et al. "Dynamics of the Accumulation of Biologically Active Agents in *Lysichitum camtsochatcense* and *Symplocarpus foetidus*," *Uch Zap Khabarovsk Gos Pedagog Inst* 26:59-62, 1970.

Slippery elm

A member of the Ulmaceae (Elm) family, slippery elm grows throughout North America. Herbalists typically use the inner bark of *Ulmus rubra* Muhl. The pieces of bark are flat and oblong, measuring about 2 to 4 millimeters thick.

Some people have used Essiac, a multiherbal decoction that contains slippery elm powdered bark, in an attempt to treat cancer. The herb was once listed in the *U.S. Pharmacopoeia,* a compendium of drug standards.

Why people use this herb

- Cough
- Digestive ailments
- Skin irritation

Common doses

Slippery elm comes as:

- powdered bark
- liquid extract (1:1 in 60% alcohol).

Some experts recommend the following doses for digestive discomfort:

- As *powdered bark,* 4 to 16 milliliters of a 1:8 decoction taken orally three times daily, or 4 grams of herb in 500 milliliters of boiling water taken orally three times daily.
- As *liquid extract,* 5 milliliters taken orally three times daily.

For topical use, some experts recommend the following dose:

- As a *skin emollient*, make a poultice of coarse powdered bark in boiling water.

Side effects

Call your health care practitioner if you experience unusual symptoms when using slippery elm. Whole bark preparations of slippery elm may increase the risk of miscarriage.

Interactions

Combining herbs with certain drugs may alter their action or produce unwanted side effects. Tell your health care practitioner about any prescription or nonprescription drugs you're taking.

Important points to remember

- Don't use slippery elm if you're pregnant or breast-feeding.
- Avoid this herb if you've ever had an allergic reaction to it or its components.

- Don't use whole-bark slippery elm preparations because no evidence shows that they're effective.

WHAT THE RESEARCH SHOWS

No clinical data support the use of slippery elm. Until convincing evidence is available, medical experts say you're better off using proven therapies instead of this herb.

Other names for slippery elm

Other names for slippery elm include American elm, Indian elm, moose elm, red elm, and sweet elm.

No known products containing slippery elm are available commercially.

Selected reference

Locock, R.A. "Essiac," *Canadian Pharmacy Journal* 14:18-19, 51, 1997.

Soapwort

Soapwort is a common ingredient in herbal shampoos because its chief components, called saponins, produce foam or suds in water. (The term *saponification* refers to the soap-making process.) Plants that contain a lot of saponins reportedly taste much like soap. Soapwort is also known as *fuller's herb* because the textile industry once used it as a fulling (cleaning and sizing) agent.

Medicinal soapwort is extracted from the root and leaves *of Saponaria officinalis.* Native to Asia, this plant has become naturalized to eastern North America. The Egyptian soapwort root, *Gypsophila struthium,* occasionally is used in place of soapwort because it contains saponin and some of the same components as *S. officinalis.*

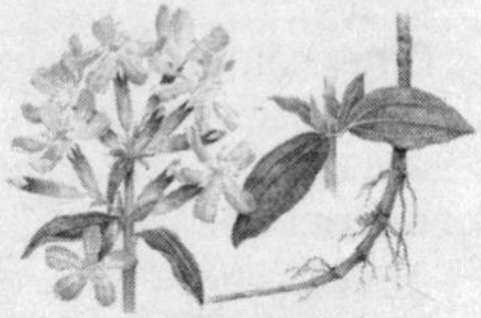

Common doses

Soapwort comes as dried root, dried leaves, decoction, extract, fluid extract, and juice. Some experts recommend the following doses:

- As a *decoction,* 2 to 4 fluid ounces taken orally three or four times daily.
- As an *extract* or a *juice,* 10 to 20 grains taken orally.
- As *fluid extract,* 0.25 to 1 dram taken orally.

Side effects

Call your health care practitioner if you experience any of these possible side effects of soapwort:

- nausea
- upset stomach
- vomiting.

This herb also can cause:

- digestive tract ulcers
- kidney damage
- liver damage
- nerve damage.

Why people use this herb

- Acne
- As a shampoo
- Boils
- Constipation
- Dandruff
- Gout
- Intestinal problems
- Jaundice
- Rheumatism
- Skin problems, including psoriasis (scaly, raised skin patches) and eczema (a type of skin inflammation)
- Skin reactions caused by syphilis
- To help expel mucus from the lungs

Interactions

Combining herbs with certain drugs may alter their action or produce unwanted side effects. Tell your health care practitioner about any prescription or nonprescription drugs you're taking.

Important points to remember

- Don't use soapwort if you're pregnant or breast-feeding.
- Don't use high doses of this herb for more than 2 weeks because it may damage your digestive tract.
- Know that most people can't or shouldn't use soapwort because ingesting it can cause toxic reactions and intense bowel evacuation.
- Be aware that your health care practitioner may recommend periodic liver and kidney function tests while you're using soapwort.

Other names for soapwort

Other names for soapwort include bouncing bet, bruisewort, crowsoap, fuller's herb, latherwort, soap root, sweet Betty, and wild sweet William.

No known products containing soapwort are available commercially.

Selected references

Chan, T.Y., et al. "Neurotoxicity Following the Ingestion of a Chinese Medicinal Plant, *Alocasia macrorrhiza,*" *Human and Experimental Toxicology* 14:727-28, 1995.

Siena, S., et al. "Activity of Monoclonal Antibody-Saporin-6 Conjugate Against B-Lymphoma Cells," *Cancer Research* 49:3328-32, 1989.

Stripe, F., et al. "Hepatotoxicity of Immunotoxins Made with Saporin, a Ribosome-Inactivating Protein from *Saponaria officinalis,*" *Virchows Archiv* 53: 259-71, 1987.

Tecce, R., et al. "Saporin 6 Conjugated to Monoclonal Antibody Selectivity Kills Human Melanoma Cells," *Melanoma Research* 1:115-23, 1991.

WHAT THE RESEARCH SHOWS

In test tube studies, purified components of soapwort called saponins have harmed cancer cells. However, we have no evidence that the herb helps cure cancer in people. Because other treatments are effective against cancer, medical experts favor them over soapwort. The same goes for other ailments—not only because virtually no clinical data are available but also because soapwort could be toxic.

Sorrel

In the 16th century, people took sorrel to treat fever—a use that continued into the late 19th century. However, concern that it was poisonous limited its use.

The type of sorrel popular for medicinal use is *Rumex acetosella*, commonly called sheep sorrel. Another type, *R. acetosa*, is more common as a garden plant. Both plants as well as related sorrel species belong to the Polygonaceae family, which is native to Europe and northern Asia and has been naturalized in North America.

Herbalists use the leaves, flowers, roots, and seeds of the sorrel plant. Concentration of active ingredients in the leaves varies with the season and the plant's geographic location.

Common dose

Sorrel comes as tea and as juice from fresh plants. Leaves and flowers can be made into tea, and juice from the plant can be diluted in water and taken orally. Experts disagree on what dose to take.

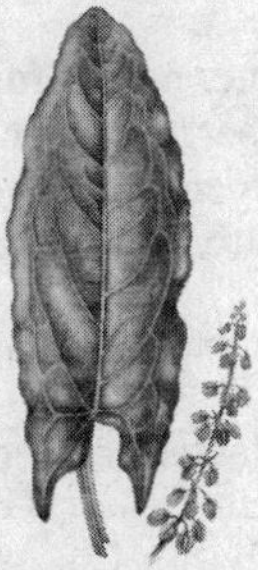

Side effects

Call your health care practitioner if you experience any of these possible side effects of sorrel:

- gastroenteritis (stomach inflammation leading to nausea, vomiting, abdominal discomfort, and diarrhea)
- jaw tightness
- skin rash.

This herb also can cause:

- brain damage
- heart damage
- kidney damage
- liver damage.

Why people use this herb

- As an antiseptic
- Diarrhea
- Fluid retention
- Scurvy

Interactions

Combining herbs with certain drugs may alter their action or produce unwanted side effects. Tell your health care practitioner about any

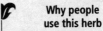

prescription or nonprescription drugs you're taking, because sorrel can cause kidney or liver problems when taken with drugs that the kidney or liver processes.

Don't use sorrel while taking a diuretic.

Important points to remember

- Don't take sorrel if you're pregnant or breast-feeding.
- Don't give this herb to a child.
- Don't take sorrel if you've had a kidney stone.
- If you cook sorrel leaves, be sure to change the cooking water at least once to decrease the herb's potency. Otherwise, the herb is toxic.
- Keep sorrel away from children and pets.
- Know that it takes very little sorrel to make you sick or even to kill you. The estimated fatal dose of oxalic acid, sorrel's major component, is 15 to 30 grams. As little as 5 grams could be fatal.

Other names for sorrel

Other names for sorrel include cuckoo sorrow, cuckoo's meate, dock, garden sorrel, greensauce, green sorrel, sour dock, sourgrass, sour sauce, and soursuds.

No known products containing sorrel are available commercially.

Selected references

Crellin, J.K., and Philpott, J. *A Reference Guide to Medicinal Plants: Herbal Medicine Past and Present.* Durham and London: Duke University Press, 1990.

Farre, M., et al. "Fatal Oxalic Acid Poisoning from Sorrel Soup," *Lancet* 2:1524, 1989.

Sanz, P., and Reig, R. "Clinical and Pathological Findings in Plant Oxalosis: A Review," *American Journal of Forensic Medicine and Pathology* 13:342-45, 1992.

WHAT THE RESEARCH SHOWS

Herbalists' claims for sorrel lack supporting evidence and the herb's toxic effects have been shown in both animals and people. For these reasons, medical experts warn against using sorrel.

Southernwood

Southernwood has an obnoxious odor that fends off moths and insects. Some people apply it to their skin and clothes for this effect—a use that explains the plant's unofficial name, *Garde Robe*.

A perennial shrub, southernwood is native to southern Europe. Some people think its genus name, *Artemisia*, comes from Artemis, the Greek goddess of hunting and chastity. Artemis was identified with Diana, the goddess of nature, the forests, and the moon. The genus has more than 180 species, including *A. absinthium* (wormwood), *A. vulgaris* (mugwort), and *A. abrotanum* (southernwood).

Southernwood's leaves, tops, shoots, and seeds are used medicinally. The branches and leaves produce a yellow dye sometimes used for coloring wool.

Why people use this herb

- As an antiseptic
- Digestive problems
- Fever
- Hair loss
- Pinworms, tapeworms, and other worm infections
- To promote menstruation
- To stimulate the uterus
- Wounds

Common doses

Southernwood is available as tea, oil, and extract. Some experts recommend the following doses:

- As *dried herb*, 2 to 4 grams in hot water taken orally three times daily.
- As an *extract* (1:1 in 25% alcohol), 2 to 4 milliliters taken orally three times daily.

Side effects

Call your health care practitioner if you experience unusual symptoms while using southernwood.

Interactions

Combining herbs with certain drugs may alter their action or produce unwanted side effects. Tell your health care practitioner about any prescription or nonprescription drugs you're taking.

Important points to remember

- Don't use southernwood if you're pregnant or breast-feeding.
- Know that little information on this herb's benefits or dangers exists.

WHAT THE RESEARCH SHOWS

Clinical trials don't support southernwood's medicinal use. Also, related herbs used for the same purposes have gained popularity over southernwood. Although some herbalists still recommend this herb to stimulate menstruation, medical experts say you're better off avoiding it until researchers gather more information.

Other names for southernwood

Other names for southernwood include appleringie, boy's love, God's tree, lad's love, maiden's ruin, and old man.

No known products containing southernwood are available commercially.

Selected references

Bergendorff, O., and Sterner, O. "Spasmolytic Flavonols from *Artemisia abrotanum,*" *Planta Medica* 61: 370-71, 1995.

Nieschulz, V.O., and Schmersahl, P. "Uber choleretische Wirkstoffe aus *Artemisia abrotanum* L.," *Arzneimittel-Forschung* 18:1330-36, 1968.

Spirulina

Spirulina is a microscopic, corkscrew-shaped alga that lives in high-salt, alkaline waters in subtropical and tropical areas. The bluish-green color of the roughly 35 *Spirulina* species stems from the chlorophyll (green) and phycocyanin (blue) pigments in the plant's cells. Some people find spirulina's color less than appetizing. Fortunately, the color can easily be changed.

Algae have a high nutritional value and have been used as protein sources during food shortages. Even now, developing countries such as Peru, India, Vietnam, and some African countries use spirulina to help fight protein deficiency and vitamin A malnutrition. Spirulina doesn't have wider nutritional use because it is expensive to produce and contains heavy metals (arsenic, cadmium, lead, and mercury) and, sometimes, radioactive ions.

Nonetheless, some advocates promote spirulina as an aid to dieting and weight loss, claiming it curbs the appetite. Spirulina also contains gamma-linolenic acid (GLA), a rich source of omega-6 essential fatty acid that may help prevent heart disease.

Why people use this herb

- Anemia
- Diabetes
- Glaucoma
- Hair loss
- Liver disease
- Pancreas inflammation
- Peptic ulcers
- Stress
- To curb the appetite
- To promote weight loss

Common doses

Spirulina comes as:

- capsules (500 and 750 milligrams)
- tablets (250, 380, 500, and 750 milligrams)
- powder (20 milligrams)
- fruit drink (20 milligrams)
- fresh plant.

Some experts recommend the following doses:

- 3 to 5 grams daily taken orally before meals.
- To *promote rapid weight gain in malnourished infants*, 3 to 15 grams daily taken orally.

Side effects

Nutritional tests have found no side effects from spirulina, but you should call your health care practitioner if you experience unusual symptoms while using it.

Interactions

Combining herbs with certain drugs may alter their action or produce unwanted side effects. Tell your health care practitioner about any prescription or nonprescription drugs you're taking.

Important points to remember

- Use spirulina cautiously if you're pregnant or breast-feeding.
- Know that spirulina may contain significant amounts of mercury depending on where it's grown. Eating 20 grams daily may give you more mercury than the maximum 180-microgram safety limit. Spirulina also may contain arsenic, cadmium, and lead.
- Consult your health care practitioner before using spirulina. For some people, the risk of heavy-metal poisoning exceeds the benefits obtained from the herb.
- Be aware that this herb may contain tiny amounts of radioactive ions, depending on where it was produced.
- Keep in mind that spirulina has a slight marine odor but a mild taste.
- Know that spirulina's GLA content is 25% to 30% compared with other sources, such as evening primrose oil or black currant berries, which contain 10% to 15%.

WHAT THE RESEARCH SHOWS

Unquestionably, spirulina has nutritional value. However, it's more expensive than other protein and nutrient sources. Also, unlike commercial vitamin and nutrient supplements, it carries the risk of heavy metal poisoning and exposure to radioactive ions. Official recommendation of spirulina as a medical remedy won't come until additional supportive data are available.

Other names for spirulina

Other names for spirulina include blue-green algae, dihe, and tecuitlatl.

A product containing spirulina is sold as Spirulina.

Selected references

Dillon J.C., et al., "Nutritional Value of the Alga Spirulina," *World Review of Nutrition and Diet* 77:32-46, 1995.

Hayashi, T., et al. "Calcium Spirulan, an Inhibitor of Enveloped Virus Replication, from a Blue-Green Alga *Spirulina platensis*," *Journal of Natural Products* 59:83-87, 1996.

Squaw vine

Native Americans were the first people to use squaw vine as a way to make childbirth safer and easier. Squaw vine is the dried plant of *Mitchella repens* Linne (Rubiaceae family), common to the woodlands of the central and eastern United States. It blooms in July and usually is harvested in late summer.

Common doses

Squaw vine comes as whole leaves, dried plant (powder), liquid extract, and tincture. Some experts recommend the following doses:

- As *dried plant,* 2 to 4 grams taken orally.
- As *fluid extract,* 0.25 to 1 teaspoon taken orally three times daily.
- As a *tincture,* 1 to 2 milliliters taken orally three times daily.

Side effects

Call your health care practitioner if you experience mucous membrane irritation when taking squaw vine. This herb also can cause:

- burning sensation in the digestive tract
- liver damage.

Interactions

Combining herbs with certain drugs may alter their action or produce unwanted side effects. Tell your health care practitioner about any prescription or nonprescription drugs you're taking, especially:

- alkaloid-related drugs, such as atropine or Transderm-Scōp
- digoxin
- iron-containing products.

Don't use squaw vine when taking Antabuse. The herbal preparation could contain alcohol and cause a reaction.

Why people use this herb

- Abdominal pain from menstruation
- Abnormal menstruation
- Diarrhea
- Fluid retention
- Frequent urination
- Gonorrhea
- Heavy menstrual bleeding
- Hysteria
- Kidney stones
- Lack of menstruation
- Painful urination
- Sore nipples
- To aid labor and childbirth
- Vaginitis

Important points to remember

- Don't use squaw vine during the first 6 months of pregnancy.
- Tell your health care practitioner if you plan to get pregnant or suspect you're pregnant.

- Use squaw vine cautiously if you have liver disease or related problems.
- If you take this herb, be aware that your health care practitioner may recommend periodic liver function tests. If those tests show changes, you'll need to stop taking squaw vine right away.
- Call your health care practitioner immediately if you develop pain in the upper right part of your abdomen, yellowish skin, or a fever. These symptoms could reflect liver damage.
- Know that squaw vine tastes bitter and can irritate the mucous membranes.
- Keep in mind that many health care practitioners consider squaw vine potentially dangerous.
- If you take Antabuse, don't take a form of squaw vine that contains alcohol.

WHAT THE RESEARCH SHOWS

Although squaw vine has long been used as a medicinal herb, none of its effects have been studied or proven in animals or people.

Other names for squaw vine

Other names for squaw vine include checkerberry, deerberry, *Mitchella repens, Mitchella undulata,* one-berry, partridge berry, running box, squawberry, twin berry, two-eyed berry, two-eyed checkerberry, and winter clover.

Products containing squaw vine are sold under such names as *Mitchella repens,* Partridge Berry, and Squaw Vine.

Selected references

Budavari, S. *The Merck Index: An Encyclopedia of Chemicals, Drugs, and Biologicals,* 12th ed. Whitehouse Station, N.J.: Merck & Co., 1996.

Chevallier, A. *The Encyclopedia of Medicinal Plants*, 1st ed. New York: DK Publishing, Inc., 1996.

Duke, J.A. *CRC Handbook of Medicinal Herbs*. Boca Raton, Fla.: CRC Press, 1985.

Squill

Squill's active components come from the bulb and dried bulb scales of *Urginea maritima*. Red squill, rich in a chemical called scilliroside, is a highly effective rat poison.

Common doses

Squill comes as dried root, extract, and tincture. Some experts recommend the following doses:

- As *dried root,* 0.06 to 0.25 gram of bulb taken orally three times daily.
- As a *decoction,* 0.5 to 1 teaspoon of bulb mixed in hot water, steeped for 10 to 15 minutes, chilled, and taken orally 1 cup at a time, three times daily.
- As a *tincture,* 0.5 to 1 milliliter taken orally three times daily.

Why people use this herb

- Fluid retention
- Heart failure symptoms
- To help expel mucus from the lungs

Side effects

Call your health care practitioner if you experience any of these possible side effects of squill:

- nervous stimulation, including nervousness, inability to sleep, and irritability
- stomach irritation
- vomiting.

Taking too much squill may lead to seizures and life-threatening heart problems.

Interactions

Combining herbs with certain drugs may alter their action or produce unwanted side effects. Tell your health care practitioner about any prescription or nonprescription drugs you're taking, especially:

- digoxin
- drugs for irregular heartbeats
- heart drugs called beta blockers (such as Inderal) or calcium channel blockers (such as Calan or Procardia).

Don't use squill while taking:

- Antabuse
- drugs that stimulate the central nervous system, such as Adipex-P, amphetamines, caffeine, Desoxyn, Dexedrine, or Tenuate

- glucocorticoids, such as Aristocort, Cortone, Decadron, Delta-Cortef, Deltasone, Depo-Medrol, Haldone, Hydeltrasol, Hydeltra-TBA Hydrocortone, Kenalog, Medrol, Predcor-25, or Solu-Medrol.

Important points to remember

- Don't take squill if you're pregnant or breast-feeding.
- Tell your health care practitioner if you're planning to get pregnant or suspect you're pregnant.
- Don't take squill if you have problems with a low potassium level.
- Use this herb cautiously, if at all, if you have heart problems or take drugs to treat a heart problem.
- Tell your health care practitioner if you become nervous or irritable, have trouble sleeping, or develop other symptoms of excessive nervous stimulation.
- Don't drive or perform other dangerous activities until you know how squill affects you.
- If you take Antabuse, don't use a squill form that contains alcohol.
- Keep squill away from children and pets.

WHAT THE RESEARCH SHOWS

Today, squill is used mainly to help expel mucus from the lungs. It has not been used to treat heart problems since a class of drugs called cardiac glycosides was developed. Medical experts don't recommend squill for heart problems.

Other names for squill

Other names for squill include European squill, Indian squill, Mediterranean squill, red squill, sea onion, sea squill, and white squill.

No known products containing squill are available commercially.

Selected references

Orita, Y. "Diuretics," *Nippon Jinzo Gakkai Shi Japanese Journal of Nephrology* 38:1-7, 1996.

Stauch M, et al. "Effect of Proscillaridin-4í-methylether on Pressure Rise Velocity in the Left Ventricle of Patients with Coronary Heart Disease," *Klinische Wochenschrift* 55:705-06, 1977.

Tuncok, Y., et al. "*Urginea maritima* (Squill) Toxicity," *Journal of Toxicology Clinical Toxicology* 33:83-86, 1995.

Stoneroot

Stoneroot comes from the rhizome (underground stem) and root of *Collinsonia canadensis*, a member of the Labiatae family. Native to North America, this plant grows wild from Massachusetts and Vermont west to Wisconsin and south to Florida and Arkansas. An advisory review panel of the Food and Drug Administration found little scientific evidence to support stoneroot's use.

Why people use this herb

- Diarrhea
- Fluid retention
- Generalized swelling
- Headache
- Hemorrhoids
- Indigestion
- Menstrual discomfort
- Varicose veins

Common dose

Stoneroot is available as tincture of the root. Some experts recommend the following dose:

- As a *diuretic* and *to treat bladder stones,* 15 to 60 drops of tincture taken orally three times daily.

Side effects

Call your health care practitioner if you experience unusual symptoms while taking stoneroot. Keep in mind that chronic use of this herb can raise your blood pressure.

Interactions

Combining herbs with certain drugs may alter their action or produce unwanted side effects. Tell your health care practitioner about any prescription or nonprescription drugs you're taking, especially drugs that lower blood pressure.

Important points to remember

- Don't use stoneroot if you're pregnant or breast-feeding.
- Don't take this herb to treat high blood pressure or swelling unless your health care practitioner approves.
- Know that your health care practitioner may recommend periodic liver function tests because prolonged stoneroot use may cause liver damage.

Other names for stoneroot

Other names for stoneroot include heal-all, horse balm, horseweed, knob root, knob weed, knot root, ox balm, rich leaf, and rich weed.

WHAT THE RESEARCH SHOWS

Medicinal claims for stoneroot focus on its astringent and diuretic actions. However, these claims aren't supported by controlled studies in animals or people. Medical experts don't consider this herb safe or effective.

A product containing stoneroot is sold as Tincture Collinson.

Selected reference

Tyler, V.E., et al. *Pharmacognosy*, 9th ed. Philadelphia: Lea & Febiger, 1988.

Sundew

Sundew comes from a carnivorous plant *(Drosera rotundifolia)* named for the sticky, dewlike substance on its leaves. After the sticky substance traps insects, the plant digests them. Herbalists use all plant parts except the roots for medicinal purposes.

Common doses

Sundew comes as tincture and fluid or solid dried extract. Some experts recommend an average daily dose of 3 grams, taken as follows:

- As an *infusion,* 1 teaspoon of dried herb in 1 cup of boiling water for 15 minutes, taken orally three times daily.
- As a *tincture,* 1 to 2 milliliters taken orally three times daily.

Why people use this herb

- Asthmatic cough
- Bronchitis
- Stomach ulcers
- Tuberculosis
- Whooping cough

Side effects

Call your health care practitioner if you experience unusual symptoms while using sundew.

Interactions

Combining herbs with certain drugs may alter their action or produce unwanted side effects. Tell your health care practitioner about any prescription or nonprescription drugs you're taking.

Important points to remember

- Don't use sundew if you have a persistent cough, low blood pressure, or tuberculosis. Instead, have your health care practitioner evaluate your condition and then get appropriate standard treatment.
- Be aware that this herb may turn your urine a harmless brownish orange.
- If you take Antabuse, don't use a sundew form that contains alcohol.

Other names for sundew

Other names for sundew include common sundew, dew plant, red rot, round-leaved sundew, and great sundew.

No known products containing sundew are available commercially.

WHAT THE RESEARCH SHOWS

Medical experts don't have enough clinical data about sundew to support its medicinal use.

Selected reference

Vinkenborg, J., et al. "The Presence of Hydroplumbagin Glucoside in *Drosera rotundifolia* L.," *Pharmaceutisch Weekblad* 104:45-49, 1969.

Sweet cicely

The roots, leaves, and seeds of sweet cicely *(Myrrhis odorata)* are used for medicinal and culinary purposes. The plant's soft, green, fernlike leaves have a myrrh-like scent. Its small white flowers bloom in late spring. (A similar plant, *Ozmorrhiza longistylis,* is called American sweet cicely.)

Why people use this herb

- Fluid retention
- Gout pain
- Intestinal gas
- Small bites
- To expel mucus from the lungs
- To stimulate the digestive tract
- Ulcers

Common dose

Sweet cicely comes as an extract and an ointment. Experts disagree on what dose to take.

Side effects

Call your health care practitioner if you experience unusual symptoms while using sweet cicely.

Interactions

Combining herbs with certain drugs may alter their action or produce unwanted side effects. Don't use sweet cicely while taking a diuretic because the herb could make the drug's effects too strong.

Important points to remember

- Don't take high doses of sweet cicely if you're pregnant or breast-feeding.
- Don't use this herb if you're taking a diuretic.
- Use sweet cicely cautiously if you have peptic ulcer disease or ulcerative colitis.

Other names for sweet cicely

Other names for sweet cicely include British myrrh, (sweet) chervil, cow chervil, Roman plant, shepherd's needle, smooth cicely, sweet bracken, sweet fern, and sweet humlock.

No known products containing sweet cicely are available commercially.

WHAT THE RESEARCH SHOWS

All parts of the sweet cicely plant are edible and considered safe, so medicinal use of this herb is probably harmless. Whether it's helpful is another matter—no controlled studies have been done. Researchers must identify the plant's active ingredients, determine standard doses, and verify its effectiveness before medical experts can recommend this herb.

Selected references

Bunney, S., ed. *The Illustrated Book of Herbs. Their Medicinal and Culinary Uses*. London: Octopus Books Ltd., 1984.

Heinerman, J. *Heinerman's Encyclopedia of Healing Herbs & Spices*. Englewood Cliffs, N.J.: Prentice Hall, 1996.

Sweet flag

Sweet flag has been used for 2,000 years worldwide to treat certain health problems. Ayurvedic medicine uses the herb mostly for digestive disorders. Native Americans of the Cree tribe chewed the plant's roots during religious ceremonies for stimulant, euphoric, and hallucinogenic effects. They also used this plant as a painkiller and to treat diabetes. Western herbalists recommend sweet flag to quiet intestinal spasms. Because sweet flag has hallucinogenic potential, it has the potential for abuse.

Sweet flag comes from the dried rhizome (underground stem) and roots of *Acorus calamus*. A member of the Araceae family, this plant probably originated in India but now grows in most parts of the world in wet soil or shallow water.

Common doses

Sweet flag comes as dried rhizome powder, liquid extract, and tincture. Some experts recommend the following doses:

- As *dried powder,* 1 to 3 grams taken orally three times daily.
- As a *liquid extract,* 1 to 3 milliliters taken orally three times daily.
- As a *tincture,* 2 to 4 milliliters taken orally three times daily.

Side effects

Call your health care practitioner if you experience any of these possible side effects of sweet flag:

- confusion
- disorientation
- hallucinations
- nausea
- vomiting.

Why people use this herb

- Digestive problems
- Pain
- To help control diabetes
- To induce hallucinations and euphoria

This herb also can cause genetic mutations.

Interactions

Combining herbs with certain drugs may alter their action or produce unwanted side effects. Tell your health care practitioner about any prescription or nonprescription drugs you're taking, especially drugs that change your mental function or stimulate your central nervous system (causing such symptoms as nervousness or irritation).

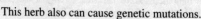

Don't use sweet flag while taking:
- Antabuse
- drugs that slow the central nervous system, such as alcohol, cold and allergy drugs, sedatives, tranquilizers, narcotic pain relievers, barbiturates, seizure drugs, or muscle relaxants.

Important points to remember

- Don't take sweet flag if you're pregnant.
- Tell your health care practitioner if you plan to get pregnant or suspect you're pregnant.
- Don't use this herb if you've been diagnosed with a psychiatric disorder.
- Use sweet flag cautiously, if at all, if you have liver problems.
- Don't drive or perform other dangerous activities until you know how sweet flag affects you.
- Report unpleasant mental or nervous side effects to your health care practitioner.
- If you take Antabuse, don't take a form of sweet flag that contains alcohol.
- Know that sweet flag components called asarones have caused liver cancer in animals.

Other names for sweet flag

Other names for sweet flag include bee wort, calamus, rat root, sweet myrtle, sweet root, and sweet sedge.

No known products containing sweet flag are available commercially.

Selected references

Hasheninejad, G., and Caldwell, J. "Genotoxicity of the Alkylbenzenes Alpha- and Beta-Asarone, Myristin and Elmicin as Determined by the UDS Assay in Cultured Rat Hepatocytes," *Food and Chemical Toxicology* 32:223-31, 1994.

Sugimoto, N., et al. "Mobility Inhibition and Nematocidal Activity of Asarone and Related Phenylpropanoids on Second-Stage Larvae of *Toxocara canis,*" *Biological and Pharmaceutical Bulletin* 18:605-09, 1995.

WHAT THE RESEARCH SHOWS

In the United States, sweet flag has been banned as a food additive and supplement because it can cause genetic mutations.

Sweet violet

Herbalists use the roots, seeds, flowers, stems, and leaves of sweet violet *(Viola odorata)* to treat certain disorders. *V. tricolor*, a closely related species known as wild pansy, has been used to treat eczema and several other skin conditions. Some perfumes contain extracts of the plant's leaves and flowers.

Why people use this herb

- Constipation
- Cough
- Inflammation
- Nervousness
- To induce vomiting

Common dose

Sweet violet comes as dried and fresh flowers, leaves, and stems. Experts disagree on what dose to take.

Side effects

Call your health care practitioner if you experience unusual symptoms while taking sweet violet, especially frequent, loose bowel movements.

Interactions

Combining herbs with certain drugs may alter their action or produce unwanted side effects. Tell your health care practitioner about any prescription or nonprescription drugs you're taking, especially laxatives.

Important points to remember

- Don't use sweet violet if you're pregnant or breast-feeding.
- Be aware that researchers know little about this herb's effectiveness.

Other names for sweet violet

Other names for sweet violet include English violet, flor de prosepina, viola, *Viola suavis*, violeta, *Violeta cheirosa*, and *Violeta comun*.

WHAT THE RESEARCH SHOWS

Researchers have little data on sweet violet, although animal studies suggest leaf extracts may reduce fever as effectively as aspirin. Nonetheless, medical experts can't recommend this herb until they see more study results.

No known products containing sweet violet are available commercially.

Selected reference

Khattak, S.G., et al. "Antipyretic Studies on Some Indigenous Pakistani Medicinal Plants," *Journal of Ethnopharmacology* 14:45-51, 1985.

Tansy

The ancient Greeks used tansy *(Tanacetum vulgare)* as an embalming preservative. The Micmac and Malecite Indians of eastern Canada used it as a diuretic and to induce abortions. Now tansy serves mainly as a food flavoring.

A member of the Compositae family, tansy is a common perennial weed with flat clusters of button-sized, yellow flowers. Active compounds come from the dried leaves and flowering tops.

Common dose

Tansy comes as essential oil, fluid extract, and tea. Experts disagree on what dose to take because the plants and preparations made from them vary greatly in the amount of active compounds they contain.

Side effects

Call your health care practitioner if you experience these possible side effects of tansy:

- nasal allergy
- personality changes
- skin inflammation
- sneezing.

Long-term tansy use can cause kidney damage. Thujone, a toxic compound in tansy, may cause poisoning. People have died from ingesting just 10 drops of tansy oil. Symptoms of tansy poisoning include a fast, weak pulse; seizures; severe gastritis (inflammation of the stomach lining); and violent muscle spasms.

Why people use this herb

- Bruises
- Diarrhea
- Fever
- Headache
- Inflammation
- Muscle spasms
- Pinworms, tapeworms, and other worm infections
- Sore throat
- Swelling
- To stimulate menstruation

Interactions

Combining herbs with certain drugs may alter their action or produce unwanted side effects. Tell your health care practitioner about any prescription or nonprescription drugs you're taking.

Important points to remember

- Don't use tansy if you're pregnant or breast-feeding.
- If you suspect you're pregnant or plan to become pregnant, tell your health care practitioner right away.

- Don't take this herb if you're allergic to it or its components.
- Know that tansy preparations may contain toxic amounts of thujone, which can be fatal.
- Don't confuse tansy with plants of similar names, such as tansy ragwort *(Senecio jacobaea)*.

WHAT THE RESEARCH SHOWS

Scientific studies don't support medicinal tansy use. The herb's main role in folk medicine is to repel insects and to expel worms from the digestive tract. However, safer and more effective products are available for these uses. What's more, tansy may contain toxic compounds and cause skin rashes in some people.

Other names for tansy

Other names for tansy include bitter buttons, golden buttons, and yellow buttons.

Products containing tansy are sold under such names as Tansy Extract and Tansy Oil.

Selected references

Chandler, R.F., et al. "Herbal Remedies of the Maritime Indians: Sterols and Triterpenes of *Tanacetum vulgare* L. (Tansy)," *Lipids* 17:102-106, 1982.

Guin, J.D., and Skidmore, G. "Compositae Dermatitis in Childhood," *Archives of Dermatology* 123:500-02, 1987.

Paulsen, E., et al. "Compositae Dermatitis in a Danish Dermatology Department in One Year," *Contact Dermatitis* 29:6-10, 1993.

Tea tree

Tea tree (melaleuca) oil is an essential oil distilled from the leaves and branches of *Melaleuca alternifolia.* A member of the myrtle family (Myrtaceae), this tree is native to Australia. Australian aborigines have long used melaleuca extracts for burns, cuts, insect bites, and other skin problems. Scientists are studying melaleuca as a possible treatment for various bacterial and fungal infections.

Common doses

Tea tree comes as creams, ointments, lotions, and soaps. It's also found in cosmetics, toiletries, and other household products. Concentrations of melaleuca oil in these products range from less than 1% to 100%. Depending on the type of product and the nature and location of the skin disorder, some experts recommend applying the oil locally in concentrations of 0.4% to 100%.

Why people use this herb

- Acne
- As an antiseptic
- Bacterial and fungal infections of the skin and mouth tissues
- Bladder inflammation
- Boils
- Eczema (a type of skin inflammation)
- Lice
- Psoriasis (scaly, raised skin patches)
- Vaginal infections
- Wounds

Side effects

Call your health care practitioner if you experience any of these possible side effects of tea tree:

- central nervous system depression, such as excessive drowsiness, sleepiness, and inability to coordinate muscles
- diarrhea
- skin irritation (in sensitive people)
- vomiting.

Tea tree also can irritate the mouth and digestive tract.

Interactions

Combining herbs with certain drugs may alter their action or produce unwanted side effects. Tell your health care practitioner about any prescription or nonprescription drugs you're taking.

Important points to remember

- Don't use tea tree preparations if you're pregnant or breast-feeding.
- Avoid tea tree if you've experienced an allergy to any of its components.

- Be aware that many commercially available products contain tea tree oil and that concentration of the oil varies greatly.
- Avoid taking tea tree products internally. Even small amounts of the oil taken internally may cause drowsiness and muscle incoordination.
- Keep tea tree products away from small children.

WHAT THE RESEARCH SHOWS

Scientists believe tea tree oil has some value in treating acne and psoriasis (scaly, raised skin patches). It may also help combat certain antibiotic-resistant bacterial skin infections. More research is needed to determine if tea tree is effective against other skin problems or vaginal infections.

Other names for tea tree

Other names for tea tree include Australian tea tree oil, *Melaleuca alternifolia,* melaleuca oil, and tea tree oil.

Products containing tea tree oil include Jason Winter's Tea Tree Oil, Swanson Ultra Tea Tree Oil, and Thursday Plantation Tea Tree Oil.

Selected references

Bassett, I.B., et al. "A Comparative Study of Tea-Tree Oil Versus Benzoylperoxide in the Treatment of Acne," *Medical Journal of Australia* 153:455-58, 1990.

Jacobs, M.R., et al. "Melaleuca Oil Poisoning," *Clinical Toxicology* 32:4:461-64, 1994.

Nelson, R.R.S. "In-Vitro Activities of Five Plant Essential Oils Against Methicillin-Resistant *Staphylcoccus aureus* and Vancomycin-Resistant *Enterococcus faecium,*" *Journal of Antimicrobial Chemotherapy* 40:305-06, 1997.

Nenoff, P., et al. "Antifungal Activity of the Essential Oil of *Melaleuca alternifolia* (Tea Tree Oil) Against Pathogenic Fungi In Vivo," *Skin Pharmacology* 9:388-94, 1996.

Thuja

Some people believe thuja tree extracts may be a cancer remedy. Active components of thuja come from the needles and young twigs of the white cedar, *Thuja occidentalis*. This common, cone-bearing evergreen is native to eastern North America.

Common doses

Thuja comes as liquid extract and tincture. Some experts recommend the following doses:

- As an *infusion*, place 1 teaspoon of dried herb in 1 cup of boiling water. Let stand 10 to 15 minutes and take orally three times daily.
- As a *tincture*, 1 to 2 milliliters taken orally three times daily.

Side effects

Call your health care practitioner if you experience any of these possible side effects of thuja:

- asthma
- digestive upset
- excitability
- intestinal gas
- seizures
- stomach irritation.

Thuja also can stimulate the uterus, possibly leading to miscarriage.

Why people use this herb

- AIDS
- As an antiseptic
- Cancer
- Fluid retention
- To help expel mucus from the lungs

Interactions

Combining herbs with certain drugs may alter their action or produce unwanted side effects. Tell your health care practitioner about any prescription or nonprescription drugs you're taking, especially caffeine or other stimulants.

Don't use thuja if you take drugs to treat seizures.

Important points to remember

- Don't use thuja if you're pregnant—it may cause miscarriage.
- Avoid thuja if you're breastfeeding.
- Be aware that thuja may increase the risk of seizures if taken with a drug used to control seizures.

- Don't use thuja if you have ulcers or gastritis (irritation of the stomach lining).

Other names for thuja

Other names for thuja include Eastern white cedar, false white cedar, hackmatack, tree-of-life, and yellow cedar.

No known products containing thuja are available commercially.

WHAT THE RESEARCH SHOWS

Scientific evidence doesn't back up medicinal claims for thuja. More studies must be done to evaluate the herb's effects in people with cancer and AIDS. As for thuja's traditional uses as a diuretic and an expectorant, medical experts point out that safer alternatives are available.

Selected references

Cartier, A., et al. "Occupational Asthma Caused by Eastern White Cedar *(Thuja occidentalis)* with Demonstration that Plicatic Acid is Present in this Wood Dust and is the Causal Agent," *Journal of Allergy and Clinical Immunology* 77: 639-45, 1986.

Elsasser-Beile, U., et al. "Cytokine Production in Leukocyte Cultures During Therapy with *Echinacea* Extract," *Journal of Clinical Laboratory Analysis* 10: 441-45, 1996.

Offergeld, R., et al. "Mitogenic Activity of High Molecular Polysaccharide Fractions Isolated from the Cuppressaceae *Thuja occidentalis* L. Enhanced Cytokine-Production by Thyapolysaccharide, G-Fraction (TPSg)," *Leukemia* 6(Suppl 3):189S-91S, 1992.

Vomel, T. "Effect of a Plant Immunostimulant on Phagocytosis of Erythrocytes by the Reticulohistiocytary System of Isolated Perfused Rat Liver," *Arzneimittel-Forschung* 35:1437-39, 1985.

Thyme

People have used thyme to treat various diseases for centuries. The herb is a common food flavoring and seasoning agent and is found in toothpastes and mouthwashes.

Active components (mainly thymol) come from the dried leaves and flowering tops of *Thymus vulgaris*, a member of the mint family (Labiatae). Native to Spain and Italy, the plant is widely cultivated worldwide.

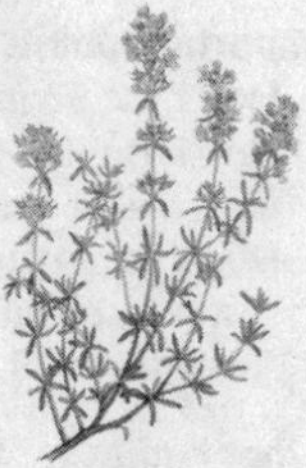

Common doses

Thyme comes as:

- extract (12% to 14%)
- ointment (1% to 2% thymol)
- tea
- essential oil.

Some experts recommend the following doses:

- As an *ointment*, apply topically for itchy skin as needed.
- As *cough syrup,* 1 teaspoon taken orally every 2 hours as needed.
- As an *essential oil,* 5 to 10 drops in water taken orally two or three times daily.
- As a *tea,* 1.5 to 2 grams of dried herb taken orally three times daily.

Why people use this herb

- Cough
- Fungal infections
- Headache
- Hysteria
- Indigestion
- Intestinal gas
- Painful menstruation
- To induce sweating
- Worm infections
- Wounds

Side effects

Call your health care practitioner if you experience any of these possible side effects of thyme:

- cracked, inflamed lips
- diarrhea
- dizziness
- headache
- muscle weakness
- nausea
- skin inflammation
- slow breathing

- slow pulse
- tongue irritation (from toothpaste)
- vomiting.

Thyme can cause allergic reactions when used as a flavoring agent. Symptoms include itching and swelling of the lips and tongue, difficulty swallowing or speaking, low blood pressure, nausea, vomiting, and shortness of breath.

Interactions

Combining herbs with certain drugs may alter their action or produce unwanted side effects. Tell your health care practitioner about any prescription or nonprescription drugs you're taking.

Important points to remember

- Don't use thyme if you're pregnant or breast-feeding.
- Don't use skin preparations containing thyme if you are allergic to grasses and other plants or have sensitive skin.
- Don't use thyme if you suffer from stomach irritation or other digestive problems.
- Avoid thyme if you have heart trouble.

Other names for thyme

Other names for thyme include common thyme, garden thyme, rubbed thyme, thymi herba, and timo.

Products containing thyme are sold under such names as Autussan "T," Olbas, Pertussin, and Pertussin N.

Selected references

Benito, M., et al. "Labiatae Allergy: Systemic Reactions Due to Ingestion of Oregano and Thyme," *Annals of Allergy, Asthma, and Immunology* 76:416-18, 1996.

Myers, H.B. "Thymol Therapy in Actinomycosis," *JAMA* 108:1875, 1937.

van Den Broucke, C.O., and Lemli, J.A. "Pharmacological and Chemical Investigation of Thyme Liquid Extracts," *Planta Medica* 41:129-35, 1981.

WHAT THE RESEARCH SHOWS

Although thyme preparations have been used for centuries to treat diseases, little scientific evidence supports these claims. Thymol, a thyme component, may hold promise as an antiseptic in dental products, but more studies are needed.

Tonka bean

Tonka bean is used mainly as a food flavoring and a scent (resembling vanilla) in pharmaceutical products. Some people regard it as an aphrodisiac or use it to prevent nausea and cramping.

Tonka's active component (coumarin) comes from the fruits and seeds of *Dipteryx odorata*. Native to Brazil and Venezuela, this tree belongs to the legume family (Leguminosae).

Why people use this herb

- As an aphrodisiac
- Lymphedema (a lymphatic disorder that causes arm or leg swelling)
- Nausea
- Stomach cramps

Common dose

Tonka bean isn't widely available commercially. Some experts recommend a dose of 60 milligrams (coumarin) taken orally once daily. (In some studies, doses were based on the product's coumarin content.)

Side effects

Call your health care practitioner if you experience unusual symptoms when using tonka bean. The herb may damage the liver.

Interactions

Combining herbs with certain drugs may alter their action or produce unwanted side effects. Especially if you're being treated for a liver problem, avoid tonka bean while taking:

- blood thinners, such as Coumadin
- drugs that can cause liver damage, such as some antibiotic, antiviral, antiseizure, and chemotherapy drugs.

Important points to remember

- Don't use tonka bean if you're pregnant or breast-feeding.
- Know that using tonka bean with a drug that may damage the liver increases the risk of such damage.
- Keep in mind that you may experience increased internal bleeding if you take tonka bean with a blood thinner.
- Be aware that the Food and Drug Administration considers this herb unsafe.

WHAT THE RESEARCH SHOWS

Several tonka bean components—especially coumarin and 7-hydroxycoumarin—show promise in treating certain lymphatic system disorders. However, more research must be done to establish if these components are safe and effective. For nausea and stomach cramps, medical experts recommend established remedies over tonka bean.

Other names for tonka bean

Other names for tonka bean include cumaru, tonka seed, tonquin bean, and torquin bean.

A product containing tonka bean is sold as Tonka Bean.

Selected references

Marshall, M.E., et al. "Growth-Inhibitory Effects of Coumarin (1,2-Benzopyrone) and 7-Hydroxycoumarin on Human Malignant Cell Lines In Vitro," *Journal of Cancer Research and Clinical Oncology* 120(Suppl):S3-S10, 1994.

Overvik, E., et al. "Activation and Effects of the Food-Derived Heterocyclic Amines in Extrahepatic Tissues," *Princess Takamatsu Symposia* 23:123-33, 1995.

Vettorello, S., et al. "Contribution of a Combination of Alpha and Beta Benzpyrones, Flavonoids and Natural Terpenes in the Treatment of Lymphedema of the Lower Limbs at the 2d Stage of Surgical Classification," *Minerva Cardioangiologica* 44:447-55, 1996.

Tormentil

In ancient Athens, Hippocrates used tormentil to treat malaria. Nicholas Culpeper, the 17th-century British herbalist, recommended packing tormentil root into a painful tooth. Before the discovery of dental plaque, the herb was used to dry up the "flux of humors" thought to cause toothaches. Today, some people use tormentil to treat inflammation and diarrhea.

Active components come mainly from the rootstock of *Potentilla tormentilla*. A perennial in the rose family (Rosaceae), the plant is native to Europe and Asia.

Why people use this herb

- Burns
- Diarrhea
- Mouth and throat inflammation
- Skin rashes
- Sunburn
- Wounds

Common doses

Tormentil comes as rootstock, tincture, and powder. Some experts recommend the following doses:

- As a *powder*, ¼ to ½ teaspoon taken orally three times daily.
- As a *tea*, place 1 tablespoon of rootstock in 1 cup of water, steep for 30 minutes, strain, and drink during the day in "mouthful" doses.
- As a *tincture*, 20 to 30 drops taken orally two or three times daily.
- As a *gargle*, boil 2 ounces of bruised rootstock in 50 ounces of water until it's reduced by one third. Strain the cooled liquid and use as gargle.
- For *diarrhea*, mix 1 ounce each of powdered tormentil, powdered galangal, and powdered marshmallow root with 240 grains of powdered ginger and 1 pint of boiling water. Strain the mixture, and take 5 to 10 milliliters (3 teaspoons) orally two or three times daily for no more than 4 days.

Side effects

Call your health care practitioner if you experience unusual symptoms when taking tormentil. Using large amounts of this herb may cause:

- abdominal pain
- nausea
- constipation (with possible fecal impaction)
- gastroenteritis symptoms (nausea, vomiting, abdominal discomfort, and diarrhea)
- vomiting.

Tormentil also can cause liver damage.

Interactions

Combining herbs with certain drugs may alter their action or produce unwanted side effects. Don't use tormentil while taking:

- alkaloids such as Quinaglute Dura-tabs or ephedrine
- Antabuse
- digitalis drugs used to treat heart failure or certain irregular heartbeats.

Important points to remember

- Don't use tormentil if you're pregnant or breast-feeding.
- If you're taking Antabuse, avoid tormentil tincture that contains alcohol because you may experience a reaction.

WHAT THE RESEARCH SHOWS

Some preliminary studies hint that tormentil may stimulate the immune system, but little scientific evidence supports any therapeutic claims for this herb. Because researchers know little about its toxic effects, medical experts caution against using it. They emphasize that you can find safer and more effective remedies for treating diarrhea and skin problems.

Other names for tormentil

Other names for tormentil include biscuits, bloodroot, earthbank, English sarsaparilla, ewe daisy, five-fingers, flesh and blood, septfoil, seven leaves, shepherd's knapperty, shepherd's knot, and thormantle.

No known products containing tormentil are available commercially.

Selected references

Bos, M.A., et al. "Procyanidins from Tormentil: Antioxidant Properties Towards Lipoeroxidation and Anti-Elastase Activity," *Biological and Pharmaceutical Bulletin* 19:146-48, 1996.

Carr, A., et al. *Encyclopedia of Herbs.* Emmaus, Pa.: Rodale Press, 1987.

Grieve, M. *A Modern Herbal.* London: Tiger Books International, 1997.

Stodola, J. *The Illustrated Book of Herbs*. London: Octopus Books Ltd., 1984.

Tragacanth

Tragacanth gets its name from the Greek words *tragos* (goat) and *akantha* (horn)—probably because the dried plant sap is curved or twisted. African folk medicine regards tragacanth as a mild laxative and uses its leaves to prepare a first-aid lotion. The pharmaceutical industry once added the herb to pills and suspensions as a binding agent. Some bookbinders still use tragacanth as a glue and cloth stiffener.

Now you can find tragacanth in some foods, candies, toothpastes, and dental adhesives. The Food and Drug Administration (FDA) lists tragacanth as a generally safe food additive.

Tragacanth is obtained by drying the gummy sap that oozes from the cut tap root and branches of *Astragalus gummifer* or other *Astragalus* species. These low thorny shrubs, members of the legume family (Leguminosae), are native to the Middle East.

Why people use this herb

- As a skin lubricant
- Constipation

Common dose

Tragancath comes as a gum, gel, syrup, tablets, and powder. The FDA allows concentrations of 0.2% and 1.3% as a thickener, stabilizer, and flavoring agent in foods. As a *laxative*, some experts recommend the following dose:

- As *tablets*, 0.42 to 100 milligrams taken orally two or three times daily.

Side effects

Call your health care practitioner if you experience any of these possible side effects of tragacanth:

- allergic reactions, such as skin rash, itching, hives, abdominal pain, swelling of the face and throat, difficulty breathing, asthma, sneezing, joint pain, or fever
- skin inflammation (with topical gel).

Interactions

Combining herbs with certain drugs may alter their action or produce unwanted side effects. Don't use tragacanth while taking fat-soluble nutrients, such as vitamin A, D, E, or K.

Important points to remember

- Avoid this herb if you're pregnant or breast-feeding.
- Don't use tragacanth if you're allergic to any natural gum used in food or pharmaceutical products.
- Know that tragacanth gum may be contaminated by coliform or *Salmonella* bacteria, which may cause infection.

WHAT THE RESEARCH SHOWS

Tragacanth is safe for use in foods and other products, and no one has reported side effects in nonallergic persons. Although medical experts say the herb may be used as a mild bulk-forming laxative, they point out that safe, effective alternatives are available.

Other names for tragacanth

Other names for tragacanth include adrilel, E413, gum dragon, goma alatira, gum tragacanth, hog gum, shagal el ketira, Syrian tragacanth, and tragacanth tree.

Products containing tragacanth are sold as Tragacanth and Gum Tragacanth.

Selected references

Eastwood, M.A., et al. "The Effects of Dietary Gum Tragacanth in Man," *Toxicology Letters* 21:73-81, 1984.

Iwu, M.M. *Handbook of African Medicinal Plants.* Boca Raton, Fla.: CRC Press, 1993.

Smolinske, S.C. *Handbook of Food, Drug, and Cosmetic Excipients.* Boca Raton, Fla.: CRC Press, 1992.

True unicorn root

Native Americans once used true unicorn root *(Aletris farinosa)* to stimulate digestion and induce menstruation. A member of the lily family (Liliaceae), this perennial herb is native to the eastern United States. Active components come from the roots and rhizomes (underground stems).

Why people use this herb

- Diarrhea
- Fluid retention
- Intestinal gas
- Menstrual problems
- Rheumatism
- Sharp intestinal pains
- Snakebite
- To induce vomiting
- To prevent habitual miscarriage
- To promote sleep
- To relieve spasms or convulsions

Common dose

True unicorn root comes as a liquid or tea. Experts disagree on what dose to take.

Side effects

Call your health care practitioner if you experience any of these possible side effects of true unicorn root:

- difficulty keeping your balance
- stupor.

Large doses can cause:

- diarrhea
- nausea
- vomiting.

Interactions

Combining herbs with certain drugs may alter their action or produce unwanted side effects. Don't use true unicorn root while using alcohol or other drugs that slow the nervous system, such as:

- barbiturates
- cold and allergy drugs
- muscle relaxants
- narcotic pain relievers
- sedatives
- seizure drugs
- tranquilizers.

Important points to remember

- Don't use true unicorn root if you're pregnant or breast-feeding.
- Avoid this herb if you have stomach or intestinal disorders.
- Don't drive or perform other dangerous activities until you know how true unicorn root affects you.

- Don't confuse true unicorn root with false unicorn root *(Chamaelirium luteum)*, which differs in chemical composition and purported uses. (See page 203, "False unicorn root.")

WHAT THE RESEARCH SHOWS

Researchers know little about the chemical components of true unicorn root. However, small doses have caused side effects. All in all, no medical evidence supports using this herb.

Other names for true unicorn root

Other names for true unicorn root include ague grass, ague root, aloe root, colic root, crow corn, devil's-bit, star grass, unicorn root, and whitetube stargrass.

Products containing true unicorn root are sold as Aletris-Heel and True Unicorn Root.

Selected references

Duke, J.A., ed. *Handbook of Medicinal Herbs.* Boca Raton, Fla.: CRC Press, 1985.

Horn, V., and Weil, C., eds. *The Encyclopedia of Medicinal Plants.* New York: DK Publishing Inc., 1996.

Lewis, W.H. *Medical Botany: Plants Affecting Man's Health.* New York: John Wiley and Sons, 1977.

Turmeric

Turmeric has a long and varied history in traditional Chinese medicine and Indian (Ayurvedic) medicine. More recently, the herb has shown promise in treating certain types of cancer. The food industry uses this bright yellow herb to color butter, margarine, cheese, curry powder, mustard, and other products. Its main active ingredient, curcumin, is an antioxidant that retards food spoilage.

Active turmeric components come from the rhizome (underground stem) of *Curcuma longa,* a perennial of the ginger family (Zingiberaceae). Turmeric is harvested commercially in India, China, Indonesia, and other tropical countries.

Why people use this herb

- Atherosclerosis (plaque buildup in the arteries)
- Bacterial infections
- Bloody urine
- Bruises
- Chest pain
- Gallstones
- Gastritis (inflammation of the stomach lining)
- Hemorrhage
- Intestinal gas
- Irritable bowel syndrome
- Jaundice
- Liver disorders
- Local pain and inflammation
- Menstrual problems
- Osteoarthritis
- Parasite infestations
- Rheumatoid arthritis
- Sharp intestinal pains
- Toothache
- Ulcers
- Viral infections

Common doses

Turmeric comes as capsules, curry and turmeric spices, dried rhizome, extract, oil, and tincture. You should take it on an empty stomach. Some experts recommend the following doses:

- As the *active component* (curcumin), 400 to 600 milligrams taken orally three times a day.
- As *turmeric*, a dose equivalent to 8 to 60 grams taken orally three times daily.

Side effects

Call your health care practitioner if you experience allergic skin inflammation when using turmeric. High doses or prolonged use of turmeric can cause stomach ulcers.

Interactions

Combining herbs with certain drugs may alter their action or produce unwanted side effects. Don't use turmeric while taking:

- blood thinners such as Coumadin
- drugs that suppress the immune system, such as Imuran or Sandimmune
- nonsteroidal anti-inflammatory drugs such as Advil.

Important points to remember

- Don't use turmeric if you're pregnant or breast-feeding because it may cause miscarriage. (The American Herbal Products Association classifies turmeric as a menstrual stimulant.)
- Avoid this herb if you have a bleeding disorder, bile duct obstruction, or a stomach ulcer.
- Report unusual bleeding or bruising to your health care practitioner.
- Keep turmeric preparations away from children and pets.

WHAT THE RESEARCH SHOWS

According to the American Institute for Cancer Research, curcumin (turmeric's active component) helps prevent certain cancers of the stomach, colon, mouth and throat, breast, and skin. The herb also shows anti-inflammatory potential: It seems to be as effective as such nonsteroidal anti-inflammatory drugs as Advil while causing fewer side effects. However, medical experts believe more research is needed to define the herb's specific role in treating medical conditions.

Other names for turmeric

Other names for turmeric include *curcuma,* Indian saffron, Indian valerian, jiang huang, radix, red valerian, and tumeric.

A medicinal product containing turmeric is sold as Turmeric Root.

Selected references

Broadhurst, L. "Curcumin, A Powerful Bioprotectant Spice, or…Curry Cures!" Botanical Medicine Conference. Philadelphia: May 15, 1997.

Hastak, K., et al. "Effect of Turmeric Oil and Turmeric Oleoresin on Cytogenic Damage in Patients Suffering from Oral Submucous Fibrosis," *Cancer Letters* 116:265-69, 1997.

Kiso, Y., et al. "Antihepatotoxic Principles of *Curcuma longa* Rhizome," *Planta Medica* 49:185-87, 1983.

Selvam, R., et al. "The Anti-oxidant Activity of Turmeric *(Curcuma longa),*" *Journal of Ethnobotany* 47:59-67, 1995.

Valerian

In Europe, valerian is used widely as a sedative and a treatment for muscle spasms. Active components come from the rhizomes (underground stems) and roots of *Valeriana officinalis,* a perennial that's native to Eurasia and naturalized worldwide.

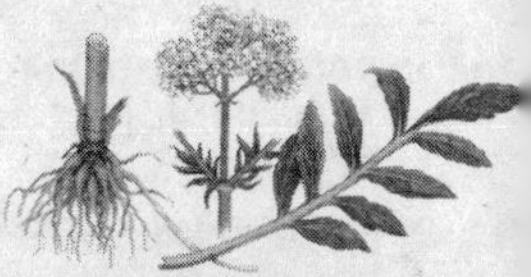

Why people use this herb

- Muscle spasms
- Restlessness
- Sleep disorders
- Tension

Common doses

Valerian comes as:

- standardized capsules (250, 400, 450, 493, 530, and 550 milligrams)
- tablets (0.8% valerenic acid; 250, 400, 450, 493, 530, and 550 milligrams)
- standardized tincture containing 2% essential oil
- teas containing crude dried herb.

Valerian also is available in combination with other dietary supplements. The composition and purity of valerian preparations vary greatly.

Some experts recommend the following doses for sleep disorders:

- As *capsules* or *tablets,* 400 to 900 milligrams of standardized valerian extract taken orally 30 minutes to 1 hour before bedtime.
- As a *tea,* 2 to 3 grams (1 teaspoon) of crude dried herb taken orally several times daily.
- As a *tincture*, 3 to 5 milliliters (½ to 1 teaspoon) taken orally several times daily.

Side effects

Call your health care practitioner if you experience unusual symptoms when using valerian. Chronic use or acute overdose may cause:

- allergic reactions
- blurred vision
- excitability
- headache
- insomnia
- irregular heartbeats
- nausea.

Combination products containing valerian and overdoses of 2.5 grams may result in liver damage.

Interactions

Combining herbs with certain drugs may alter their action or produce unwanted side effects. Don't use valerian while taking:

- alcohol or other drugs that depress the central nervous system
- Antabuse.

Important points to remember

- Avoid this herb if you're pregnant or breast-feeding.
- Don't take valerian if you've experienced an allergy to valerian preparations.
- If you're taking Antabuse, don't take a valerian tincture that contains alcohol because you may experience a reaction. (Many extract products contain 40% to 60% alcohol.)
- Don't use valerian if you have a liver disease.
- Don't drive or perform other dangerous activities until you know how valerian affects you.
- Be aware that valerian's safety and effectiveness in children are unknown.

Other names for valerian

Other names for valerian include all heal, amantilla, baldrianwurzel, great wild valerian, herba benedicta, katzenwurzel, phu germanicum, phu parvum, *Pinnis dentatis,* setewale, capon's tail, setwell, theriacaria, valeriana, *Valeriana foliis pinatus,* and *Valeriana radix.*

Products containing valerian are sold as Valerian Extract, Valerian Root, and Valerian Root Extract.

WHAT THE RESEARCH SHOWS

A few small studies have shown that valerian can induce sleepiness. The German Commission E (similar to the U.S. Food and Drug Administration) recommends valerian for restlessness and nervous sleep disturbances. However, American medical experts believe more research is needed to define the herb's role in treating sleep disorders. They also point out that other sleep aids with no liver-damaging potential are available.

Selected references

Chan, T.Y.K., et al. "Poisoning Due To an Over-The-Counter Hypnotic, Sleep-Qik (Hyoscine, Cyprohepatadine, Valerian)," *Post Graduate Medical Journal* 71:227-28, 1995.

Petkov, V. "Plants with Hypotensive Antiatheromatous and Coronarodilating Action," *American Journal of Chinese Medicine* 7:197-236, 1979.

Schulz, V., et al. *Rational Phytotherapy: A Physicians' Guide to Herbal Medicine,* 3rd ed. New York: Springer Publishing Co., 1998.

Shepard, C. "Sleep Disorders. Liver Damage Warning with Insomnia Remedy," *BMJ* 306:1472, 1993.

Vervain

Vervain has been used as a folk remedy for a wide range of disorders, even though the Food and Drug Administration calls its safety "undefined." Active components come from the leaves and flowering heads of European vervain, *Verbena officinalis*, a member of the verbena family (Verbenaceae). Native to the Mediterranean area, the plant now grows throughout Europe, Asia, and North America. A related species, American vervain, *V. hastata*, also is used medicinally.

Why people use this herb

- As an aphrodisiac
- Bronchitis
- Common cold
- Cramps
- Difficult or painful urination
- Fluid retention
- Eye diseases
- Fever
- Hemorrhoids
- Inflammation of the lung cavity
- Insomnia
- Itchy skin
- Kidney stones
- Muscle spasms
- Pain along nerve trunks
- Parasite infestations
- Red blood cell deficiency
- Rheumatism
- Swelling
- To cause sweating
- To help expel mucus from the lungs
- To induce vomiting
- To relieve pain
- Tumors
- Ulcers
- Uterine disorders
- Whooping cough

Common doses

Vervain comes as capsules (350 milligrams). Some experts recommend the following doses:

- As *capsules*, 360 milligrams (1 capsule) orally as a sedative at bedtime.
- As a *purgative* and for *bowel pain*, a decoction of 2 ounces to 1 quart taken orally once daily.

Side effects

Call your health care practitioner if you experience skin inflammation when using vervain. Large doses may paralyze the central nervous system and cause stupor and seizures.

Interactions

Combining herbs with certain drugs may alter their action or produce unwanted side effects. Don't use vervain while taking blood thinners such as Coumadin.

Important points to remember

- Don't take vervain if you have asthma or have experienced an allergy to vervain preparations.
- Avoid this herb if you have a seizure disorder because it may induce seizures.

- Be aware that, although vervain has been used in folk medicine to slow blood clotting, people who take a blood thinner should avoid the herb.

Other names for vervain

Other names for vervain include American vervain, blue vervain, enchanter's herb, European vervain, herba veneris, herbe sacrée, herb of the cross, holy herb, pigeon grass, purvain, simpler's joy, and wild hyssop.

A product containing vervain is sold as Blue Vervain.

WHAT THE RESEARCH SHOWS

Scientific evidence doesn't support vervain's many traditional uses. One study of vervain in treating kidney stones concluded that more effective drug treatments are available.

Selected references

Almeida, C.E., et al. "Analysis of Antidiarrheic Effects of Plants Used in Popular Medicine," *Revista De Saude Publica* 29:428-33, 1995.

Auf'Mkolk, M., et al. "Inhibition by Certain Plant Extracts of the Binding and Adenylate Cyclase Stimulatory Effect of Bovine Thyrotropin in Human Thyroid Membranes," *Endocrinology* 115:527-34, 1984.

Grases, F., et al. "Urolithiasis and Phytotherapy," *International Urology and Nephrology* 26:507-11, 1994.

Wahoo

The active components of wahoo, such as euonymin, come from the dried root bark and sometimes the stem of *Euonymus atropupureus*. This shrub or tree is native to the central eastern parts of the United States and Canada. Researchers have studied the bark of a related species, *E. sieboldianus*, as a possible cancer treatment.

Why people use this herb

- Fever
- Fluid retention
- Head lice
- Indigestion
- To cause a productive cough
- To induce vomiting
- To stimulate menstruation
- To stimulate the liver

Common doses

Wahoo comes as tablets, extracts, tinctures, dried powders, syrups, and teas. Some experts recommend the following doses:

- As *dried root,* 1 ounce added to 1 pint of water, simmered slowly. Drink 1 cup two or three times daily.
- As *euonymin extract*, 1 to 4 grains.

Side effects

Call your health care practitioner if you experience any of these possible side effects of wahoo:

- chills
- diarrhea
- fainting
- seizures
- vomiting
- weakness.

Interactions

Combining herbs with certain drugs may alter their action or produce unwanted side effects. If you're taking wahoo, tell your health care practitioner about any prescription or nonprescription drugs you're taking.

Important points to remember

- Don't use wahoo if you're pregnant or breast-feeding.
- Be aware that this herb may be poisonous.

WHAT THE RESEARCH SHOWS

Although wahoo has been used to treat various internal and external conditions, little evidence supports these claims. What's more, taking large amounts of the herb may be hazardous, so medical experts don't recommend it. However, one wahoo species may help fight cancer, which of course merits further investigation.

Other names for wahoo

Other names for wahoo include arrowwood, bitter ash, bleeding heart, burning-bush, bursting heart, fish-wood, Indian arrowwood, pegwood, prickwood, skewerwood, spindletree, strawberry bush, and strawberry tree.

Products containing wahoo are sold as GB Tablets, Indigestion Mixture, Jecopeptol, Ludoxin, Stago, and Stomachiagil.

Selected references

Baek, N.I., et al. "Euonymoside: A New Cytotoxic Cardenolide Glycoside from the Bark of *Euonymus sieboldianus,*" *Planta Medica* 60:26-29, 1994.

Grieve, M. *A Modern Herbal*. London: Tiger Books International, 1997.

Watercress

Researchers are studying certain watercress compounds as possible cancer treatments. A popular salad green, this herb comes from *Nasturtium officinale*. All parts of the plant, which grows in running water, have been used medicinally. Because it contains vitamin C, it was once used to prevent scurvy.

Why people use this herb

- Acne
- Eczema (a type of skin inflammation)
- Inflammation
- Rashes
- Scurvy
- Skin infections

The plant belongs to the mustard family (Cruciferae or Brassicaceae). Native to Europe, it's naturalized as a weed in the United States.

Common dose

Watercress is available as the whole plant, a tea, and juice expressed from the leaves. Some experts recommend the following dose:

- As *fluid extract* (juice), 2 ounces taken orally three times daily.

Side effects

Call your health care practitioner if you experience unusual symptoms while using watercress, especially as a salad green. Several reports of liver infection by a parasitic worm have been reported in people who ate the wild plant.

Interactions

Combining herbs with certain drugs may alter their action or produce unwanted side effects. Don't use watercress while taking a nonsteroidal anti-inflammatory drug, such as Advil.

Important points to remember

- Don't use watercress if you're pregnant or breast-feeding.
- If you collect wild watercress, wash it carefully before using because it may contain water-borne parasites or pathogens.
- Be aware that drug interactions with watercress are largely unknown.
- Don't confuse watercress with the garden nasturtium or Indian cress *(Tropaeolum majus)*, a popular annual flower in a different plant family.

Other names for watercress

Other names for watercress include garden cress, scurvy grass, and wasserkresse.

No known medicinal products containing watercress are available commercially.

WHAT THE RESEARCH SHOWS

Many people eat watercress as a salad green, and few problems have been reported. This suggests that it's generally safe to consume—provided it's washed properly.

Although scientists believe certain watercress compounds may hold promise as cancer treatments, more research is needed. The herb has no apparent activity against existing tumors.

Selected references

Chen, L., et al. "Decrease of Plasma and Urinary Oxidative Metabolites of Acetaminophen after Consumption of Watercress by Human Volunteers," *Clinical Pharmacology and Therapeutics* 60:651-60, 1996.

Chung, F.L., et al. "Chemopreventative Potential of Thiol Conjugates of Isothiocyanates for Lung Cancer and a Urinary Biomarker of Dietary Isothiocyanates," *Journal of Cellular Biochemistry Supplement* 27:76-85, 1997.

Hecht, S.S., et al. "Effects of Watercress Consumption on Metabolism of a Tobacco-Specific Lung Carcinogen in Smokers," *Cancer Epidemiology, Biomarkers, and Prevention* 4:877-84, 1995.

Rivera, J.V., et al. "Radionuclide Imaging of the Liver in Human Fascioliasis," *Clinical Nuclear Medicine* 9:450-53, 1984.

Wild cherry

Active components of wild cherry come from the dried bark of *Prunus virginiana* or *P. serotina,* mid-sized trees found throughout the northern United States. The tree's fruits are edible, but the seeds and all other parts should be avoided because they contain poisonous compounds that turn into hydrogen cyanide (HCN) in the digestive tract.

Why people use this herb

- Cancer
- Common cold
- Cough
- Diarrhea
- Respiratory problems

Common dose

Wild cherry comes as:

- fluid extract (1 or 2 ounces)
- tea.

Some experts recommend the following dose:

- As *fluid extract,* 1 to 2 grams in 1 cup of boiling water taken orally twice daily.

Side effects

Call your health care practitioner if you experience any of these possible side effects of wild cherry, which may indicate cyanide poisoning:

- headache
- muscle weakness
- nausea
- spasms or tremors
- vomiting.

Wild cherry also can cause stomach ulcers, respiratory failure, stupor, coma, and death.

Wild cherry is considered toxic because all plant parts except the fruits contain HCN. Children have died from eating the seeds or leaves or from drinking tea made from the plant. Livestock have died from eating the leaves. Symptoms of HCN poisoning include difficulty breathing or speaking, twitching, spasms, stupor, and coma leading to death. In mild cases, symptoms include nausea, vomiting, headache, muscle weakness, and irregular heartbeats.

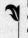

Interactions

Combining herbs with certain drugs may alter their action or produce unwanted side effects. If you're taking wild cherry, tell your health care practitioner about any prescription or nonprescription drugs you're taking.

Important points to remember

- Don't use wild cherry if you're pregnant or breast-feeding.
- Know that consuming wild cherry extracts can be dangerous and may cause death from cyanide poisoning. The fatal adult dose of HCN is 50 milligrams. (Fatal doses for plants containing cyanide can't be predicted.)
- Keep wild cherry plant parts out of children's reach.

WHAT THE RESEARCH SHOWS

Even though people use wild cherry for various conditions, the bark, seeds, and leaves can be poisonous. Little medical evidence exists to support medicinal claims for this herb.

Other names for wild cherry

Other names for wild cherry include black choke, chokecherry, and rum cherry.

Products containing wild cherry are sold as Wild Cherry Bark and Wild Cherry Bark Compound.

Selected references

Ellenhorn, M.J., ed. *Ellenhorn's Medical Toxicology: Diagnosis and Treatment of Human Poisoning*. Baltimore: Williams & Wilkins, 1997.

Selby, L.A., et al. "Outbreak of Swine Malformations Associated with the Wild Black Cherry, *Prunus serotina*," *Archives of Environmental Health* 22:496-501, 1971.

Williams, M.C., and James, L.F. "Effects of Herbicides on the Concentration of Poisonous Compounds in Plants: A Review," *American Journal of Veterinary Research* 44:2420-22, 1983.

Wild ginger

Essential oils in the wild ginger plant can kill certain bacteria and fungi. Dentists use one such oil, methyl eugenol, as a painkiller. Another oil, geraniol, inhibited growth of pancreatic cancer cells in tests on animals.

Active components of wild ginger come from the dried rhizome (underground stem) and roots of *Asarum canadense.* A low-growing perennial, this herb is native to the northern and central parts of the United States and southern Canada.

Common dose

Wild ginger comes as the whole root. Experts disagree on what dose to take.

Why people use this herb

- Angina (chest pain caused by heart problems)
- Intestinal gas
- Irregular heartbeats

Side effects

Call your health care practitioner if you experience any of these possible side effects of wild ginger:

- cracked, inflamed lips
- mouth inflammation
- skin inflammation.

Interactions

Combining herbs with certain drugs may alter their action or produce unwanted side effects. Tell your health care practitioner about any prescription or nonprescription drugs you're taking. Certain wild ginger components may impede the liver's ability to process other drugs.

Important points to remember

- Don't use wild ginger if you're pregnant or breast-feeding.
- Avoid this herb if you've experienced an allergic skin reaction to any of its volatile oils.

Other names for wild ginger

Other names for wild ginger include Canada snakeroot, colic root, false coltsfoot, Indian ginger, and Vermont snakeroot.

No known medicinal products containing wild ginger are available commercially.

WHAT THE RESEARCH SHOWS

Preliminary research findings on wild ginger warrant further study of some of its components in treating certain infections and cancer. But to date, little evidence supports medicinal claims.

Selected references

Burke, Y.D., et al. "Inhibition of Pancreatic Cancer Growth by the Dietary Isoprenoids Farnesol and Geraniol," *Lipids* 32:151-56, 1997.

Pattnaik, S., et al. "Antibacterial and Antifungal Activity of Aromatic Constituents of Essential Oils," *Microbios* 89:39-46, 1997.

Roffey, S.J., et al. "Hepatic Peroxisomal and Microsomal Enzyme Induction by Citral and Linalool in Rats," *Food and Chemical Toxicology* 28:403-08, 1990.

Wild indigo

Wild indigo *(Baptisia tinctoria)* serves mainly as an antiseptic in folk medicine. A few studies hint that it may have some action on the immune system. The herb sometimes is confused with true indigo, used for centuries as a dye plant.

A perennial that belongs to the legume family (Leguminosae), wild indigo is native to the central and eastern United States and Canada. Active components come from the leaves and dried roots, which may be toxic to livestock.

Why people use this herb

- As an antiseptic
- As a purgative
- Constipation
- Scarlet fever
- Typhus

Common dose

Wild indigo comes as a tincture. Some experts recommend the following dose:

- 10 to 20 drops taken orally three times daily.

Side effects

Call your health care practitioner if you experience unusual symptoms when using wild indigo. High doses may cause vomiting.

Interactions

Combining herbs with certain drugs may alter their action or produce unwanted side effects. Tell your health care practitioner about any prescription or nonprescription drugs you're taking.

Important points to remember

- Don't use wild indigo if you're pregnant or breast-feeding.
- Avoid wild indigo if you've experienced an allergy to any of the plant's components.
- Know that researchers suspect certain wild indigo components may be toxic, despite lack of reports of human poisonings.

Other names for wild indigo

Other names for wild indigo include false indigo, horse fly weed, indigo weed, *Podalyria tinctoria,* rattlebush, rattlesnake weed, *Sophora,* and yellow indigo.

A product containing wild indigo is sold as Wild Indigo.

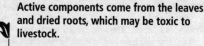

WHAT THE RESEARCH SHOWS

Clinical evidence doesn't bear out herbalists' reports that wild indigo aids in the treatment of scarlet fever or typhus. Although recent studies hint that the herb may affect the immune system, this finding must be investigated further.

Selected references

Beuscher, N., and Kopanski, L. "Stimulation of Immunity by the Contents of *Baptisia tinctoria,*" *Planta Medica* Oct(5):381-84, 1985.

Beuscher, N., et al. "Immunologically Active Glycoproteins of *Baptisia tinctoria,*" *Planta Medica* 55:358-63, 1989.

Egert, D., and Beuscher, N. "Studies on Antigen Specificity of Immunoreactive Arabinogalactan Proteins Extracted from *Baptisia tinctoria* and *Echinacea purpurea,*" *Planta Medica* 58:163-65, 1992.

Wagner, H., and Jurcic, K. "Immunologic Studies of Plant Combination Preparations. In-Vitro And In-Vivo Studies on the Stimulation of Phagocytosis," *Arzneimittel-Forschung* 41:1072-76, 1991.

Wild lettuce

Ancient Egyptians thought wild lettuce *(Lactuca virosa)* could induce sleep. According to some sources, a few *L. virosa* species contain tiny amounts of morphine—although too little to have a noticeable drug effect. Nonetheless, during the 1970s some people rolled the dried leaves of wild lettuce with tobacco or other additives into a cigarette and smoked it to achieve a sense of euphoria. Some herbalists take the stem juice directly from the plant and use it for various medicinal purposes.

Why people use this herb

- Cough
- To cause euphoria
- To induce sleep

Common doses

Wild lettuce comes as the dried latex (sap) from stems, dried leaves, lettuce leaf cigarettes, and tincture. Some experts recommend the following doses:

- As a *tea*, 0.5 to 3 grams taken orally three times daily.
- As *dried latex extract,* 0.3 to 1 gram taken orally twice daily.
- As *fluid extract* (1:1 in 25% alcohol), 0.5 to 30 milliliters taken orally three times daily.
- As a *tincture*, 2 to 4 milliliters taken orally three times daily.

Side effects

Call your health care practitioner if you experience unusual symptoms when using wild lettuce. This herb can cause skin inflammation.

Smoking large amounts of wild lettuce may cause stupor, shallow breathing, coma, and even death.

Interactions

Combining herbs with certain drugs may alter their action or produce unwanted side effects. Tell your health care practitioner about any prescription or nonprescription drugs you're taking.

Important points to remember

- Don't use wild lettuce if you're pregnant or breast-feeding.

- Avoid this herb if you've experienced an allergy to any plant in the lettuce family.
- Be aware that smoking wild lettuce leaves may produce hallucinogenic effects.
- Don't confuse wild lettuce with garden lettuce *(L. sativa).*

Other names for wild lettuce

Other names for wild lettuce include bitter lettuce, German lactucarium, and lettuce opium.

Products containing wild lettuce are sold as Lactucarium, Lettuce Hash, Lettucine, and Lopium.

WHAT THE RESEARCH SHOWS

Research doesn't validate claims that smoking wild lettuce leaves produces hallucinogenic effects. Some evidence suggests that the plant sap may fight fungal infections, but we need more research in this area.

Because we know little about the herb's potential toxicity, medical experts can't recommend it. As for its use as a sleep aid, experts stress that more effective products are available, both by prescription and over the counter.

Selected references

Huang, Z.J., et al. "Studies on Herbal Remedies I: Analysis of Herbal Smoking Preparations Alleged To Contain Lettuce (*Lactuca sativa* L.) and Other Natural Products," *Journal of Pharmaceutical Sciences* 71:270-71, 1982.

Krook, G. "Occupational Dermatitis from *Lactuca sativa* (Lettuce) and *Cichorium* (Endive): Simultaneous Occurrence of Immediate and Delayed Allergy as a Cause of Contact Dermatitis," *Contact Dermatitis* 3:27-36, 1977.

Roman-Ramos, R., et al. "Anti-hyperglycemic Effect of Some Edible Plants," *Journal of Ethnopharmacology* 48:25-32, 1995.

Wild yam

Wild yam *(Dioscorea villosa)* is a deciduous perennial vine that grows wild in the damp woodlands of North America and Central America. It has heart-shaped leaves and tiny green flowers, and commonly climbs to 20 feet.

Why people use this herb

- Adrenal gland malfunction
- Asthma
- Diverticulosis (pouchlike projections in the colon)
- Dysentery
- Gallstones
- Inflammatory rheumatism
- Intermittent claudication (severe calf muscle pain)
- Menopause symptoms
- Muscle spasms
- Pain in the uterus and ovaries
- Rheumatoid arthritis
- Stomach and muscle cramps
- To induce sweating

This herb once was the only source of raw manufacturing materials for contraceptive hormones, cortisone, and certain other drugs. Wild yam also contains a steroid hormone called dihydroepiandrosterone (DHEA), which may be useful in treating various diseases.

Common doses

Wild yam comes as:

- liquid extract
- tincture
- topical oil
- tea
- powder
- DHEA powder for compounding in 25- and 50-milligram capsules
- chewing gum containing 25 milligrams of DHEA.

The average dose is 2 to 4 grams or fluid equivalent taken orally three times daily. Some experts recommend the following doses:

- As a *food supplement*, DHEA dose shouldn't exceed 50 milligrams daily. Medical approval is needed for higher doses.
- As *fluid extract,* 2 to 4 milliliters in water taken orally three times daily, or 5 to 30 drops taken orally three times daily.
- As a *tincture* (1:5 in 45% alcohol), 2 to 10 milliliters in water taken orally twice daily.
- As a *tea,* add ¼ teaspoon to 1 cup of boiling water, and steep 15 minutes. Drink ¼ to 1 cup twice daily.
- As a *powder*, 0.5 to 2 grams taken orally twice daily.

Side effects

Call your health care practitioner if you experience any of these possible side effects of wild yam:

- acne
- hair loss (in men)
- headache
- excessive body hair (in women)
- menstrual irregularities
- oily skin.

Wild yam also may promote prostate cancer growth.

Interactions

Combining herbs with certain drugs may alter their action or produce unwanted side effects. If you're using wild yam, tell your health care practitioner about any prescription or nonprescription drugs you're taking.

Important points to remember

- Don't use wild yam if you're pregnant or breast-feeding.
- Avoid this herb if you have liver disease or a family history of hormone-related cancer (such as breast, ovarian, uterine, or prostate cancer).
- Know that in women, taking over 25 milligrams of DHEA daily may cause masculinizing effects (irreversible voice changes and increased body hair).
- Obtain DHEA and other natural products only from reliable sources to ensure their quality, purity, and strength.

Other names for wild yam

Other names for wild yam include colic root, Mexican wild yam, and rheumatism root.

WHAT THE RESEARCH SHOWS

Preliminary studies suggest that the hormone DHEA in wild yam may hold promise in treating such conditions as AIDS, multiple sclerosis, and lupus erythematosus. However, until more studies are done, the evidence doesn't warrant medicinal use of wild yam.

No known medicinal products containing wild yam are available commercially.

Selected references

Morales, A.J., et al. "Effects of Replacement Dose Dihydroepiandrosterone in Men and Women of Advancing Age, " *Journal of Clinical Endocrinology and Metabolism* 78:1360-67, 1994.

Salvato, P., et al. "Viral Load Response to Augmentation of Natural Dihydroepiandrosterone (DHEA)." XI International Conference on AIDS, 1996.

Willow

The ancient Egyptians used willow bark extracts to treat inflammatory conditions. Beethoven's autopsy reports suggest that the great composer's long habit of using powdered willow bark may have led to or worsened his kidney disease.

Active components of this herb, which is related chemically to aspirin, come from the bark of various willows, including white willow *(Salix alba)* and black willow *(S. nigra)*. White willow is native to Europe and naturalized in the United States. Black willow is native to North America.

Why people use this herb

- Fever
- Flu
- Inflammation
- Pain
- Rheumatism

Common doses

Willow comes as:

- dried bark
- capsules (379 and 400 milligrams)
- liquid extract (1 ounce).

Some experts recommend the following doses:

- As a *tea from the dried bark,* 1 to 3 grams taken orally twice daily.
- As *liquid extract* (1:1 in 25% alcohol), 1 to 3 milliliters taken orally three times daily.

Side effects

Call your health care practitioner if you experience any of these possible side effects of willow:

- asthma attacks and sneezing (from airborne willow pollen)
- severe allergic reaction (chest tightness, wheezing, hives, itching, and rash).
- skin inflammation
- symptoms of salicylate (aspirin) toxicity, such as nausea, vomiting, dizziness, ringing in the ears, confusion, lethargy, and diarrhea.

Willow also can cause:

- digestive tract bleeding
- kidney damage
- liver dysfunction
- prolonged bleeding.

Interactions

Combining herbs with certain drugs may alter their action or produce unwanted side effects. Don't use willow while taking:

- blood thinners such as Coumadin
- diuretics
- drugs that lower blood pressure
- nonsteroidal anti-inflammatory drugs such as Advil.

Important points to remember

- Don't use willow if you're pregnant or breast-feeding.
- Avoid this herb if you've had an allergic reaction to willow preparations or aspirin.
- Don't take willow if you have heart disease or stomach ulcers, if you bruise or bleed easily, or if you've had a stroke.

WHAT THE RESEARCH SHOWS

Advocates have long claimed that willow relieves pain and inflammation, but little hard evidence supports these claims. With many safe and effective remedies on the market, medical experts see little need for willow preparations.

Other names for willow

Other names for willow include black willow and white willow.

Products containing willow are sold as Aller g Formula 25, White Willow Bark, and Willowprin.

Selected reference

Schwarz, A. "Beethoven's Renal Disease Based on His Autopsy: A Case of Papillary Necrosis," *American Journal of Kidney Diseases* 21:643-52, 1993.

Wintergreen

As a folk remedy, children with chest colds wore a paper "jacket" made from a brown paper bag coated with wintergreen oil and camphor. Today, synthetic wintergreen oil is a well-known remedy for irritation. It's also used to flavor candies and other foods.

Wintergreen is a low-growing woodland plant with pleasant-tasting, red berries. The herb's active component (methyl salicylate) comes from the leaves and bark of *Gaultheria procumbens.* A member of the heath family (Ericaceae), this plant is native to parts of Canada and the eastern United States.

Common dose

Wintergreen comes as teas, lotions, liniments, ointments, lozenges, creams, and as oil. Some experts recommend the following dose:

- As *topical oil,* apply 10% to 30% wintergreen oil or methyl salicylate product to the skin no more than three or four times daily.

Side effects

Call your health care practitioner if you experience any of these possible side effects of wintergreen:

- abnormally fast or deep breathing
- lack of energy
- upset stomach
- vomiting.

Why people use this herb

- Joint pain
- Muscle strain
- Sciatica (pain along nerves in the lower back)
- Trigeminal neuralgia (a condition that causes facial pain)

Small children who ingest as little as 4 milliliters of wintergreen oil may be poisoned or may die.

Applying too much wintergreen oil to the skin may cause salicylate poisoning (from methyl salicylate in the oil). Heat and physical activity increase its absorption through the skin. Symptoms of salicylate poisoning include nausea and vomiting, body fluid and salt imbalances, bleeding, pulmonary edema, improper blood clotting, hepatitis, muscle tissue deterioration, ringing in the ear, central nervous system toxicity, and even death.

Interactions

Combining herbs with certain drugs may alter their action or produce unwanted side effects. Don't use wintergreen while taking:

- aspirin
- blood thinners such as Coumadin.

Important points to remember

- Don't use wintergreen if you're pregnant or breast-feeding.
- Don't take wintergreen products internally if you have acid reflux disease.
- To avoid skin irritation, don't use external wintergreen products with heating devices or warmed towels.
- To avoid toxic effects, don't use external wintergreen products after strenuous exercise or in hot, humid weather.
- Keep wintergreen products out children's reach.

> **WHAT THE RESEARCH SHOWS**
>
> Wintergreen can cause poisoning if taken internally or applied too liberally to the skin. Medical experts see no reason to use this herb, and point out that most commercial products containing methyl salicylate use a synthetic form of wintergreen.

Other names for wintergreen

Other names for wintergreen include boxberry, Canada tea, checkerberry, deerberry, gaultheria oil, mountain tea, oil of wintergreen, partridgeberry, and teaberry.

Products containing wintergreen are sold as Koong Yick Hung Fa Oil (KYHFO), Wintergreen Altoids, and Wintergreen Sucrets.

Selected references

Chan, T.Y. "Potential Dangers from Topical Preparations Containing Methyl Salicylate," *Human and Experimental Toxicology* 15:747-50, 1996.

Howrie, D.L., and Moriarty, R. "Candy Flavoring as a Source of Salicylate Poisoning," *Pediatrics* 75:869-71, 1985.

Watson, R. "Senna-Pod and Wintergreen," *Nursing Times* 88:64, 1992.

Yip, A.S.B., et al. "Adverse Effects of Topical Methyl Salicylate Ointment on Warfarin Anticoagulation: An Unrecognized Potential," *Postgraduate Medical Journal* 66:367-69, 1990.

Witch hazel

Witch hazel comes from the leaves and bark of *Hamamelis virginiana*, a shrub native to North America. It's prepared by distilling the plant's twigs and adding alcohol to the distillate.

Witch hazel water distillate (prepared from wintergreen twigs) contains 13% to 15% alcohol in water. In this country, most commercial sources of witch hazel are from Tennessee, the Blue Ridge Mountains (Virginia), and North Carolina.

Why people use this herb

- Anal itching and irritation
- Bruises
- Discomfort after episiotomy or hemorrhoid surgery
- Hemorrhoids
- Local swelling
- To ease oral inflammation
- Varicose veins
- Vaginal itching and irritation

Common doses

Witch hazel comes as:

- liquid extract
- witch hazel water (a milder form of the extract)
- cream
- medicated pads.

Some experts recommend the following doses:

- As a *tea from dried leaves,* gargle with 2 grams twice daily.
- As a *liquid extract* (1:1 in 45% alcohol), 2 to 4 milliliters taken as a gargle or applied topically twice daily.
- As *witch hazel water,* apply topically two or three times daily.

Side effects

Call your health care practitioner if you experience any of these possible side effects of witch hazel:

- nausea, vomiting, and constipation (with doses over 1,000 milligrams)
- skin inflammation.

Witch hazel also may cause liver toxicity. Some researchers believe it may cause cancer.

Interactions

Combining herbs with certain drugs may alter their action or produce unwanted side effects. If you're using witch hazel, tell your health care practitioner about any prescription or nonprescription drugs you're taking.

Important points to remember

- Don't use witch hazel if you're pregnant or breast-feeding.
- Don't take witch hazel internally.
- Consult a health care practitioner if your skin condition gets worse or doesn't improve after a few days of applying witch hazel.
- Keep witch hazel products out of children's reach.

> **WHAT THE RESEARCH SHOWS**
>
> Witch hazel products reduce bleeding and serve as effective astringents. Some studies show that witch hazel distillate relieves skin swelling and inflammation after exposure to ultraviolet-B radiation. According to medical experts, witch hazel is safe for external use but shouldn't be taken internally.

Other names for witch hazel

Other names for witch hazel include *Hamamelis,* snapping hazel, spotted alder, tobacco wood, and winterbloom.

Products containing witch hazel are sold as Witch Doctor, Witch Hazel Cream, Witch Hazel Liquid, Witch Hazel Pads, and Witch Stik.

Selected references

Dauer, A., et al. "Proanthocyanidins from the Bark of *Hamamelis virginiana* Exhibit Antimutagenic Properties Against Nitroaromatic Compounds," *Planta Medica* 64:324-27, 1998.

Duwieja, M., et al. "Anti-inflammatory Activity of *Polygonum bistorta, Guaiacum officinale* and *Hamamelis virginiana* in Rats," *Journal of Pharmacy and Pharmacology* 46:286-90, 1994.

Hughes-Formella, B.J., et al. "Anti-inflammatory Effects of Hamamelis Lotion in a UV-B Erythema Test," *Dermatology* 196:316-22, 1998.

Masaki, H., et al. "Protective Activity of Hamamelitannin on Cell Damage of Murine Skin Fibroblasts Induced By UVB Irradiation," *Journal of Dermatological Sciences* 10:25-34, 1995.

Wormwood

Wormwood extract is the main ingredient in absinthe, an emerald-green liqueur that was popular a century ago. Vincent van Gogh was thought to be an absinthe addict, and some experts suspect his addiction profoundly influenced his art. Absinthe was banned in the early 20th century for its toxic effects but is now making a comeback.

Active wormwood components come from the leaves and flowering tops of *Artemisia absinthium,* a shrubby perennial native to Europe, northern Africa, and western Asia. Wormwood shouldn't be confused with other herbal substances called "wormwood." For instance, sweet wormwood or Chinese wormwood, from *A. annua,* has been used in China for almost 2,000 years to treat fever and its active component shows promise in treating malaria. A wormwood extract lacking the thujone component is used to flavor alcoholic beverages such as vermouth.

Why people use this herb

- As an insect repellent
- As a sedative
- Fever
- To expel parasitic worms

Common dose

Wormwood comes as an essential oil. Experts disagree on what dose to take.

Side effects

Call your health care practitioner if you experience any of these possible side effects of wormwood:

- allergic reactions (with topical use)
- seizures.

Wormwood also can cause:

- kidney failure
- porphyria, a disease that leads to unusual light sensitivity, abdominal pain, and nerve pain
- rhabdomyolysis, a condition marked by deterioration of muscle tissue
- xanthopsia, a vision defect that makes objects appear to be tinged with yellow.

Long-term wormwood use may cause absinthinism, which can lead to hallucinations, nervousness, mental deterioration, and other symptoms.

Interactions

Combining herbs with certain drugs may alter their action or produce unwanted side effects. If you're taking wormwood, tell your health care practitioner about any prescription or nonprescription drugs you're taking.

Important points to remember

- Don't use wormwood if you're pregnant or breast-feeding.
- Don't take wormwood internally.

WHAT THE RESEARCH SHOWS

Several wormwood components show promise in treating inflammation, fever, parasitic worms, and liver damage caused by certain drugs. However, we need more research to establish the herb's safety and effectiveness. Because wormwood extract can damage the central nervous system, it shouldn't be taken internally.

Other names for wormwood

Other names for wormwood include absinthe and absinthium.

No known products containing wormwood are available commercially.

Selected references

Arnold, W.N., and Loftus, L.S. "Xanthopsia and van Gogh's Yellow Palette," *Eye* 5:503-10, 1991.

Bonkovsky, H.L., et al. "Porphyrogenic Properties of the Terpenes Camphor, Pinene, and Thujone (with a Note on Historic Implications for Absinthe and the Illness of Vincent van Gogh)," *Biochemical Pharmacology* 43:2359-68, 1992.

Sherif, A., et al. "Drugs, Insecticides and Other Agents from *Artemisia*," *Medical Hypotheses* 23:187-93, 1987.

van Geldre, E., et al. "State of the Art Production of the Antimalarial Compound Artemisinin in Plants," *Plant Molecular Biology* 33:199-209, 1997.

Weisbord, S.D., et al. "Poison on Line: Acute Renal Failure Caused by Oil of Wormwood Purchased Through the Internet," *New England Journal of Medicine* 337:825-27, 1997.

Woundwort

Active components of woundwort come from the leaves and stems of *Stachys palustris* and *S. sylvatica*. These plants belong to the mint family (Labiatae).

Common doses

Woundwort comes as tea, ointment, and tincture. Some experts recommend the following doses:

- As a *tea,* steep 1 teaspoon of dried herb in 1 cup of boiling water for 10 to 15 minutes, and drink twice daily.
- As a *tincture,* 1 to 2 milliliters taken orally twice daily for stomach cramps or diarrhea.
- As a *poultice,* apply bruised leaves to wounds.
- As an *ointment,* mix dried leaves into an ointment base and apply to the skin.

Why people use this herb

- As an antiseptic
- Cramps
- Diarrhea
- Dysentery
- Joint pain
- To stop bleeding
- Vertigo
- Wounds

Side effects

Call your health care practitioner if you experience unusual symptoms while using woundwort.

Interactions

Combining herbs with certain drugs may alter their action or produce unwanted side effects. If you're taking woundwort, tell your health care practitioner about any prescription or nonprescription drugs you're taking.

Important points to remember

- Don't use woundwort if you're pregnant or breast-feeding.
- Be aware that scientific evidence doesn't support taking woundwort for any medical condition.

Other names for woundwort

Other names for woundwort include hedge woundwort and marsh woundwort.

WHAT THE RESEARCH SHOWS

Scientific evidence doesn't prove that woundwort aids wound healing or has other medicinal uses. However, researchers did find that a related species, *Stachys sieboldii*, may contain a compound useful in treating a kidney disease called glomerulonephritis. More studies are needed to evaluate the herb's effects in this condition and other diseases.

No known products containing woundwort are available commercially.

Selected reference

Hayashi, K., et al. "Acteoside, a Component of *Stachys sieboldii* MIQ, May Be a Promising Antinephritic Agent (3): Effect of Acteoside on Expression of Intercellular Adhesion Molecule-1 in Experimental Nephritic Glomeruli in Rats and Cultured Endothelial Cells," *Japanese Journal of Pharmacology* 70:157-68, 1996.

Yarrow

Yarrow's botanical name, *Achillea,* comes from Achilles, Homer's legendary warrior. At the battle of Troy, a Greek god showed Achilles how to stop bleeding from a wound by applying yarrow leaves.

Yarrow's active components come from the dried leaves and flowering tops of *Achillea millefolium*. This member of the daisy family (Compositae) is native to Europe and Asia and naturalized in North America.

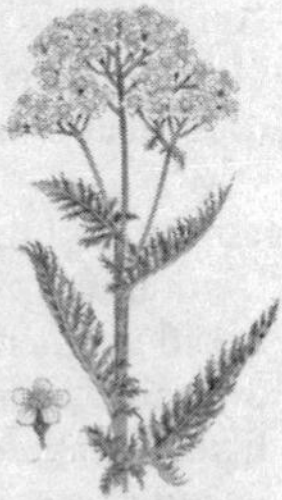

Why people use this herb

- Digestive disorders
- Eczema (a type of skin inflammation)
- Female reproductive disorders
- To reduce phlegm and relieve other symptoms of respiratory infections
- To stop bleeding of skin wounds
- Urinary tract problems

Common doses

Yarrow comes as:

- capsules (320 and 340 milligrams)
- liquid extract (1 or 2 ounces)
- tincture
- powder.

Some experts recommend the following doses:

- As *dried herb,* 2 to 4 grams boiled as a tea, taken twice daily.
- As *liquid extract* (1:1 in 25% alcohol), 2 to 4 milliliters taken orally twice daily.
- As a *tincture* (1:5 in 45% alcohol), 2 to 4 milliliters taken orally twice daily.

Side effects

Call your health care practitioner if you experience any of these possible side effects of yarrow:

- allergic skin inflammation or rash
- bleeding
- increased light sensitivity.

High doses of yarrow may stimulate the uterus.

Interactions

Combining herbs with certain drugs may alter their action or produce unwanted side effects. Tell your health care practitioner about any prescription or nonprescription drugs you're taking, especially:

- alcohol and other drugs that slow the nervous system, such as cold and allergy drugs, sedatives, tranquilizers, narcotic pain relievers, barbiturates, seizure drugs, and muscle relaxants
- Antabuse
- blood thinners such as Coumadin
- drugs that lower blood pressure.

Important points to remember

- Don't use yarrow if you're pregnant or breast-feeding.
- Avoid this herb if you've experienced a skin allergy after using it or similar plants.
- If you're taking Antabuse, don't take an alcohol-containing yarrow tincture because it may cause a reaction.
- Avoid driving and other dangerous activities until you know how the herb affects you.

WHAT THE RESEARCH SHOWS

Although yarrow has been used to treat various internal and external conditions, no clinical evidence supports these uses. Medical experts emphasize that yarrow should be used cautiously because of the risk of allergic skin inflammation.

Other names for yarrow

Other names for yarrow include *Achillea millefolium,* bloodwort, gordaldo, milfoil, nosebleed, old man's pepper, sanguinary, soldier's woundwort, stanchgrass, and thousand-leaf.

Products containing yarrow are sold as Diacure, Lasadoron, Rheumatic Pain Remedy, and Yarrow Flowers.

Selected references

Hausen, B.M., et al. "Alpha-Peroxyachifolid and Other New Sensitizing Sesquiterpene Lactones from Yarrow (*Achillea millefolium* L., Compositae)," *Contact Dermatitis* 24:274-80, 1991.

Rucker, G., et al. "Peroxides As Plant Constituents. 8. Guaianolide-Peroxides from Yarrow, *Achillea millefolium* L., a Soluble Component Causing Yarrow Dermatitis." *Archiv der Pharmazie* 324:979-81, 1991.
Tozyo, T., et al. "Novel Antitumor Sesquiterpenoids in *Achillea millefolium,*" *Chemical and Pharmaceutical Bulletin (Tokyo)* 42:1096-1100, 1994.

Yellow dock

Europeans cultivate yellow dock as a vegetable, and Himalayan natives use it to treat rash caused by stinging nettles. A dried extract is prepared from the roots of *Rumex crispus,* a common and troublesome perennial weed native to Europe and Asia and naturalized in the United States. You can spot this weed along many roadsides and in gravelly soils of pastures and meadows.

Why people use this herb

- Allergy symptoms
- Chronic liver congestion
- Constipation
- Fluid retention
- Intermittent fever
- Rash caused by stinging nettles
- Scabies and other skin diseases
- Sore throat
- Stomach upset
- Swollen glands
- Syphilis
- Tonsillitis (tonsil inflammation)

Common dose

Yellow dock comes as capsules (470 or 500 milligrams). In studies, people received a single oral dose of 2.5 to 5 milligrams.

Side effects

Call your health care practitioner if you experience any of these possible side effects of yellow dock:

- abdominal pain
- diarrhea
- nausea
- vomiting.

Consuming excessive amounts of yellow dock can cause metabolic acidosis (a blood acid disorder) and a severe calcium deficiency in the blood, resulting in death.

Interactions

Combining herbs with certain drugs may alter their action or produce unwanted side effects. Tell your health care practitioner about any prescription or nonprescription drugs you're taking.

Important points to remember

- Don't use yellow dock if you're pregnant because it may cause miscarriage.
- If you get pregnant or think you might have become pregnant while using yellow dock, notify your health care practitioner promptly.
- Avoid this herb while breast-feeding.

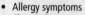

- Don't use yellow dock if you have kidney dysfunction or kidney failure, diabetes, liver disease, or a severe body salt (electrolyte) abnormality.
- Use yellow dock cautiously if you have heart failure, newly diagnosed diabetes, malnutrition, or a disease related to alcoholism or if you've had recent thyroid or parathyroid surgery. Also use caution if you're taking drugs that decrease blood calcium, such as diuretics, Dilantin, Miacalcin, or Mithracin.
- Watch for symptoms of low blood calcium, including fatigue, seizures, confusion, muscle spasms, and numbness or tingling around the mouth.
- Be sure to tell your health care practitioner you're using yellow dock. He or she may recommend periodic blood calcium tests and may want to check for symptoms of low blood calcium.
- Report sudden onset of nausea, vomiting, or abdominal pain.
- Use yellow dock in very small portions, if any, in food.
- Don't use yellow dock instead of prescribed antiviral drugs to treat herpes or HIV.
- If you continue to experience allergy symptoms while using yellow dock, notify your health care practitioner.
- Be aware that boiling the root too long reduces yellow dock's chemical activity.

WHAT THE RESEARCH SHOWS

Although clinical data on yellow dock come from animals, medical experts believe the herb relieves itching to some extent and reduces the extent of certain skin inflammations (although they don't know exactly how or why). However, because of the poisoning risk, experts advise people to take established antihistamine or antiallergy products instead of yellow dock.

Other names for yellow dock

Other names for yellow dock include chin ch'iao mai, curled or curly dock, garden patience, hualtata, hummaidh, kivircik labada, narrow dock, niu she t'ou, oseille marron (sauvage), sour dock, and surale di bierdji.

Products containing yellow dock are sold under such names as LC Tone, Detox, and Rumex Crispus.

Selected references

Aggarwal, M., et al. "Effect of *Rumex nepalensis* Extracts on Histamine, Acetylcholine, Carbachol, Bradykinin, and PGs Evoked Skin Reactions in Rabbits," *Annals of Allergy* 56:177-82, 1986.

el-Mekkawy S., et al. "Inhibitory Effects of Egyptian Folk Medicines on Human Immunodeficiency Virus (HIV) Reverse Transcriptase," *Chemical and Pharmaceutical Bulletin (Tokyo)* 43:641-48, 1995. Abstract.

Farr, M., et al. "Fatal Oxalic Acid Poisoning from Sorrel Soup" *Lancet* 23:1524, 1989. Letter.

Panciera, R., et al. "Acute Oxalate Poisoning Attributable to Ingestion of Curly Dock *(Rumex crispus)* in Sheep," *Journal of the American Veterinary Medical Association* 196:1981-90, 1990.

Taylor, R.S. et al. "Antiviral Activities of Medicinal Plants of Southern Nepal," *Journal of Ethnopharmacology* 53:97-104, 1996.

Yerba maté

Yerba maté is a popular beverage in Brazil, Paraguay, and Argentina. Originally it was served in a small gourd (maté) and sipped through a filter straw to strain out plant material. Some people add burnt sugar, lemon juice, or milk to the drink.

Aside from its popularity as a drink in South America, yerba maté has inspired many therapeutic claims. Herbal preparations come from the dried leaves of an evergreen tree, *Ilex paraguariensis,* which belongs to the holly family (Aquifoliaceae).

Common doses

Yerba maté comes as leaves, tea, and liquid extract. Some experts recommend the following doses:

- As *fluid extract* (1:1 in 25% alcohol), 2 to 4 milliliters taken orally twice daily.
- As a *tea,* 2 to 4 grams dried leaf taken orally twice daily.

Why people use this herb

- Depression
- Diabetes
- Fluid retention
- Fatigue (mental and physical)
- Heart disease
- High blood pressure
- Joint pain
- Nervous disorders
- Pain
- Stomach disorders
- To curb the appetite
- To induce vomiting

Side effects

Call your health care practitioner if you experience any of these possible side effects of yerba maté:

- flushed skin
- irregular heartbeats
- irritability
- muscle twitching
- nausea
- nervousness
- vomiting
- withdrawal headache.

This herb also may cause liver toxicity, leading to unusual bleeding or bruising, extreme drowsiness or weakness, appetite loss, vomiting, yellow-tinged eyes and skin, trembling, and fever.

Prolonged yerba maté consumption has been linked to an increased cancer risk.

Interactions

Combining herbs with certain drugs may alter their action or produce unwanted side effects. Tell your health care practitioner about any prescription or nonprescription drugs you're taking, especially:

- alcohol and other drugs that slow the nervous system, such as cold and allergy drugs, sedatives, tranquilizers, narcotic pain relievers, barbiturates, seizure drugs, and muscle relaxants
- Antabuse
- caffeine, cigarettes, and other central nervous system stimulants
- Calan (used to treat angina, high blood pressure, and certain arrhythmias)
- Cipro (used to treat urinary tract infections)
- diuretics
- Tagamet (used to treat ulcers and acid reflux disease).

Important points to remember

- Don't use yerba maté if you're pregnant or breast-feeding.
- Avoid using this herb if you have high blood pressure or suffer from anxiety.
- If you're taking Antabuse, avoid using an herbal form that contains alcohol because this may cause a reaction.
- Keep yerba maté products out of children's reach because they may be especially vulnerable to toxic effects.
- Avoid caffeine and other central nervous system stimulants while taking this herb.
- Be aware that heavy yerba maté consumption may increase the risk of liver disease, upper digestive tract cancers, and bladder cancer.
- Report unusual symptoms to your health care practitioner.

WHAT THE RESEARCH SHOWS

The risks of taking yerba maté clearly outweigh the possible—and unproven—benefits. Medical experts point out that long-term consumption has been linked to an increased risk of bladder and esophagus cancer.

Other names for yerba maté

Other names for yerba maté include armino, Bartholomew's tea, boca juniors, campeche, el agricultor, elacy, flor de lis, gaucho, jaguar, Jesuit's tea, la hoja, la mulata, la tranquera, lonjazo, madrugada, maté,

maté bulk loose tea, nobleza gaucha, oro verde, Paraguay tea, payadito, rosamonte, safira, union, yerba-de-maté, yi-yi, and zerboni.

No known products containing yerba maté are available commercially.

Selected references

De Stefani, E., et al. "Black Tobacco, Maté, and Bladder Cancer. A Case-Control Study from Uruguay," *Cancer* 67:536-40, 1991.

McGee, I., et al. "A Case of Veno-Occlusive Disease of the Liver in Britain Associated With Herbal Tea Consumption," *Journal of Clinical Pathology* 29:788-94, 1976.

Pintos, J., et al. "Maté, Coffee, and Tea Consumption and Risk of Cancers of the Upper Aerodigestive Tract in Southern Brazil," *Epidemiology* 5:583-90, 1994.

Yerba santa

Native Americans used yerba santa externally for bruises and inflammation and smoked or chewed the leaves to treat asthma. Some bitter drugs contain yerba santa to mask their taste. The fluid extract is used in foods and beverages.

Why people use this herb

- Asthma
- Bronchitis
- Bruises
- Common cold
- Cough
- Fever
- Hay fever
- Inflammation
- Rheumatism
- To help expel mucus from the lungs
- Tuberculosis

Active components come from the leaves and roots of *Eriodictyon californicum*. This evergreen shrub, which belongs to the waterleaf family (Hydrophyllaceae), is native to the mountains of California and northern Mexico.

Common doses

Yerba santa comes as:

- liquid extract (1 ounce)
- liniment
- powder
- syrup
- tea.

It's also available in several nonprescription herbal preparations.

Some experts recommend the following doses:

- For *coughs, colds, asthma,* and *tuberculosis,* make a tea from the leaves.
- As an *expectorant to loosen chest secretions,* use the powdered leaves.
- To *reduce fever,* make a liniment from the leaves and apply to the skin.
- To treat *bruises* and *rheumatism,* apply fresh leaves to the skin as a poultice.

Side effects

Call your health care practitioner if you experience unusual symptoms while using yerba santa. Chewing the herb leaves a gummy residue on the teeth.

Interactions

Combining herbs with certain drugs may alter their action or produce unwanted side effects. If you're taking yerba santa, tell your health care practitioner about any prescription or nonprescription drugs you're taking.

Important points to remember

- Don't use yerba santa if you're pregnant or breast-feeding.
- Don't rely on yerba santa to treat asthma or tuberculosis.

Other names for yerba santa

Other names for yerba santa include bear's weed, consumptive's weed, gum plant, holy weed, mountain balm, and tarweed.

A product containing yerba santa is sold as Respirtone.

WHAT THE RESEARCH SHOWS

Several yerba santa components show some promise as cancer treatments, but no clinical data are available and we know little about the herb's safety and effectiveness. Also, you can easily obtain safer preparations to treat cough, fever, and pain—the most common conditions for which people take yerba santa.

Selected reference

Liu, Y.L., et al. "Isolation of Potential Cancer Chemopreventative Agents from *Eriodictyon californicum*," *Journal of Natural Products* 55:357-63, 1992.

Yew

Native Americans used yew extracts to treat rheumatism, fever, and arthritis. However, all plant parts except the seed's bright-red outer covering are poisonous.

Active components of the herb, especially paclitaxel, come from the branch tips and bark of the Pacific or Western Yew *(Taxus brevifolia),* an evergreen tree native to the northwestern United States and British Columbia. Paclitaxel occurs in lesser amounts in other yew species, such as the American yew and the Japanese yew *(T. cuspidata).* The English yew contains a similar compound called docetaxel (also known as taxotere).

Paclitaxel (under the name Taxol) is labeled by the Food and Drug Administration as a treatment for metastatic ovarian cancer after failure of first-line chemotherapy. Many studies have shown that paclitaxel is effective against metastatic ovarian and breast cancers.

Why people use this herb

- Arthritis
- Breast cancer
- Fever
- Leukemia
- Lung cancer
- Malignant melanoma
- Ovarian cancer
- Rheumatism

Common doses

Yew comes as an extract (concentrated tincture), salve, and capsules (with olives). Because consuming yew can be dangerous, you should use it only under the supervision of a qualified health care practitioner.

Some experts recommend the following doses:

- As a *tincture,* 10 to 60 drops taken orally two to four times daily.
- As a *tea,* 1 cup taken orally once daily.
- As a *salve,* apply as needed.

Side effects

Call your health care practitioner if you experience unusual symptoms while using yew. Use of paclitaxel and long-term use of other yew products have caused the following symptoms:

- allergic reactions
- hair loss
- irregular heartbeats

- joint pain
- low blood pressure
- muscle pain
- nausea
- rash
- vomiting.

Yew also can cause:
- high blood fat levels
- elevated liver function tests
- low platelet and white and red blood cell levels
- peripheral nerve degeneration.

Interactions

Combining herbs with certain drugs may alter their action or produce unwanted side effects. Tell your health care practitioner about any prescription or nonprescription drugs you're taking, especially:
- cancer chemotherapy drugs
- drugs for fungal infections such as Nizoral.

Important points to remember

- Don't use yew if you're pregnant or breast-feeding.
- Know that although paclitaxel (and its derivative, docetaxel) are effective in treating cancer, other products containing yew are highly toxic and untested. Don't use nonpharmaceutical yew products.

WHAT THE RESEARCH SHOWS

Taxol and other yew components are effective against cancer but must be used only under strict medical supervision. Other yew products (from the entire plant or whole plant extracts) haven't been studied as treatments for any medical condition. What's more, these products are toxic. Medical experts caution people not to use nonstandardized products containing yew.

Other names for yew

Other names for yew include American yew, California yew, chinwood, globe-berry, ground hemlock, Oregon yew, and western yew.

A product containing yew is sold as Yew Tea.

Selected references

Howard, R.A., and DeWolf, G. "Poisonous Plants," *Arnoldia* 34:41-96, 1974.
Huxtable, R.J. "Regional Sources of Natural Products: *Taxomyces andreanae*," *Proceedings of the Western Pharmacology Society* 38:1-4, 1995.
O'Leary, J., et al. "Taxanes in Adjuvant and Neoadjuvant Therapies for Breast Cancer," *Oncology* 12:23-27, 1998.
von Hoff, D.D. "The Taxoids: Same Roots, Diffèrent Drugs," *Seminars in Oncology* 24:S13:3-10; 1997.

Yohimbe

Some people use yohimbe as an aphrodisiac or a hallucinogen. Researchers are studying it as a possible treatment for male erectile impotence and certain types of low blood pressure. In male erectile impotence, it may work by improving blood flow to the penis and improving smooth muscle relaxation (although clinical studies have produced contradictory results).

Active herbal components come from the bark of *Pausinystalia yohimbe*, a West African tree native to Congo, Cameroon, and Gabon. Since 1977, the U.S. Department of Agriculture has listed yohimbe as unsafe.

Why people use this herb

- As an aphrodisiac
- For hallucinogenic effects
- Low blood pressure caused by rising too quickly from a sitting or lying position
- Male erectile impotence
- Overdose of Capoten (a drug used to lower blood pressure)

Common doses

Yohimbe comes as tablets (3 milligrams and 5.4 milligrams). Some experts recommend the following doses:

- For *male impotence,* 5.4 milligrams taken orally twice daily. If side effects occur, reduce the dose to 2.7 milligrams twice daily and then gradually increase it to 5.4 milligrams. Daily doses of 20 to 30 milligrams may cause a fast pulse and high blood pressure.
- For *low blood pressure when rising from a sitting or lying position,* 12.5 milligrams taken orally once daily. (However, be aware that more research is needed on yohimbe's use for this condition.)

Side effects

Call your health care practitioner if you experience any of these possible side effects of yohimbe:

- anxiety
- appetite loss
- diarrhea
- dizziness
- flushed skin
- genital pain
- headache
- high blood pressure symptoms, such as headache or blurred vision

- irritability
- nausea
- nervousness
- painful urination
- rapid pulse
- tremors.

Yohimbe also can cause kidney failure. Manic reactions have occurred in people receiving an average daily dose of 12.5 milligrams.

Interactions

Combining herbs with certain drugs may alter their action or produce unwanted side effects. Don't use yohimbe while taking:

- drugs used to treat depression, including selective serotonin reuptake inhibitors (such as Prozac) and tricyclic antidepressants (such as Norpramin or Tofranil)
- foods containing tyramine, such as aged cheese, wine, and liver
- nonprescription stimulant products, such as caffeine or cold medicines that contain phenylephedrine or phenylpropanolamine.

Important points to remember

- Don't use yohimbe if you're pregnant or breast-feeding.
- Avoid this herb if you're being treated for a psychiatric disorder or if you have kidney or liver disease, ulcers, or other digestive problems.
- Avoid caffeine when using yohimbe.
- Don't take yohimbe if you've had an allergic reaction to a yohimbe preparation.
- Keep yohimbe products out of children's reach.
- If you're taking this herb along with a drug that lowers blood pressure, rise slowly from a sitting or lying position to minimize dizziness.
- Be aware that the effects of long-term yohimbe use (more than 10 weeks) aren't known.

Other names for yohimbe

Other names for yohimbe include aphrodien, *Corynanthe yohimbe,* corynine, *Pausinystalia yohimbe,* quebrachine, yohimbehe, yohimbene, yohimbime, and yohimbine.

WHAT THE RESEARCH SHOWS

Some research suggests that yohimbe may help treat male organic impotence caused by diabetes. However, the herb hasn't been compared against currently available impotence treatments. More research must be done to define its specific role in this or any other medical condition.

Products containing yohimbe are sold as Aphrodyne, Dayto Himbin, Potensan, Vikonon Combination, Yobinol, Yocon, Yohimbine HCl, and Yohimex.

Selected references

Knoll, L.D., et al. "A Randomized Crossover Study using Yohimbine and Isoxsuprine versus Pentoxifylline in the Management of Vasculogenic Impotence," *Journal of Urology* 155:144-46, 1996.

Morales, A., et al. "Nonhormonal Pharmacological Treatment of Organic Impotence," *Journal of Urology* 128:45-47, 1982.

Price, H.L., et al. "Three Cases of Mania Symptoms Following Yohimbine Administration," *American Journal of Psychiatry* 141:1267-68, 1984.

Roberge, R.J., et al. "Yohimbine as an Antidote for Clonidine Overdose," *American Journal of Emergency Medicine* 14:7:678-80, 1996.

Siegel, R.K. "Herbal Intoxication: Psychoactive Effects from Herbal Cigarettes, Tea, and Capsules," *JAMA* 236:473-76, 1976.

Teloken, C., et al. "Therapeutic Effects of High Dose Yohimbine Hydrochloride on Organic Erectile Dysfunction," *Journal of Urology* 159:124, 1998

NONHERBAL ALTERNATIVE MEDICINES

Acidophilus

A bacterium, *Lactobacillus acidophilus* is used for various skin problems and for intestinal and other internal disorders. It's usually sold as concentrated, dried, viable cultures. Many dairy products, especially milk and yogurts, contain some acidophilus cultures. However, some have questionable *L. acidophilus* levels. Such products also may contain other bacteria of dubious benefit and may vary widely in potency and stability.

Why people use acidophilus

- Acne
- Bacterial vaginosis
- Canker sores
- Diarrhea (especially when caused by antibiotic use)
- Diverticulitis
- Fever blisters
- Hives
- Irritable bowel syndrome
- Stomach ulcers caused by the bacterium *Helicobacter pylori*
- To lower cholesterol
- Ulcerative colitis
- Vaginal yeast infections

Common dose

Acidophilus comes in various doses, in cultures ranging from 500 million to 4 billion viable organisms of *L. acidophilus,* including:

- capsules
- granules
- powders
- softgels
- suppositories
- tablets
- milk
- yogurt.

Doses are based on the number of live organisms in a commercial acidophilus culture. Some experts recommend the following dose:

- For *most reported uses,* 1 to 10 billion viable organisms taken daily in three or four equal doses.

Side effects

Call your health care practitioner if you experience intestinal gas when taking acidophilus. However, keep in mind that this side effect usually subsides with continued use.

Interactions

Combining acidophilus products with certain drugs may alter their action or produce unwanted side effects. Tell your health care practitioner about any prescription or nonprescription drugs you're taking.

Important points to remember

- Know that if you're lactose-sensitive, you may have trouble tolerating dairy products that contain acidophilus cultures.
- Remember that acidophilus products aren't effective unless they're manufactured, packaged, and stored properly. Some manufacturers require refrigeration of their products.
- Be aware that some dairy sources of acidophilus, particularly yogurt and milk, may not contain viable cultures. Also, some dairy products may be unreliable culture sources because of dramatic temperature swings during transport.
- Know that the Food and Drug Administration doesn't consider acidophilus products safe and effective in treating diarrhea.

WHAT THE RESEARCH SHOWS

Scientific studies on people haven't shown that acidophilus is effective in treating diarrhea or vaginal infections. However, the quality of the acidophilus cultures used in these studies varied, which may have influenced the results. Medical experts say acidophilus products can't be evaluated properly until they're standardized.

Other names for acidophilus

Other names for acidophilus include acidophilus milk, lactobacillus acidophilus, probiotics, and yogurt.

Products containing acidophilus are sold under such names as Bacid, DDS-Acidophilus, Florajen Acidophilus Extra Strength, Kyo-Dophilus, Lactinex, MoreDophilus, Probiata, Pro-Bionate, and Superdophilus.

Selected reference

Fredricsson, B., et al. "Bacterial Vaginosis Is Not a Simple Ecological Disorder," *Gynecologic and Obstetric Investigation* 28:156, 1989.

Agar

A jelly-like substance, agar comes from various species of red marine algae, including *Gelidium cartilagineum* and *Gracilaria confervoides*. Bacteriologists use agar as a culture medium, and some herbalists recommend it as a laxative. Many pharmaceutical and food products contain agar as an emulsifying and suspending agent.

Common dose

Agar comes as dry powder and in flakes and strips. Some experts recommend the following dose:

- As a *bulk-forming laxative,* 4 to 16 grams taken orally once or twice daily.

Why people use agar

- Constipation
- High bilirubin in newborns

Side effects

Call your health care practitioner if you experience any of these possible side effects of agar:

- abdominal pain
- chest pain or tightness
- choking (from taking agar without enough liquid)
- difficulty swallowing or breathing
- vomiting.

Agar can also cause:

- decreased absorption of vitamins, minerals, and nutrients (especially calcium, iron, zinc, copper, chromium, and cobalt)
- obstruction of the bowel or esophagus.

Interactions

Combining agar products with certain drugs may alter their action or produce unwanted side effects. Don't use agar while taking:

- electrolyte solutions
- products that contain alcohol or tannic acid.

Important points to remember

- Don't use agar if you're pregnant or breast-feeding.
- Avoid agar if you've had throat problems, difficulty swallowing, or bowel or esophageal obstruction.
- Take agar products on an empty stomach to improve vitamin and mineral absorption from foods.

WHAT THE RESEARCH SHOWS

No long-term studies have evaluated agar's effects on mineral and nutrient absorption in people. With more effective bulk-forming laxatives such as psyllium available, medical experts see no need to use agar to treat constipation.

Other names for agar

Other names for agar include agar-agar, Chinese gelatin, colle du japon, E406, gelose, Japanese gelatin, Japanese isinglass, layor carang, and vegetable gelatin.

Products containing agar are sold under such names as Agarbil, Agoral, Agoral Plain, Demosvelte-N, Falqui, Lexat, Paragar, and Pseudophage.

Selected references

Harmuth-Hoene, A. E., et al. "Effect of Dietary Fiber on Mineral Absorption in Growing Rats," *Journal of Nutrition* 110:1774-84, 1980.

Kondo, H., et al. "Influence of Dietary Fiber on the Bioavailability of Zinc in Rats," *Biomedical and Environmental Sciences* 9:204-08, 1996.

Vales, T.N., et al. "Pharmacologic Approaches to the Prevention and Treatment of Neonatal Hyperbilirubinemia," *Clinics in Perinatology* 17:245-73, 1990.

Bee pollen

Bee pollen consists of flower pollen and nectar mixed with digestive enzymes (saliva) from worker honeybees. The pollen is harvested at the entrance of a beehive as bees travel through a wire mesh, which forces them to brush their legs against a collection vessel. Commercial pollen quantities can be obtained directly from flowers.

Bee pollen achieved new popularity during the late 1970s after several famous athletes made therapeutic claims for it. Some people use it as a nutritional supplement and to treat allergies and other disorders.

Why people use bee pollen

- Allergies
- Asthma
- Atherosclerosis (plaque buildup in the arteries)
- Hemorrhoids
- High blood pressure
- Impotence
- Inflammatory conditions
- Poor circulation
- Prostate inflammation
- To help prevent cancer and heart disease
- Varicose veins

Common dose

Bee pollen comes as:
- tablets (500 and 1,000 milligrams)
- capsules (500 and 1,000 milligrams)
- granules (300 milligrams).

It's also added to liquids, candy bars, and wafers. Some experts recommend the following dose:
- 500 to 1,000 milligrams taken orally three times a day, 30 minutes before meals.

Side effects

Call your health care practitioner if you experience an allergic reaction, which can range from self-limited nausea and vomiting to life-threatening anaphylaxis (chest tightness, wheezing, hives, itching, and rash).

Interactions

Combining bee pollen products with certain drugs may alter their action or produce unwanted side effects. If you have diabetes, don't use bee pollen while taking insulin or other drugs that lower blood sugar.

Important points to remember

- Don't take bee pollen if you've experienced an allergy to pollen preparations.

- Avoid bee pollen if you have diabetes.
- Refrigerate fresh bee pollen to maintain its quality.
- Be aware that many imported flower pollens are sterilized during customs inspections and therefore lack many enzymes and nutrients.
- Know that bee pollen products aren't standardized. Typically, they contain pollens from many kinds of plants. Also, pollen composition varies from week to week and hive to hive. This lack of standardization means that product effectiveness can vary from one dose to the next.

WHAT THE RESEARCH SHOWS

The argument that bee pollen prevents allergies resembles the theory behind allergy shots. Both techniques introduce an allergen into the body, stimulating an immune response.

But bee pollen must be taken orally, and you'd have to take 10,000 times the amount of allergen in a typical allergy shot to obtain an immune response from bee pollen.

Overall, we need more research to define bee pollen's specific role in treating any medical condition. Until studies are done, medical experts say it's best to avoid bee pollen.

Other names for bee pollen

Other names for bee pollen include buckwheat pollen, maize pollen, pine pollen, pollen pini, puhuang, rape pollen, songhuafen, and typha pollen.

A product containing bee pollen is sold as Aller G Formula 25.

Selected references

Broadhurst, L. "*Information About Bee Pollen.*" Botanical Medicine Conference. Philadelphia, 1997.

Griffith, H.W. "Bee Pollen," in *The Complete Guide to Vitamins, Minerals, and Supplements.* Tucson, Ariz.: Fisher Books, 1988.

Chondroitin

A byproduct of meat processing, chondroitin is extracted from cartilage. Public interest in chondroitin has ballooned since the 1997 publication of *The Arthritis Cure*, a book claiming that a combination of chondroitin sulfates and glucosamine sulfate is "the medical miracle that can halt, reverse, and may even cure osteoarthritis." Unfortunately, this enthusiasm is premature.

Why people use chondroitin

- During eye surgery
- Heart disease
- Osteoarthritis and related disorders
- Pain
- To preserve a cornea for transplantation

Common doses

Chondroitin comes as capsules (200 and 400 milligrams, usually in combination with glucosamine sulfate) and an injection (available only in Europe). Some experts recommend the following doses, usually based on weight:

- *For people weighing less than 120 pounds,* 1,000 milligrams of glucosamine sulfate plus 800 milligrams of chondroitin sulfates taken orally.
- *For people weighing 120 to 200 pounds,* 1,500 milligrams of glucosamine sulfate plus 1,200 milligrams of chondroitin sulfates.
- *For people weighing more than 200 pounds,* 2,000 milligrams of glucosamine sulfate plus 1,600 milligrams of chondroitin sulfates.

Usually, the total daily dosage is taken with food in two to four equal doses. Recent studies evaluating chondroitin sulfates alone used doses of 400 milligrams taken orally two or three times daily, and 1,200 milligrams taken orally once daily.

Side effects

Call your health care practitioner if you experience any of these possible side effects of chondroitin:

- headache
- indigestion
- irritability
- nausea
- pain (after chondroitin injection)
- unusual sense of well-being.

Animal studies show that chondroitin carries a risk of internal bleeding because it's similar to a blood-thinning drug called heparin. However, internal bleeding hasn't been reported in people.

Interactions

Combining chondroitin with certain drugs may alter their action or produce unwanted side effects. Don't use chondroitin while taking blood thinners, such as Coumadin or heparin.

Important points to remember

- Don't use chondroitin if you're pregnant or breast-feeding.
- Avoid chondroitin if you have a bleeding disorder.

WHAT THE RESEARCH SHOWS

Most human studies on chondroitin have been flawed, and we have little clinical trial data on the combination of glucosamine sulfate and chondroitin sulfates. Defining chondroitin's role in medical treatment will take larger long-term clinical trials with better study design. In the meantime, the Arthritis Foundation doesn't recommend chondroitin sulfates and glucosamine sulfate for osteoarthritis or any other arthritis form.

Other names for chondroitin

Other names for chondroitin include CAS, chondroitin sulfate-A or chondroitin-4-sulfate, chondroitin-C or chondroitin-6-sulfate, and CSS.

Products containing chondroitin are sold under such names as 100% CSA, Chondroitin-4 Sulfate, and Purified Chondroitin Sulfate.

Selected references

Kerzberg, E.M., et al. "Combination of Glycosaminoglycans and Acetylsalicylic Acid in Knee Osteoarthrosis," *Scandinavian Journal of Rheumatology* 16:377-80, 1987.

McNamara, P.S., et al. "Hematologic, Hemostatic, and Biochemical Effects in Dogs Receiving an Oral Chondroprotective Agent for Thirty Days," *American Journal of Veterinary Research* 57:1390-94, 1996.

Morreale, P., et al. "Comparison of the Anti-inflammatory Efficacy of Chondroitin Sulfate and Diclofenac Sodium in Patients with Knee Osteoarthritis," *Journal of Rheumatology* 23:1385-91, 1996.

Theodosakis, J. *The Arthritis Cure.* New York: St. Martin's Press, 1997.

Coenzyme Q10

An antioxidant, coenzyme Q10 (Co-Q10) occurs in all human cells. It's most abundant in the heart, liver, kidneys, and pancreas. Some people claim Co-Q10 protects muscle cells from damage caused by impaired blood supply or other conditions. This claim rests on the theory that people with significant heart disease have abnormally low Co-Q10 levels in their heart muscle.

Japan retains all patents for Co-Q10 products and is the major supplier of the world's Co-Q10.

Common dose

Co-Q10 comes as:

- tablets (25, 50, 100, and 200 milligrams)
- capsules (10, 30, 60, and 100 milligrams).

In studies, people received doses of 50 to 300 milligrams orally daily.

Why people use coenzyme Q10

- Angina pectoris (chest pain caused by a heart condition)
- Bell's palsy (partial facial paralysis)
- Deafness
- Diabetes
- Gum disease
- Heart failure
- High blood pressure
- Immune deficiency
- Irregular heartbeats
- Ischemic heart disease (insufficient blood supply to the heart)
- Mitral valve prolapse
- To counter Adriamycin's toxic effects on the heart

Side effects

Call your health care practitioner if you experience any of these possible side effects of Co-Q10:

- appetite loss
- burning sensation in the stomach
- diarrhea
- mild nausea.

Co-Q10 can damage heart tissue during intense exercise.

Interactions

Combining Co-Q10 with certain drugs may alter their action or produce unwanted side effects. Tell your health care practitioner about any prescription or nonprescription drugs you're taking, especially:

- Coumadin
- drugs that lower blood sugar.

Important points to remember

- Don't take Co-Q10 if you're allergic to it or its formulation.
- Don't perform intense physical exercise while taking this substance.
- If you have heart failure, report changes in your condition to your health care practitioner.

WHAT THE RESEARCH SHOWS

Researchers found that adding coenzyme Q10 (Co-Q10) to other therapies can shorten hospital stays and help prevent serious complications in heart failure patients. Despite these preliminary findings, Co-Q10 hasn't been shown to reduce death from heart failure. More studies are needed to compare it with other standard drug treatments (such as beta blockers, ACE inhibitors, and aspirin) to determine survival rates.

We also need more research to define a specific role for Co-Q10 in treating other medical conditions. Until the results are in, medical experts won't recommend it.

Other names for coenzyme Q10

Other names for Co-Q10 include mitoquinone, ubidecarenone, and ubiquinone.

Products containing Co-Q10 are sold under such names as Adelir, Co-Q10, Heartcin, Inokiton, Neuquinone, Taidecanone, Ubiquinone, and Udekinon.

Selected references

Sinatra, S.T., et al. "Coenzyme Q10: A Vital Therapeutic Nutrient for the Heart with Special Application in Congestive Heart Failure," *Connecticut Medicine* 65:707-11, 1997.

Vasankari, T.J., et al. "Increased Serum and Low-Density-Lipoprotein Antioxidant Potential After Antioxidant Supplementation in Endurance Athletes," *American Journal of Clinical Nutrition* 65:1052-56, 1997.

Creatine monohydrate

Creatine monohydrate comes from such dietary sources as red meat, milk, and fish and is produced by the kidney, liver, and pancreas. An amino acid, creatine plays an important role in the reactions that allow muscle cells to store energy. Recently, it has become popular as a muscle-building nutritional supplement. Athletes in resistance-training programs may find that taking creatine supplements allows them to complete workouts at a higher level of intensity and strength. Although creatine was discovered nearly 160 years ago, its effect on human exercise performance wasn't studied until 1992.

Common doses

Creatine monohydrate comes as:
- tablets (2.5 and 5 grams)
- powder (1 teaspoon contains 5 grams).

Why people use creatine monohydrate
- To enhance exercise performance

Some experts recommend the following doses:
- As a *loading dose,* 15 to 20 grams taken orally daily for the first 5 days, then 5 to 10 grams taken orally daily as a maintenance dose.
- As a *long-term supplement,* 2 to 4 grams taken orally daily.

In most clinical trials, people received a dose of 20 to 25 grams daily for 5 days, and then their exercise performance was measured.

Side effects

Call your health care practitioner if you experience any of these possible side effects of creatine monohydrate:
- dehydration symptoms, such as pronounced thirst
- digestive upset (stomach pain, bloating, diarrhea)
- muscle cramps
- weight gain.

Interactions

Combining creatine monohydrate with certain drugs may alter their action or produce unwanted side effects. Tell your health care practitioner about any prescription or nonprescription drugs you're taking, especially:
- caffeine
- glucose.

Important points to remember

- Don't use creatine monohydrate if you're pregnant or breast-feeding.
- Be aware that this substance is useful only for intense exercise of short duration or when you need short bursts of strength (such as in weightlifting, sprinting, or ice hockey).
- If you experience muscle cramps, stop taking creatine or take smaller daily amounts.
- Be aware that although creatine isn't on the International Olympic Committee Drug list, some consider it in a gray zone between doping and substances allowed as performance enhancers.
- Know that because the kidney quickly excretes creatine, doses exceeding 20 grams a day are ineffective.
- Keep in mind that a single 5-gram dose of oral creatine monohydrate has the creatine content of about 2.4 pounds (1 kilogram) of uncooked steak.

WHAT THE RESEARCH SHOWS

Studies found that adding creatine to the diet improved high-intensity, intermittent exercise performance. However, creatine's use in enhancing aerobic exercise or endurance exercise performance is unclear and probably insignificant.

Because a muscle's normal creatine content varies, response to creatine supplements also varies. It seems that people who start out with low muscle creatine levels benefit more from creatine supplements than do those who have higher creatine levels to begin with.

Medical experts point out that creatine's long-term safety remains unknown. Consequently, they can't recommend it.

Other names for creatine monohydrate

Another name for creatine monohydrate is creatine.

Products containing creatine monohydrate are sold under such names as Advanced Genetics, Bio-Tech, Champion's Choice, GNC Pro Performance Labs, ISP Nutrition, Joe Weider, Labrada, Metaform, Muscle Tribe, Nature's Best, Universal Nutrition, and VitaLife Sport Products.

Selected references

Earnest, C.P., et al. "The Effect of Oral Creatine Monohydrate Ingestion on Anaerobic Power Indices, Muscular Strength, and Body Composition," *Acta Physiologica Scandinavica* 153:207-09, 1995.

Greenhaff, P.L., et al. "Influence of Oral Creatine Supplementation of Muscle Torque During Repeated Bouts of Maximal Voluntary Exercise in Man," *Clinical Science* 84:565-71, 1993.

Harris, R.C., et al. "Elevation of Creatine in Resting and Exercised Muscle of Normal Subjects by Creatine Supplementation," *Clinical Science* 83:367-74, 1992.

Harris, R.C., et al. "The Effects of Oral Creatine Supplementation on Running Performance During Maximal Short Term Exercise in Man," *Journal of Physiology* 467:P74, 1993.

Glucosamine

An amino sugar, glucosamine is found in chitin—a substance in some plants and in the hard outer husk of insects, spiders, scorpions, mites, lobsters, shrimps, crabs, and barnacles. Glucosamine sulfate is synthetically manufactured.

In some studies, glucosamine helped to repair damaged joint cartilage. Researchers have been intensively studying the use of glucosamine sulfate and chondroitin sulfates since the 1997 book, *The Arthritis Cure,* claimed that this combination can halt or perhaps even cure osteoarthritis. However, much more research is needed to support this claim.

Why people use glucosamine

- Osteoarthritis
- To aid regeneration of damaged cartilage

Common doses

Glucosamine comes in various molecular forms. Most experts seem to prefer glucosamine sulfate, which comes as:

- capsules (250, 375, 500, 600, and 1,000 milligrams)
- tablets (63, 87, 375, 500, 600, and 750 milligrams).

In some studies, patients received 500 milligrams orally twice daily. Other doses have been based on weight:

- *In people weighing less than 120 pounds,* 1,000 milligrams of glucosamine plus 800 milligrams of chondroitin sulfates.
- *In people weighing 120 to 200 pounds,* 1,500 milligrams of glucosamine plus 1,200 milligrams of chondroitin sulfates.
- *In people weighing over 200 pounds,* 2,000 milligrams of glucosamine plus 1,600 milligrams of chondroitin sulfates.

Side effects

Call your health care practitioner if you experience any of these possible side effects of glucosamine:

- constipation
- diarrhea
- drowsiness
- headache
- heartburn

- nausea
- skin rash
- stomach pain or discomfort.

Interactions

Combining glucosamine with certain drugs may alter their action or produce unwanted side effects. If you use this compound, tell your health care practitioner about any prescription or nonprescription drugs you're taking.

Important points to remember

- Don't use glucosamine if you're pregnant or breast-feeding.
- Keep glucosamine products out of children's reach.
- Don't take glucosamine if you have any form of diabetes.
- Know that the Arthritis Foundation doesn't recommend glucosamine for osteoarthritis or any other arthritis forms because too little is known about its effectiveness.

WHAT THE RESEARCH SHOWS

Some research has found that glucosamine sulfate improved osteoarthritis symptoms. Unfortunately, those studies were poorly designed and analyzed. Defining glucosamine's role in treating bone and joint disorders will require long-term, carefully designed and controlled studies.

WIth inadequate information about its effectiveness, the Arthritis Foundation doesn't recommend glucosamine for osteoarthritis or any other arthritis form. What's more, animal studies suggest glucosamine may impede insulin secretion, posing a potential risk for anyone with diabetes.

Other names for glucosamine

Other names for glucosamine include chitosamine, glucosamine sulfate, and GS.

Products containing glucosamine are sold under such names as Arth-X Plus, Enhanced Glucosamine Sulfate, Flexi-Factors, Glucosamine Complex, Glucosamine Mega, Joint Factors, Nutri-Joint, and Ultra Maximum Strength Glucosamine Sulfate.

Selected references

Anon. "Glucosamine sulfate treatment." Public information memo #96-05. Atlanta, GA: Arthritis Foundation. March 4, 1996.

Drovanti, A., et al. "Therapeutic Activity of Oral Glucosamine Sulfate in Osteoarthrosis: A Placebo-Controlled Double-Blind Investigation," *Clinical Therapeutics* 3:260-72, 1980.

Reichelt, A., et al. "Efficacy and Safety of Intramuscular Glucosamine Sulfate in Osteoarthritis of the Knee," *Arzneimittel-Forschung* 44:75-80, 1994.

Theodosakis, J. *The Arthritis Cure.* New York: St. Martin's Press, 1997.

Vaz, A.L. "Double-Blind Clinical Evaluation of the Relative Efficacy of Ibuprofen and Glucosamine Sulphate in the Management of Osteoarthrosis of the Knee in Outpatients," *Current Medical Research and Opinion* 8:145-49, 1982.

Melatonin

Melatonin is a hormone produced by the pineal gland, a tiny organ located at the base of the brain. Melatonin regulates sleep cycles and the hormonal changes that trigger sexual maturity during adolescence. Studied for many conditions, it has been promoted most widely for preventing and treating jet lag and other forms of insomnia.

Why people use melatonin

- Birth control
- Cancer
- Insomnia
- Jet lag
- Other sleep disorders
- To slow weight loss in a person with cancer

Common doses

Melatonin comes as:

- extended-release capsules (3 milligrams)
- tablets (500 micrograms and 1, 1.5, or 3 milligrams)
- liquid (500 micrograms per milliliter)
- injectable forms.

Some experts recommend the following doses:

- For *cancer (solid tumors) as a single agent,* 20 milligrams injected into muscle for 2 months, then 10 milligrams taken orally once daily.
- For *cancer (given with interleukin-2 [IL-2]),* 40 to 50 milligrams taken orally at bedtime, starting 7 days before IL-2.
- For *chronic insomnia,* 75 milligrams taken orally at bedtime.
- For *delayed sleep phase syndrome,* 5 milligrams taken orally at bedtime.
- For *jet lag,* 5 milligrams taken orally once daily, starting 3 days before and ending 3 days after departure.
- To *normalize nocturnal melatonin levels,* 4 micrograms per hour for 5 hours by intravenous injection.
- For *insomnia in blind people,* 5 milligrams taken orally at bedtime.
- For *insomnia in elderly people,* 1 to 2 milligrams of an extended-release form taken orally 2 hours before bedtime.

Side effects

Call your health care practitioner if you experience any of these possible side effects of melatonin:

- altered sleep patterns
- chills

- confusion
- drowsiness
- headache
- itching
- rapid pulse.

Interactions

Combining melatonin with certain drugs may alter their action or produce unwanted side effects. Don't use melatonin while taking:

- DHEA (a steroid hormone)
- magnesium or zinc supplements
- methamphetamines such as Desoxyn.

Use caution when taking melatonin along with tranquilizers such as benzodiazepines (for instance, Klonopin, Librium, or Xanax).

Important points to remember

- Don't take melatonin if you have kidney or liver disease.
- Avoid melatonin if you have a history of stroke, depression, or a neurologic disorder.
- Before surgery, tell the anesthesiologist that you've been taking melatonin. This information may influence the type of muscle relaxant he or she administers.
- Know that comprehensive therapy for sleep disorders may include behavior modification, light therapy, drugs, and counseling.

WHAT THE RESEARCH SHOWS

Melatonin seems to be a promising treatment for jet lag, although more controlled trials must be done to find the best administration schedule. Melatonin also may benefit people with other sleep disorders and aid blind people with abnormal body rhythms.

More research may tell if melatonin has a role in treating cancer or preventing pregnancy. For now, medical experts are withholding judgment.

Other names for melatonin

Other names for melatonin include Mel and n-acetyl-5-methoxytryptamine.

Products containing melatonin are sold under such names as Bevitamel, Melatonin, Rapi-Snooze, and Tranzone.

Selected references

Claustraut, B. "Melatonin and Jet Lag: Confirmatory Result Using a Simplified Protocol," *Biological Psychology* 32:705-11, 1992.

Haimov, I., et al. "Melatonin Replacement Therapy of Elderly Insomniacs," *Sleep* 18:598-603, 1995.

Lissoni, P., et al. "Clinical Results with the Pineal Hormone Melatonin in Advanced Cancer Resistant to Standard Antitumor Therapies," *Oncology* 48:448-50, 1991.

Lissoni, P., et al. "Is There a Role for Melatonin in the Treatment of Neoplastic Cachexia?" *European Journal of Cancer* 32A:1340-43, 1996.

Petrie, K., et al. "Effect of Melatonin on Jet Lag after Long Haul Flights," *BMJ* 298:705-07, 1989.

Petrie, K., et al. "A Double-Blind Trial of Melatonin as a Treatment for Jet Lag in International Cabin Crew," *Biological Psychology* 33:526-30, 1993.

Octacosanol

Some people claim octacosanol enhances muscle endurance and athletic performance. Studies hint at its possible use in treating amyotrophic lateral sclerosis (Lou Gehrig's disease) and Parkinson's disease.

Octacosanol comes from sugar cane wax, other vegetable waxes, and wheat germ oil. It also has been isolated from some *Euphorbia* species, *Acacia modesta*, and other plants.

Why people use octacosanol

- Amyotrophic lateral sclerosis (Lou Gehrig's disease)
- Heart and blood vessel disease
- Parkinson's disease
- To enhance athletic performance

Common dose

Octacosanol comes as:

- regular capsules (3,000 and 8,000 micrograms)
- softgel capsules (3,000 micrograms)
- tablets (1,000 and 6,000 micrograms).

Some experts recommend the following dose:

- 40 to 80 milligrams taken orally daily.

Side effects

Call your health care practitioner if you experience any of these possible side effects of octacosanol:

- dizziness when rising from a sitting or lying position
- jerky, involuntary movements
- nervousness.

Interactions

Combining octacosanol with certain drugs may alter their action or produce unwanted side effects. Don't use octacosanol while taking Sinemet.

Important point to remember

- Don't use octacosanol if you're pregnant or breast-feeding.

Other names for octacosanol

Other names for octacosanol include octocosanol, 1-octacosanol, 14c-octacosanol, n-octacosanol, octacosyl alcohol, and policosanol.

WHAT THE RESEARCH SHOWS

Medicinal claims for octacosanol aren't backed by solid evidence. More studies are needed to evaluate its effects in Parkinson's disease, amyotrophic lateral sclerosis (Lou Gehrig's disease), and heart and blood vessel diseases.

Products containing octacosanol are sold under such names as Octacosanol Concentrate and Super Octacosanol.

Selected references

Arruzazabala, M.L., et al. "Cholesterol-Lowering Effects of Policosanol in Rabbits," *Biological Research* 27:205-8, 1994.

Kabir, Y., and Kimura, S. "Tissue Distribution of 8-14C-octacosanol in Liver and Muscle of Rats After Serial Administration," *Annals of Nutrition and Metabolism* 39:279-84, 1995.

Kato, S., et al. "Octacosanol Affects Lipid Metabolism in Rats Fed on a High-Fat Diet," *British Journal of Nutrition* 73:433-41, 1995.

Snider, S. "Octacosanol in Parkinsonism," *Annals of Neurology* 16:723, 1984. Letter.

Royal jelly

Royal jelly is a milky-white substance that worker bees make and feed to their queen bee to aid her growth and development. Some people believe royal jelly slows the human aging process, based on the observation that queen bees are twice the size of worker bees, live 5 to 8 years longer and, unlike worker bees, are fertile. Other claims for royal jelly center on its purported value in treating male pattern baldness, easing menopause symptoms, and enhancing sexual performance.

Why people use royal jelly

- Male-pattern baldness
- Skin wrinkles and blemishes
- To enhance sexual performance
- To reduce blood cholesterol
- To slow the aging process

Common doses

Royal jelly comes as:

- ampules (100 milligrams)
- capsules (100 milligrams)
- topical cream
- ointment
- lotion
- soap.

Some experts recommend the following doses:

- To *lower cholesterol,* 50 to 100 milligrams taken orally daily.
- For *cosmetic use,* royal jelly applied to the skin two or three times daily.

Side effects

Call your health care practitioner if you experience any of these possible side effects of royal jelly:

- allergic reaction (which can be severe)
- worsening of asthma.

Royal jelly also may cause:

- increased blood sugar.
- life-threatening closure of lower airway muscles in people with asthma. At least one person has died.

Interactions

Combining royal jelly with certain drugs may alter their action or produce unwanted side effects. Tell your health care practitioner about any prescription or nonprescription drugs you're taking, especially drugs that lower blood sugar.

Important points to remember

- Avoid royal jelly if you're pregnant or breast-feeding. Tell your health care practitioner if you suspect you're pregnant or are planning a pregnancy.
- Don't take royal jelly if you've had an allergic reaction to royal jelly preparations. Sudden contraction of the lower airway muscles may occur.
- Don't take royal jelly if you have diabetes.

> **WHAT THE RESEARCH SHOWS**
>
> Despite claims that royal jelly reduces the effects of aging, rejuvenates the skin, treats baldness, and improves sexual performance, the substance lacks hormonal components that promote fertility, growth, or longevity. Studies haven't completely substantiated its effectiveness in reducing wrinkles and blemishes.
>
> Other research suggests royal jelly may lower cholesterol and kill bacteria. However, safer and more effective drugs are available for these purposes.

Other names for royal jelly

Another name for royal jelly is queen bee jelly.

A product containing royal jelly is sold as Royal Jelly.

Selected references

Bullock, R.J., et al. "Fatal Royal Jelly Induced Asthma," *Medical Journal of Australia* 160:44, 1994.

Harwood, M., et al. "Asthma Following Royal Jelly," *New Zealand Medical Journal* 23:325, 1996.

Vittek, J. "Effect of Royal Jelly on Serum Lipids in Experimental Animals and Humans with Atherosclerosis," *Experientia* 51:927-35, 1995.

Shark cartilage

Shark cartilage is a dietary supplement that some people claim fights cancer. It comes from the spiny dogfish shark, *Squalus acanthias,* and the hammerhead shark, *Sphyrna lewini*.

After the 1992 publication of W. Lane's *Sharks Don't Get Cancer,* shark cartilage became the newest cancer "cure." Contributing to the media frenzy, a *60 Minutes* television segment in 1993 spotlighted shark cartilage as a promising treatment. This triggered an onslaught of calls to cancer information agencies. However, no solid scientific evidence supports claims that it works in treating cancer.

Common doses

Shark cartilage comes as:
- ampules (10 milliliters, containing 80 milligrams per milliliter)
- capsules (750 milligrams)
- tablets (750 milligrams)
- concentrate (500 milligrams per 15 milliliters).

Why people use shark cartilage
- Cancer

For cancer treatment, typical doses of commercially available shark cartilage supplements range from 500 to 4,500 milligrams daily, depending on the type of preparation and amount of "pure" shark cartilage it contains. However, many such supplements contain only binding agents or fillers.

Some experts recommend the following doses:
- As *tablets and capsules,* 2 to 6 doses taken orally daily.
- As *ampules,* 1 ampule taken orally daily.
- As a *concentrate,* 1 to 2 tablespoonfuls taken orally daily.

Side effects

Call your health care practitioner if you experience unusual symptoms when using shark cartilage. It may cause hepatitis.

Interactions

Combining shark cartilage with certain drugs may alter their action or produce unwanted side effects. Tell your health care practitioner about any prescription or nonprescription drugs you're taking.

Important points to remember

- Don't use shark cartilage if you have liver disease.
- Be aware that your health care practitioner may recommend periodic liver function tests while you're taking shark cartilage.
- Know that commercially available forms of shark cartilage contain varying amounts of the active ingredient.

> **WHAT THE RESEARCH SHOWS**
>
> Usually, the digestive tract can't absorb the large molecules in shark cartilage. So it's doubtful that taking shark cartilage orally can release usable compounds into the blood. Also, no well-controlled clinical studies have been published. In 1994, the National Cancer Institute began a trial of shark cartilage—but stopped it when they found that each batch of shark cartilage (provided by advocates) was contaminated. At this time, no evidence shows that shark cartilage offers benefits to people with cancer.

Other names for shark cartilage

Products containing shark cartilage are sold under such names as Carticin, Cartilade, GNC Liquid Shark Cartilage, Informed Nutrition Shark Cartilage, and Natural Brand Shark Cartilage.

Selected references

Ashar, B., and Vargo, E. "Shark Cartilage-Induced Hepatitis," *Annals of Internal Medicine* 125:780-81, 1996.

Hunt, T.J., and Connelly J.F. "Shark Cartilage for Cancer Treatment," *American Journal of Health-System Pharmacy* 52:1756-60, 1995.

Mathews, J. "Media Feeds Frenzy Over Shark Cartilage as Cancer Treatment," *Journal of the National Cancer Institute* 85:1190-91, 1993.

Miller, D.R., et al. "Phase I/II Trial of the Safety and Efficacy of Shark Cartilage in the Treatment of Advanced Cancer," *Journal of Clinical Oncology* 16:3649-55, 1998.

GLOSSARY

ACE inhibitor A drug that blocks the formation of a natural body chemical, thus relaxing blood vessels and decreasing water and salt retention. It's used to lower blood pressure or manage heart failure.

active ingredient The drug component that produces therapeutic effects.

alkaloid A substance found in plants that acts like a drug in the body. Examples include caffeine, morphine, nicotine, quinine, and strychnine. The term also applies to synthetic substances whose structures resemble that of plant alkaloids.

anaphylaxis A severe, life-threatening allergic reaction marked by flushing, hives, itching, swelling of the lips and eyelids, throat tightening, sudden hoarseness, nausea, and vomiting. It can start within seconds of exposure to an allergy-causing substance and can cause death within minutes unless treated immediately.

anesthetic A drug that dulls body sensations, especially pain. Its effects may be local (confined to one body part) or general (affecting the entire body).

annual A plant that completes its life cycle in one growing season.

antacid A drug that neutralizes excess stomach acid.

antibiotic A drug that kills disease-causing bacteria or prevents bacteria from reproducing.

antidepressant A drug used to prevent or relieve mental depression. Types of antidepressants include tricyclics, selective serotonin reuptake inhibitors, and monoamine oxidase inhibitors.

antidote A substance used to counteract a poison.

antihistamine A drug that blocks the action of histamine, a body chemical released by the immune system, by binding to histamine receptors in various body tissues. In the nose, it stops histamines from making the nasal blood vessels expand (the cause of runny nose).

antioxidant A substance, such as vitamin E, that works alone or in a group to destroy disease-causing substances called free radicals.

antiseptic A substance used to destroy harmful microorganisms (such as bacteria, fungi, viruses, and protozoa) or to inhibit their growth.

aphrodisiac A drug that causes sexual arousal.

astringent A substance that causes tissues to contract. It's usually used locally, as on the skin.

Ayurvedic medicine The ancient traditional Indian system of medicine based on Hindu philosophy. This system shares some fundamental concepts with traditional Chinese medicine: the interconnectedness of body, mind, and spirit; the belief that the cosmos is composed of five basic elements (earth, air, fire, water, and space); and the belief in a human energy field that must be kept in balance to maintain health. Ayurvedic medicine also stresses the importance of a person's metabolic body type (*dosha*) in determining his or her health, personality, and susceptibility to disease.

barbiturate A drug that causes sedation, a hypnotic state, or both. Barbiturates can be addictive.

benzodiazepine A drug used to treat anxiety or sleeping disorders, to relax muscles, or to control seizures.

beta blocker A drug that decreases the rate and force of heart contractions and widens blood vessels, helping to reduce blood pressure. Beta blockers typically are prescribed for people with coronary artery disease, angina (chest pain caused by heart problems), irregular heartbeats, or a history of heart attacks.

biennial A plant that completes its life cycle in 2 years. During the first year, it grows; during the second year, it fruits and dies.

binder A substance added to a drug or herbal product to hold together the product's ingredients.

bioflavonoid One of a group of naturally occurring plant compounds needed to strengthen tiny blood vessels called capillaries. Some researchers believe bioflavonoids may help protect against cancer and infection.

biomedicine A system of medicine based on the principles of the natural sciences.

blood thinner A drug that prevents blood clotting. Examples include heparin and Coumadin (also called warfarin).

botanical A substance or product derived from a plant.

calcium channel blocker A drug that helps maintain blood flow through the arteries and reduces the heart's work. It lowers the calcium concentration in heart cells and the blood vessel's smooth muscles, thus widening the vessels, slowing the heart rate, and reducing blood pressure.

capsule A powdered, granulated, or liquid drug encased in a hard or soft shell that dissolves in the stomach. Solid drug particles may be coated for sustained-release action.

chronic Long-term.

citric acid An organic acid extracted from citrus fruits (especially lemons and limes) or obtained by fermentation of sugars. Citric acid is used as a flavoring agent in drug products, foods, and carbonated beverages.

clinical trial An experiment performed on people to evaluate the effectiveness and safety of medical therapies.

colon The main part of the large intestine, which connects the small intestine with the rectum. It converts what's left of consumed food into stool by removing water and salts.

Commission E A government committee in Germany that evaluates and reviews the safety and effectiveness of herbal products.

compound A substance made up of two or more ingredients.

compress A soft pad, usually made of cloth, that's used to apply heat, cold, or drugs to the surface of a body area.

cream A thick substance that contains a paste-drug mixture of oil and water. Creams soften tissue and are designed for topical use.

crude Raw or unrefined.

decoction A drug or other substance prepared by boiling.

decongestant A drug that relieves nasal congestion by narrowing blood vessels in the nose, which serves to ease swelling. Decongestants are used to treat allergies and the common cold.

dehydration A state of deficient fluids.

dementia An organic mental syndrome marked by general loss of intellectual abilities, with chronic personality disintegration, confusion, disorientation, and stupor.

diuretic A drug that increases the amount of urine produced by the body to help the kidneys eliminate water and salt. Diuretics most commonly are used to treat high blood pressure and heart failure. Also called a water pill.

DNA Deoxyribonucleic acid; an acid found mainly in the chromosomes of the cell nucleus that serves as the primary genetic material of most living organisms.

Doctrine of Signatures In herbal medicine, the primitive method of determining which plants should be used for which ailments, based on the plant's resemblance to the ailment—for example, heart-shaped leaves for heart conditions and plants with red flowers for bleeding disorders.

dram A unit of weight equivalent to ⅛ ounce or 60 grains.

drug A pharmacologic agent capable of affecting the structure or functioning of living organisms to produce biological effects. Also called a medication.

duodenum The first part of the small intestine, measuring about 10 inches long. The duodenum plays a key role in digestion.

eczema An acute or chronic skin inflammation triggered by an allergy or by no apparent cause. It's commonly accompanied by blistering, scaling, and itching.

elixir A mixture of a drug, alcohol, water, and sugar.

enzyme A protein found in cells and digestive juices that triggers or speeds up chemical reactions.

esophagus A muscular passage measuring about 9 inches long that connects the throat to the stomach.

essential oil A naturally occurring pure oil obtained from distillation of a plant.

estrogen Any of a group of female reproductive hormones made primarily in the ovaries but present in men in small amounts. Estrogen promotes development of female secondary sex characteristics and, during the menstrual cycle, makes the female genital tract suitable for fertilization, implantation, and nutrition of the early embryo.

expectorant A drug that helps to expel mucus or phlegm from the lungs or throat. An expectorant is commonly one of several ingredients in cough medications.

extract A concentrate prepared by extracting—that is, removing all or nearly all of the solvent and adjusting the residual amount to a prescribed standard. Most extracts are solutions of essential constituents of a plant or other complex material placed in alcohol.

fiber The indigestible part of vegetable matter consisting mainly of polymers called cellulose and lignin. Fiber is found in cereals, fruits, and vegetables.

filler A substance added to a drug product to increase its weight, bulk, or thickness.

flaccid Not firm or stiff; limp; lacking in force or vigor.

Food and Drug Administration The U.S. federal agency that protects the public against health hazards from foods and food additives and ensures the safety and effectiveness of drugs, medical devices, and dietary supplements.

formulation A drug product prepared according to a specific composition.

free radical A molecule containing an odd number of electrons. Some researchers believe free radicals may play a role in cancer development by interacting with DNA (the cell's genetic material) and impairing normal cell function.

gallbladder The pear-shaped organ located just under the liver that acts as a bile reservoir.

gastroesophageal reflux disease Inflammation of the esophagus caused by backflow of acid from the stomach. Its main symptom is chronic heartburn.

glycerite A solution or mixture of a medicinal substance in glycerin. Usually sweet to the taste and warm on the tongue, glycerites are an alternative to alcohol extracts and better suited to some people.

glycoside An active component in plants that yields sugars when it decomposes.

goiter An enlargement of the thyroid gland that causes swelling in the front of the neck.

gout A metabolic disease marked by localized deposits of uric acid and its salts, causing painfully arthritic joints. Symptoms include recurrent attacks of extreme pain in one joint or several joints.

grain The smallest unit of weight in the apothecary system, equivalent to 0.06 gram. It's based on the weight of a grain of wheat.

gram The basic unit of weight in the metric system, equivalent to 1/1000 of a kilogram or three one-hundredths (0.03) of an ounce.

gum A carbohydrate of plant origin that is gel-like when moist but hardens on drying.

heart attack Sudden blockage of one or more of the arteries that supply blood to the heart, causing damage to the heart muscle.

hemorrhage Bleeding (usually rapid and significant).

hemorrhoid An abnormally swollen vein beneath the lining of the anal canal or near the anus that may cause itching, pain, or bleeding.

herbalist 1. A person who practices healing by the use of herbs. 2. A person who grows or collects herbs. 3. An herb doctor.

herbal medicine The use of plants for healing purposes, dating back to the ancient cultures of Egypt, China, and India, and possibly even prehistoric times. Today, more than a quarter of conventional drugs are derived from herbs and about 80% of the world's population uses herbal remedies.

hernia The projection or outpouching of an organ or a part of an organ through the wall that normally contains it.

histamine A chemical found in all tissues that causes tiny arteries called capillaries to widen, makes smooth muscles contract, increases the heart rate, causes blood pressure to drop, and promotes secretion of stomach acids. Histamine is formed and released during allergic reactions.

hives Itchy, raised, red areas of inflamed skin caused by an allergic reaction.

homeopathy A method of healing in which minute amounts of a substance that causes symptoms in a healthy person are given to a sick person to cure the same symptoms. Homeopathic remedies are thought to stimulate the body's ability to heal itself.

hormone A chemical produced in one body part or organ that triggers or regulates the activity of an organ or a group of cells in another part of the body.

hypnotic A medication that induces sleep, such as a benzodiazepine.

immune system The body's defense against infection and disease, which also may trigger an allergic reaction.

immunization The process of rendering the body immune (resistant) to a disease, as by inoculating with a vaccine.

impotence Inability of an adult male to achieve or maintain an erection of the penis.

infection A disease caused by a bacterium, virus, fungus, or other pathogenic organism.

infusion A method of making an herbal tea in which a dried herb is steeped in hot water for 3 to 5 minutes and then drunk.

inhalation treatment A type of herbal treatment used mainly to open congested sinuses and lung passages, help discharge mucus, and ease breathing. In one inhalation method, 2 to 5 drops of an herbal oil are placed in a sink filled with very hot water; the steam is then inhaled for 5 minutes. In another method, dried or fresh herbs (or an aromatic oil) are added to a large pot of hot water, which is then brought to a boil, allowed to simmer for 5 minutes, and removed from the heat to cool. Then the person drapes a towel over his or her head to form a tent, leans over the pot, and inhales the steam for 5 minutes.

insomnia Difficulty falling or staying asleep.

insulin A hormone produced by the pancreas that regulates the amount of glucose in the blood. Natural insulin is produced in the pancreas. Insulin prepared from the pancreatic tissue of animals is used to treat people with diabetes (who have insufficient insulin production and secretion).

interaction The relationship between drugs or other substances administered at the same time that leads to changes in the therapeutic effects or toxicity of any or all of the drugs or substances.

internal use Intended for administration through the stomach by swallowing.

iris The round, colored part of the eye that adjusts pupil size and regulates the amount of light reaching the retina in the back of the eye.

jaundice Yellowing of the skin, mucous membranes, or whites of the eyes, caused by buildup of bilirubin (a bile pigment) in the skin.

joint The juncture of two or more bones.

kidney One of a pair of bean-shaped urinary organs on either side of the spine in the lower back. The kidney filters wastes from the blood, regulates certain chemicals, and removes fluid from the body as urine, thus helping to maintain the body's water balance.

lactation Milk secretion from the breast's mammary glands.

laxative A drug that promotes bowel movements, commonly used to treat constipation.

liniment An oily liquid preparation meant to be applied to the skin.

liter A metric unit of volume equal to 1,000 cubic centimeters or 1.05 quarts liquid measure.

localized Limited to a specific area.

lozenge A medicated tablet containing sugar, made to dissolve in the mouth.

lymph node One of many rounded structures, ranging from the size of a pinhead to a grape, that filter out bacteria and other toxic substances to stop them from entering the bloodstream and causing infection. Lymph nodes also produce lymphocytes, a type of blood cell.

medicinal Used to cure disease; having healing qualities.

menopause The cessation of menstrual periods caused by loss of ovarian estrogen production. Typically, menopause occurs between ages 45 and 60 but may occur earlier because of illness or surgical removal of the uterus or both ovaries.

metabolism The sum of all biochemical reactions in the body, including anabolism (building of complex chemicals from less complex ones) and catabolism (breakdown of complex substances into simpler ones).

microgram A unit of weight in the metric system that's one-millionth of a gram or one one-thousandth (0.001) of a milligram.

milligram A unit of weight in the metric system that's one-thousandth (0.001) of a gram.

milliliter A unit of volume in the metric system that's one one-thousandth (0.001) of a liter.

minim A unit of capacity in the British imperial system that's one six-hundredth (0.06) of a milliliter.

muscle relaxant A drug that reduces tension in the muscles, commonly used to treat muscle spasms resulting from muscle, bone, or joint injury.

mutation An alteration in a cell's DNA (genetic material) caused by a disruption in cell division or by exposure to a cancer-causing substance or certain other substances.

naturopathy An alternative system of medical practice that combines a mainstream understanding of human physiology and disease with alternative remedies, such as herbal and nutritional therapies, acupuncture, hydrotherapy, and counseling. Naturopathic doctors favor natural treatments aimed at stimulating the body's own healing ability over drugs and surgery.

nonprescription drug A drug that can be obtained without a prescription (over the counter). Nonprescription drugs can be used safely without the supervision of a licensed health care practitioner, provided the person follows the directions on the product label.

nonsteroidal anti-inflammatory drug (NSAID) A drug that reduces inflammation and controls pain without the use of steroids. Examples include Advil, Indocin, Orudis, and Naprosyn.

ointment A semisolid, oil-based preparation that contains a medication for topical application.

ovary One of two female reproductive organs in the lower abdomen that produce egg cells and the hormones estrogen and progesterone.

pancreas An oblong organ located behind the stomach that secretes various substances, such as digestive enzymes and the hormones glucagon and insulin.

paralysis Inability to move a muscle or to feel sensation.

parasite Any living thing that attaches to or lives inside another organism and feeds off its host.

pathogen A microorganism, such as a fungus, virus, or bacterium, that's capable of causing disease.

perennial A plant whose life cycle exceeds 2 years.

pharmaceutical A medicinal drug.

pharmacognosy The study of the natural sources of drugs, such as plants, animals, and minerals and their products.

phenothiazine A drug used to control psychosis or ease vomiting.

phytomedicine Herbal medicine.

phytotherapy Treatment by use of plants.

plaque 1. Buildup of cholesterol and other substances on an artery wall. 2. A thin film made up of mucin (the chief ingredient in mucus) and colloidal material that adheres to the teeth.

platelet One of many small, disk-shaped cells that originate in the bone marrow and clump together for blood clotting.

postmenopausal Referring to the phase of life after menstrual periods stop.

poultice A moist paste made from crushed herbs that's applied directly to the affected area or wrapped in cloth and then applied.

powder Small particles of medication obtained by grinding a solid drug.

practitioner A person who practices a profession, such as medicine or nursing.

prescription drug A drug that can be used safely only under the supervision of a health care professional licensed to prescribe or dispense drugs according to federal and state laws.

processed Treated or made by a special process.

profuse Markedly abundant, bountiful.

prostate-specific antigen (PSA) test A blood test that measures the level of a protein produced by prostate gland cells. The PSA test is used to help detect prostate diseases.

psychosis A mental condition marked by being out of touch with reality.

pulmonary edema A condition in which fluid builds up in the spaces outside the lung's blood vessels.

pupil The dark area (actually an opening) in the middle of the iris that narrows to limit the amount of light entering the eye or widens to let more light enter.

purgative A susbstance that causes bowel evacuation.

regimen A systematic plan of therapy designed to improve and maintain a person's health.

resin A sticky substance found on trees and shrubs or made synthetically that hardens when exposed to cold.

retina The delicate, 10-layered, nervous tissue membrane of the eye that receives images and sends them for processing through the optic nerve to the brain.

rhizome A plant's underground stem, commonly thickened by deposits of reserve food material, that produces shoots above and roots below. Unlike a true root, a rhizome typically has buds, nodes, and (usually) scalelike leaves.

salivation Production of saliva, especially an excess; drooling.

salve A thick ointment.

side effect A usually undesirable but predictable drug effect, which can range from mild to severe or life-threatening. A side effect can be related to the dose or to the person's individual sensitivity to the drug.

spasm A sudden, involuntary muscle contraction, possibly causing pain and restricting movement.

spirit A volatile liquid, especially one that has been distilled; a volatile substance dissolved in alcohol.

stool softener A drug that lowers the surface tension of feces, allowing intestinal fluids to penetrate and soften the stool.

stroke A sudden condition in which blockage of an artery or rupture of a blood vessel cuts off the brain's blood supply, causing damage to the affected brain area. Also called cerebrovascular accident.

syrup A concentrated solution that contains a drug, flavoring, sugar, and water.

tablet A solid dosage form in which a drug is combined with inert ingredients and compressed into a shape.

therapeutic Providing or assisting in a cure.

thyroid gland A butterfly-shaped gland in the front of the neck that regulates the body's metabolic rate by producing thyroid hormone.

tincture A liquid preparation that contains a drug and alcohol (alcoholic solution) or a drug, alcohol, and water (hydroalcoholic solution).

tonic A drug or other remedy that restores, invigorates, refreshes, or stimulates.

topical use Application of a drug or an herbal product to the skin and surface tissues of the body. Topical drugs come in a wide range of forms, including creams, ointments, solutions, dusting powders, nasal drops, rectal and vaginal suppositories, and ear and eye drops. Topical drugs deliver medication directly to the problem area, helping to avoid the complications that systemic drugs can cause.

toxic Poisonous.

toxicity A condition caused by the presence of a poison or excess amounts of a substance that doesn't cause side effects in smaller amounts.

traditional Chinese medicine A sophisticated, complex health care system based on the belief that good health depends largely on a person's lifestyle, thoughts, and emotions. It has expanded over the centuries to embrace many theories, methods, and approaches.

The cornerstone of traditional Chinese medicine, which evolved from Taoism, Confucianism, and Buddhism, is the concept of *qi,* defined as a vital life force, or energy, that flows through the body along channels called meridians.

tuberous root A thick, fleshy storage root that lacks buds or scale leaves.

tumor New tissue growth in which cells multiply in a progressive, uncontrolled way. It may be benign or cancerous.

unprocessed Crude or raw.

vertigo The sensation of spinning or dizziness in the absence of head or body movements.

volatile oil An oil that evaporates quickly. (In contrast, a fixed oil, such as castor oil or olive oil, isn't easily evaporated.) Volatile oils occur in aromatic plants, giving them odor and other characteristics. Examples include peppermint, spearmint, and juniper. Also called distilled oil or essential oil.

WHERE TO GET MORE INFORMATION

You can learn more about herbs by contacting the organizations below. As you can see, many of them have Web addresses. Keep in mind that these addresses may change without notice. (*Note:* Follow the Web addresses carefully when entering them into your Web browser. Several do not include "www.") Inclusion in this list doesn't indicate endorsement of any organization by the authors or publisher.

All Natural Healthcare Association
PO Box 834
Clyde, NC 28721
Tel/Fax: (828) 926-9557
http://www.allnaturalhealth.org

American Association of Naturopathic Physicians
601 Valley St., Suite 105
Seattle, WA 98109
Tel: (206) 298-0126
Fax: (206) 298-0129
http://www.naturopathic.org

American Association of Oriental Medicine
433 Front St.
Catasauqua, PA 18032
Tel: (610) 266-1433
Fax: (610) 264-2768
http://www.aaom.org

American Botanical Council
PO Box 144345
Austin, TX 78714-4345
Tel: (512) 926-4900
Fax: (512) 926-2345
http://www.herbalgram.org

American Herbal Products Association
8484 Georgia Ave., Suite 370
Silver Spring, MD 20910
Tel: (301) 588-1174
http://www.ahpa.org

American Holistic Medical Association
6728 Old McLean Village Dr.
McLean, VA 22101
Tel: (703) 556-9245
http://www.holisticmedicine.org

American Nutraceutical Association
22 Inverness Center Parkway
Suite 150
Birmingham, AL 35242
Tel: (205) 980-5710
Fax: (205) 991-9302
http://www.americanutra.com

American Society of Pharmacognosy
College of Pharmacy
220 Ferris Dr.
Big Rapids, MI 49307
Contact: R.J. Krueger, Ph.D.
Tel: (231) 591-2236
Fax: (231) 591-3821
http://www.phcog.org

Association of Natural Medicine Pharmacists
P.O. Box 150727
San Rafael, CA 94915-0727
Tel: (415) 453-3534
Fax: (415) 453-4963
http://www.anmp.org

Australasian College of Herbal Studies
USA Office
530 First St.
PO Box 57
Lake Oswego, OR 97034

Tel: (503) 635-6652 or (800) 487-8839
FAX: (503) 636-0706
http://www.herbed.com

Botanical Society of America
1735 Neil Ave.
Columbus, OH 43210-1293
Tel: (614) 292-3519
http://www.botany.org

Centers for Disease Control and Prevention
Public Health Service
US Dept. of Health and Human Services
1600 Clifton Rd. NE
Atlanta, GA 30333
Tel: (404) 639-3311
http://www.cdc.gov

Citizens for Health
P.O. Box 2260
Boulder, CO 80306
Tel: (303) 417-0772 or
(800) 357-2211
Fax: (303) 417-9378
http://www.citizens.org
e-mail: cfh@ares.csd.net

Committee for Freedom of Choice in Medicine
1180 Walnut Ave.
Chula Vista, CA 91911
Tel: (619) 429-8200 or
(800) 227-4473
Fax: (619) 429-8004
http://www.americanbiologics.com
e-mail: cfcm@inetworld.net

Herb Research Foundation
1007 Pearl St., Suite 200
Boulder, CO 80302
Tel: (303) 449-2265 or
(800) 748-2617

Fax: (303) 449-7849
http://www.herbs.org

Lloyd Library
917 Plum St.
Cincinnati, OH 45202
Tel: (513) 721-3707
Fax: (513) 721-6575
http://www.libraries.uc.edu/lloyd

NAPRALERT (NAtural PRoducts ALERT)
College of Pharmacy
University of Illinois at Chicago
Chicago, IL 60680
Contact: Mary Lou Quinn
Tel: (312) 996-2246
Fax: (312) 996-7107
http://www.dna.affrc.go.jp/htdocs/LIMB/NAPRALERT.html

National Center for Complementary and Alternative Medicine
NCCAM Clearinghouse
National Institutes of Health
PO Box 8218
Silver Spring, MD 20907-8218
Tel: (888) 644-6226
TTY/TDY: (888)-644-6226
Fax: (301) 495-4957
http://nccam.nih.gov

National Council for Reliable Health Information
300 East Pink Hill Rd.
Independence, MO 64057
Tel: (816) 228-4595
http://www.ncahf.org

National Nutritional Foods Association
3931 MacArthur Blvd.
Suite 101
Newport Beach, CA 92660
Tel: (949) 622-6272

Fax: (949) 622-6266
http://www.nnfa.org

Office of Dietary Supplements
National Institutes of Health
Building 31, Room 1B25
31 Center Dr., MSC 2086
Bethesda, MD 20892-2086
Tel: (301) 435-2920
Fax: (301) 480-1845
http://odp.od.nih.gov/ods

Society for Economic Botany
Dr. Brian Boom, Secretary
New York Botanical Garden
Bronx, NY 10458-5126
Tel: (718) 817-8632
Fax: (718) 220-6783
http://www.econbot.org

US Food and Drug Administration
Public Health Service
Dept. of Health and Human Services
5600 Fishers Lane
Rockville, MD 20857
Tel: (888) INFO-FDA or (888) 463-6332
http://www.fda.gov

US National Library of Medicine
National Institutes of Health
8600 Rockville Pike
Bethesda, MD 20894
Tel: (888) 346-3656
http://www.nlm.nih.gov

INDEX